Physical Rehabilitation Laboratory Manual:
Focus on Functional Training

Physical Rehabilitation Laboratory Manual: Focus on Functional Training

SUSAN B. O'SULLIVAN, EdD, PT
Professor
Department of Physical Therapy
College of Health Professions
University of Massachusetts Lowell
Lowell, Massachusetts

THOMAS J. SCHMITZ, PhD, PT
Associate Professor
Division of Physical Therapy
Brooklyn Campus
Long Island University
New York, New York

F. A. DAVIS COMPANY • Philadelphia

F. A. Davis Company
1915 Arch Street
Philadelphia, PA 19103

ISBN 0-8036-0257-X

Printed in the United States of America

Last digit indicates print number: 10 9 8 7 6 5 4 3 2 1

Publisher: Jean-François Vilain
Developmental Editor: Marianne Fithian
Cover Designer: Louis J. Forgione

As new scientific information becomes available through basic and clinical research, recommended treatments and therapies undergo changes. The authors and publisher have done everything possible to make this book accurate, up to date, and in accord with accepted standards at the time of publication. The authors, editors, and publisher are not responsible for errors or omissions or for consequences from application of the book, and make no warranty, expressed or implied, in regard to the contents of the book. Any practice described in this book should be applied by the reader in accordance with professional standards of care used in regard to the unique circumstances that may apply in each situation. The reader is advised always to check for changes and new information regarding drugs.

PREFACE

Physical Rehabilitation Laboratory Manual: Focus on Functional Training presents an integrated treatment model applicable to a wide variety of clinical problems and diagnoses. The model integrates newer motor control and motor learning strategies with more traditional remediation and compensatory treatment interventions. The overriding emphasis of treatment is attainment of *functional outcomes*. The content follows a logical progression from learning treatment activities and techniques to solving specific clinical problems. Analysis of the underlying rationale of treatment and synthesis into a proposed plan of care is achieved through comprehensive case studies. Self-evaluation and feedback are promoted by appended sample solutions to the clinical problems and case study questions.

The Laboratory Manual is divided into three major sections. Section I addresses principles of traditional therapeutic exercise foundations and motor learning approaches. Section II focuses on facilitating skill development through specific functional training activities and techniques. Several different treatment options are typically described for each functional outcome. The treatments are sequenced by specific motor control goals, which include mobility, stability, controlled mobility, and skill-level function. The progression proceeds from a hands-on approach (assisted or facilitated patterns of movement) to promotion of active movements based on task-oriented, functional practice. Treatment suggestions are presented with recognition that they represent only a small sample of possible options and that there is no absolute prescription for all patients. Our goal is to provide useful, practical treatment examples from the repertoire of skills that can be used to enhance functional performance. Owing to the variety of treatment options available, approaches other than those suggested may be equally effective in accomplishing a desired outcome.

Students and clinicians alike will find the detailed descriptions and accompanying figures helpful in improving clinical practice skills. As with any motor skill, learning requires practice. It is our hope that readers will use this manual to practice the activities and techniques, and to build upon and improve them. Readers are encouraged to practice with several different classmates or colleagues at first in order to enhance initial learning. This practice will also assist successful adaptation of the functional training activities and techniques for use with patients.

Section III focuses on the development of clinical decision-making skills. These skills are vital to the provision of effective treatments. Fundamental changes within the health care system have created a cost-conscious environment requiring therapists to provide more efficient care in less time. Functional outcomes and functional training must be made an early priority in rehabilitation in order to optimize the available treatment allocation and achieve desired outcomes in a shorter time. The clinical problem-solving activities presented in Section III provide an opportunity to apply content from Sections I and II. Section III is divided into two segments—specific clinical problems and more detailed case studies, with sequential introduction of more comprehensive clinical management problems as the segments progress. Students and clinicians are encouraged to use the questions provided to practice making critical decisions and resolve the specific problems or address the unique needs of the patient presented. As required levels of practice will differ from learner to learner, the number of practice applications to gain mastery will also vary. Suggested answers are provided in Appendix A and Appendix B. We recognize these answers represent *only one possible solution* to a given problem or question. It is our hope that practice of clinical decision-making skills will lead to useful problem-solving dialogue and feedback from classmates and colleagues. Among our goals for preparation of

v

the manual was to create a learning format useful to both students and clinicians for augmenting and expanding their bases for clinical practice, and for providing sound rationale for the treatments provided.

As physical therapy is a growing profession with frequent and often rapid advances in theory and practice, we consider this manual a work in progress. We welcome suggestions for improvement from our colleagues and students.

Susan B. O'Sullivan, EdD, PT
Thomas J. Schmitz, PhD, PT

ACKNOWLEDGMENTS

This Laboratory Manual is a product of our combined years of experience in clinical practice and teaching physical therapy students. We gratefully acknowledge input from both our students and our patients, who have challenged us to improve our teaching and clinical decision-making skills in order to develop plans that are understandable, systematic, and effective.

The authors express sincere gratitude to several individuals who reviewed the manuscript at different points during development. Their constructive comments greatly enhanced the content and clarity of presentation. The completed manual is reflective of their collective talent, expertise, and commitment to physical therapy education.

Candy Bahner, MS, PT
Assistant Professor and Director
Physical Therapy Assistant Program
Washburn University
Topeka, Kansas

John J. Jeziorowski, PhD, PT, ATC
Associate Professor, Department of Health Sciences
Director, Physical Therapy Program
Cleveland State University
Cleveland, Ohio

Catherine Perry Wilkinson, EdD, PT
Professor and Chair, Physical Therapy Department
Division of Health Sciences
College Misericordia
Dallas, Pennsylvania

Peter Zawicki, MS, PT
Director, Physical Therapy Assistant Program
Gateway Community College
Phoenix, Arizona

Our gratitude is extended to Paul Coppens, Director of Media Services, University of Massachusetts Lowell Library, Lowell, Massachusetts, whose photography talents and skills are displayed throughout the text. Our thanks also go to John Matson and Maureen Depres, who graciously contributed their time and talents to the production of the photographs.

We would also like to thank the following people who reviewed the manuscript proposal: Suzanne R. Brown, MPH, PT, Kirksville College of Osteopathic Medicine, Phoenix, Arizona; Anne E. Ekes, MEd, PT, Universtiy of Puget Sound, Tacoma, Washington; Toby Sternheimer, PT, Cuyahoga Community College, Cleveland, Ohio.

Appreciation is extended to Jean-François Vilain, Publisher, F. A. Davis Company, for his continued encouragement, support, and commitment to excellence in expanding the physical therapy literature. Thanks are also extended to Marianne Fithian, Developmental Editor, F. A. Davis Company, to Ona Kosmos, Editorial Assistant, F. A. Davis Company, to Barbara R. Stratton, Project Coordinator, Compset Inc., Beverly, Massachusetts, and to Catherine M. Kinane, Division of Physical Therapy, Long Island University.

CONTENTS

Functional Training

Functional training uses functional postures and activities to help patients with disordered control regain motor control. Because many functional skills are first acquired during earlier developmental stages, the term **developmental skills** (or **developmental sequence**) is often applied to many of these activities and postures. Examples include rolling, lying prone on elbows, kneeling on all fours (quadruped posture), sitting, kneeling (kneel-standing), standing, and walking. Individuals can vary considerably in their ability to acquire these skills across the life span, depending on their age, body dimensions (height, weight, limb length), level of physical activity or inactivity, and environment. Functional training focuses on using a variety of different motor skills needed for everyday life, including transitions between and within postures, and skills needed for activities of daily living such as reaching, lifting, or turning. Training also focuses on showing each patient how to adapt different movements in order to respond to changing environmental demands.

Functional training uses a logical, sequential progression in terms of increasing difficulty. In general, the patient learns to control increasingly larger segments of the body against progressively increasing effects of gravity and body weight. Thus the base of support (BOS) is narrowed while the center of mass (COM) is elevated, placing increased demands on postural control and balance. Functional training helps the patient develop skill in using muscle groups in multiple axes and planes of movement. Different types and combinations of muscle contractions (concentric, eccentric, isometric, and so on) are used to impose demands that simulate normal movement.

The advantages of this type of exercise are numerous. Functional recruitment of muscles occurs, with emphasis on synergistic motor patterns. The types of contractions involved more closely represent the work muscles typically do during the execution of daily activities. There is increased proprioceptive input from the body to assist in movement control. Finally, because of the inherent use of body weight and gravity, enhanced demands for postural control are placed on the trunk and limb segments during performance of these activities. Thus functional training activities are complex movements in which the primary focus is on coordinated action, not isolated muscle or joint control.

Learning a motor skill is a complex process. For patients with a dysfunction, training in a whole task as a single unit may not achieve the desired results. In these situations the therapist is challenged to make critical decisions about how to break the task down into its component parts within a functionally relevant context. Training strategies then address mastery of the individual components of the larger motor skill before combining them as a whole.

Within the context of treatment, the individual components of a whole task are referred to as **lead-up skills.** Each lead-up skill represents a component that is required to perform a larger functional task (referred to as the **criterion skill**). A single lead-up skill typically represents part of more than one larger motor task. For example, lower trunk rotation is a lead-up skill to upright bipedal gait (as well as other motor skills such as rolling). The use of lead-up activities prepares the individual to achieve the more important criterion functional skill. Once each lead-up skill to the larger task has been identified, decisions can be made about the best way to help the patient master the individual lead-ups before practicing the whole task. For example, lower trunk rotation is a lead-up skill that can be practiced in a number of different non-weight-bearing and weight-bearing postures, including sidelying, bridging, kneeling, and standing. Gradual control of the lead-up skill is achieved within a progression of postures that make inherently greater demands on the patient. A clinical decision is then made to combine lower trunk rotation with other lead-up skills identified as necessary prerequisites to practice of the whole criterion skill, for example, walking. The transfer of learning from parts to whole, or *from lead-up skills to criterion,* can only be ensured with additional practice of the whole skill. Thus, the patient practices walking and learns to incorporate lower trunk rotation as part of the normal pattern.

Emphasis on appropriate motor learning strategies enhances motor skill acquisition. Organized practice schedules and appropriate feedback delivery are important for learning. Patients are encouraged to solve their own problems as movement challenges are presented. Patients need to be challenged to critique their own movements with questions like "How did you do that time?" or "How can you improve your next attempt?".

Functional training activities are complex and can be very difficult and frustrating for patients. For example, practicing sit-to-stand transitions involves control of large segments of the body through activities with a gradually decreased BOS and elevated COM. These are skills that are not only important to patients but were previously performed with little effort or conscious thought. It is important to motivate and support patients with effective learning strategies. For example, the therapist can begin a training session with those functional skills that the patient can master or almost master, thereby letting the patient experience success. Varying the difficulty of the tasks can then challenge skill development. It is equally important to end treatment sessions with a relatively easy task so that the patient leaves the session with a renewed feeling of success and motivation to continue rehabilitation.

Initially, the therapist may give support during the relearning of functional skills. This can include manual support (guided movement, active-assistive movement, facilitated movement) or verbal support (detailed instructions, and verbal cueing that provides augmented feedback about movement responses such as knowledge of results and knowledge of performance).

The therapist needs to anticipate patient performance with questions such as:

1. What are the critical elements necessary for success of a particular skill? How can I help the patient focus on these critical elements?
2. How much assistance is needed to ensure successful performance? When are the demands for my assistance the greatest?
3. How should I position my body to assist the patient most effectively during the beginning, middle, and end of the movement?
4. When and how can I reduce the level of my assistance?
5. What level of verbal support is needed? When should I provide verbal cues?
6. At what point can the patient become more independent and assume active control of the movement?
7. How can I foster independence and critical decision-making skills?
8. How can I foster adaptation of skills to varying environments?

The level of assistance and support should be removed gradually and systematically as the patient achieves greater independent control. It is important not to persist in excessive levels of support long after the patient needs such support. This may result in the patient becoming overly dependent on the therapist (the "my therapist" syndrome). In this situation, the patient responds to efforts of assistance from someone new with comments such as, "My therapist does it this way."

Careful assessment and clinical decision making enable the therapist to identify movement elements that are functional and those that are not. The therapist can use this knowledge to formulate an effective plan of care for each patient. For some patients, the focus of treatment may be to help restore function following injury or insult. **Remediation training strategies** are appropriate to promote recovery and function. However, an overall goal of restoration of "normal movement" is not realistic for many patients. Patients with severe movement impairments and incomplete recovery (for example, patients with complete spinal cord injury) benefit from treatment focused on **compensatory training strategies** designed to promote optimal function using their residual abilities. The therapist needs to recognize the importance of both types of training activities during rehabilitation.

This laboratory manual is intended for professional-level physical therapy students. The initial sections focus on the clinical application of functional training activities. Specific motor control goals, compatible treatment techniques, and motor learning strategies are suggested. Students are provided with specific guidelines for the application of the exercise techniques in the various positions and activities. Activities progress from the more dependent postures (supine, prone, and quadruped) to more upright postures (sitting, kneeling, modified plantigrade, and standing) and more skilled activities (walking). Adult patients with functional disabilities do not necessarily need to complete this entire sequence of treatment activities; each patient requires a treatment plan tailored to his or her needs. Some patients may require more of a hands-on approach initially whereas others can begin with active practice of functional tasks. The overall focus of this manual is on *integrated function* as opposed to close adherence to any single treatment approach.

Theoretical aspects of motor control, motor learning, and treatment are not discussed in detail. A brief review of relevant terminology is presented in Section I. For more details on the theoretical foundation for treatment, readers can consult O'Sullivan and Schmitz.[1] Additional references are provided at the end of this laboratory manual.

The final section of this manual deals with the clinical application of functional training activities to specific clinical problems and case studies. This section provides opportunities for students to practice clinical decision making in progressively more difficult clinical situations. Students are challenged to consider their treatment plans within the context of the needs and goals of the patient and family.

Therapeutic Exercise Foundations

DEVELOPMENTAL SKILLS: STAGES OF MOTOR CONTROL

Mobility

Initial mobility in a functional pattern represents discrete movements that are not well controlled. Postural or antigravity control is typically lacking.

Characteristics

- Movements may or may not be full range.
- Movements are not sustained or well coordinated.
- The reflexive base is large (primarily low-threshold receptors, phasic stretch reflexes, and fast-twitch muscle responses); for example, protective reflexes may provide the basis for initial mobilizing responses in patients recovering from traumatic brain injury.
- Movements occur in dependent postures (for example, rolling occurs in supine, side-lying, and prone positions).

Stability

Stability (static postural control) is the ability to maintain a steady position in a weight-bearing, antigravity posture. Center of mass (COM) is maintained within limits of stability.

Tonic holding. Tonic holding is an integral part of initial stability control; it is achieved primarily by postural extensors holding in the shortened range.

Co-contraction. Co-contraction during midrange holding is required to achieve stability control. Co-contraction of postural extensors and flexors stabilizes joints.

Characteristics

- Stabilization of proximal segments and trunk is important to provide a stable base for distal movements (movements of the extremities).
- Prolonged holding (endurance function) is an integral part of stability.
- Stability primarily uses high-threshold receptors (static stretch reflexes and slow-twitch muscle responses).

Controlled Mobility

Controlled mobility (dynamic postural control) is the ability to alter a position or move in a weight-bearing position while maintaining postural stability. This stage represents mobility superimposed on stability.

Characteristics

- Movement (for example, weight shifting or rocking) is added once control in a static posture is achieved.

- Distal segments are fixed; proximal segments are mobile.
- Movement normally occurs through increments of range (small to large).
- Movement through decrements of range (large to small) can be used for progression to stability control for patients with hyperkinesia (for example, patients with ataxia).
- Full range of motion and balanced control in reversing directions are expected.
- Controlled mobility includes weight shifts, independent assumption of a posture, and transitions from one posture to another. Movement occurs against maximum effects of gravity.
- A major distinguishing factor between normal and abnormal control of movement transitions is typically the degree to which rotation is incorporated into the movement.
- Dynamic balance responses (maintaining the center of mass over the base of support) are essential for success in controlled mobility and skill activities.

Static-dynamic control is a variation of controlled mobility. This stage involves the ability to shift weight onto one side and free the opposite limb for non-weight-bearing, dynamic activities.

Characteristics

- Support limbs assume full weight bearing while the dynamic limb is moving in a functional pattern; movement challenges static postural control.
- Static-dynamic control is a prerequisite for the final skill stage of motor control.
- The stronger limb is generally the initial support limb.

Skill

Skill involves highly coordinated movement that allows for adaptability to meet the demands of the individual and the environment. The term "skill" is also used to describe the quality of performance. Skill includes both investigatory and adaptive behaviors.

Investigatory behaviors increase sensory input through eye and head movements, grasp and manipulation, and oral-motor exploration.

Adaptive behaviors include interaction with the environment through body orientation, position, and movement—for example, grasp and manipulation, locomotion and exploration, and functional skills.

TERMINOLOGY

Motor skill. Motor skill is an action or task that has a goal; voluntary movement of the body and/or limbs is required to achieve the goal.

Gross motor skills are motor tasks that involve large musculature and a goal where precision of movement is not important to the successful execution of the skill (for example, running or jumping).

Fine motor skills are motor tasks that require control of small muscles of the body to achieve the goal of skill. This type of task (for example, writing, typing, or buttoning a shirt) typically requires eye-hand coordination.

Control can be *reactive* or *proactive*.

Reactive movements are adapted in response to ongoing feedback; for example, muscle stretch causes an increase in muscle contraction in response to a forward weight shift.

Proactive movements are adapted in advance of ongoing movements via feed-forward mechanisms (for example, the postural adjustments made in preparation for catching a heavy, large ball).

Skill movements are shaped to the specific environments in which they occur.

Regulatory conditions are those features of the environment to which movement must be molded in order to be successful (for example, stepping on a moving walkway or escalator).

Closed skills are movements in a stable or fixed environment.

Open skills are movements in a changing or variable environment.

Skill movements can be defined by beginning and end points.

Discrete motor skills have clearly defined beginning and end points defined by the task itself (for example, locking the brake on a wheelchair).

Serial motor skills are discrete skills put together in a series (for example, transferring from a bed to a wheelchair).

Continuous motor skills have arbitrary beginning and end points defined by the performer or some external agents (for example, swimming or running).

Skill movements can be *single* (individual) movements or *simultaneous* (dual-task) movement sequences (for example, bouncing a ball while walking).

Self-paced action is initiated at will and typically involves closed skills (for example, a voluntary movement).

Externally paced action is initiated by dictates of the external environment and typically involves open skills (for example, stepping onto an escalator).

Characteristics

- Proximal segments stabilize the body while distal segments are free for function.
- Consistency of movement is achieved in attaining a goal.
- Movements display an economy of effort.
- Movements are regulated with precise timing and direction (a high degree of temporal and spatial organization).
- Skill movement control is task specific; skill in one task does not necessarily carry over to another without practice and experience.
- Adaptation enables movements to be modified in response to changing task and environmental demands.

Part
2

Treatment Approaches

TRADITIONAL THERAPEUTIC EXERCISE APPROACHES: REMEDIATION/FACILITATION APPROACHES

In the traditional approaches described in the following discussion, the focus of treatment is on therapeutic exercises and neuromuscular facilitation techniques to reduce the effects of impairments and disability and promote motor recovery and improved function. The involved segments are targeted in rehabilitation to prevent learned nonuse and overcompensation by intact segments. For example, a person who has had a stroke learns to roll over onto the affected side and sit up using the affected upper extremity. Developmental postures and activities are used to limit the degrees of freedom and focus on function of specific body segments. For example, prone-on-elbows posture can be used to develop initial head, upper trunk, and shoulder control.

Proprioceptive Neuromuscular Facilitation

Proprioceptive Neuromuscular Facilitation (PNF) was developed in the 1950s by Herman Kabat, MD, and Margaret Knott, PT, at the Kaiser Foundation in Vallejo, California. Dorothy Voss, PT, later made significant contributions focusing on the addition of a sequence of developmental activities in collaboration with Margaret Knott. Their work led to the publication of a now-classic textbook (Voss, Ionta, and Myers).[2]

Basic Principles and Treatment Strategies

- The facilitation of total patterns of movement and posture promotes motor learning in synergistic muscle groups.
- Normal synergies are essential for skilled function; synergies are developed initially through a well-established developmental pattern or sequence.
- Weakness, incoordination, adaptive shortening, joint immobility, and alterations in muscle tone may lead to impaired patterns of posture and movement as well as functional dependency.
- Normal patterns of movement are spiral and diagonal.

Upper extremity (UE) patterns are named for motions occurring at the proximal joint (shoulder). The intermediate joint (elbow) may be straight, flexed, or extended (intermediate pivot).
  - **Flexion-Adduction-External Rotation, or Diagonal 1 Flexion (D1F):** The hand closes with wrist and finger flexion; the upper limb externally rotates and pulls up and across the face, moving into shoulder adduction and flexion.
  - **Extension-Abduction-Internal Rotation, or Diagonal 1 Extension (D1E):** The hand opens with wrist and finger extension; the upper limb internally rotates and pushes down and out, moving into shoulder abduction and extension.
  - **Flexion-Abduction-External Rotation, or Diagonal 2 Flexion (D2F):** The hand opens with wrist and finger extension; the upper limb externally rotates and lifts up and out, moving into shoulder abduction and flexion.
  - **Extension-Adduction-Internal Rotation, or Diagonal 2 Extension (D2E):** The

8

hand closes with wrist and finger flexion; the upper limb internally rotates and pulls down and across the body, moving into shoulder adduction and extension.

Lower-extremity (LE) patterns are named for motions occurring at the proximal joint (hip). The intermediate joint (knee) may be straight, flexed, or extended (intermediate pivot).

- **Flexion-Adduction-External Rotation, or Diagonal 1 Flexion (D1F):** The foot dorsiflexes and inverts; the lower limb externally rotates and pulls up and across the body, moving into hip adduction and flexion.
- **Extension-Abduction-Internal Rotation, or Diagonal 1 Extension (D1E):** The foot plantarflexes and everts; the lower limb internally rotates and pushes down and out, moving into hip abduction and extension.
- **Flexion-Abduction-Internal Rotation, or Diagonal 2 Flexion (D2F):** The foot dorsiflexes and everts; the lower limb internally rotates and lifts up and out, moving into hip abduction and flexion.
- **Extension-Adduction-External Rotation, or Diagonal 2 Extension (D2E):** The foot plantarflexes and inverts; the lower limb externally rotates and pushes down and in, moving into hip adduction and extension.

Head and trunk patterns combine flexion or extension with rotation.

- **Chop, or upper trunk flexion with rotation to right or left:** The lead arm moves in D1E; the assist arm holds on from the top of the wrist; the elbows are straight. The head and trunk flex and rotate to the right or left.
- **Lift, or upper trunk extension with rotation to right or left:** The lead arm moves in D2F; the assist arm holds on from underneath the wrist; the elbows are straight. The head and trunk extend and rotate to the right or left.
- **Lower trunk flexion with rotation to right or left:** The hips flex; the legs pull up and across the body toward one side; the knees may be extended or flexed.
- **Head and neck flexion with rotation to right or left:** The head turns and bends down, bringing the chin to the opposite side of the chest.
- **Head and neck extension with rotation to right or left:** The head turns and extends back to the opposite side.

- **Normal timing:** Timing of muscle components occurs in a distal to proximal sequence during PNF extremity patterns. Proximal motion is delayed until the distal component approaches full range.
- Effective use of **maximum resistance** and **stretch** recruits additional motor units and facilitates muscle contraction and motor control.
- Additional proprioceptive stimulation includes the use of **traction** (to promote flexor patterns) and **approximation** (to promote extensor patterns).
- **Verbal commands** (both preparatory and action commands) facilitate active movements and assist in motor learning.
- **Manual contacts** (MCs) guide movement and enhance motor control through grip and pressure.
- **Vision** is used to guide movement and enhance motor control.
- Effective motor learning is emphasized through the use of **repetition** and **practice.** Varying practice through pattern variations and combinations fosters continued learning.

PNF Techniques of Treatment

PNF techniques of treatment (described fully in Part 3) used to address problems of posture and movement control include:

Agonist reversals (ARs)
Alternating isometrics (AI)
Contract-relax (CR)
Hold-relax (HR)
Hold-relax active motion (HRAM)

Repeated contractions (RCs)
Resisted progression (RP)
Rhythmic initiation (RI)
Rhythmic rotation (RRo)
Rhythmic stabilization (RS)
Slow reversals (SRs)

Neurodevelopmental Treatment

Neurodevelopmental Treatment (NDT) is a comprehensive treatment approach developed by Berta Bobath, PT, and Karel Bobath, MD,[3] to promote motor development and recovery in patients with neurological dysfunction. Normal development is promoted in children with cerebral palsy; patients with stroke or traumatic brain injury relearn movement control through structured functional activities. The theory base has been expanded in recent years to incorporate current concepts of motor control and learning and forced recovery training. Movement control within the context of functional tasks is emphasized.

Basic Principles and Treatment Strategies

- Normal movement sequences and balance are the focus of intervention.
- Emphasis is on normalization of sensory and perceptual experiences through tactile and kinesthetic stimulation.
- Treatment is individualized. Accurate movement analysis is essential for treatment planning; this includes assessment of patterns of movement, tone, and reflexes. Emphasis is on the patient as a whole.
- Permanent changes in behavior and movement are facilitated by practice and experience.
- Abnormal tone, primitive reflex patterns such as those imposed by the tonic reflexes, and mass synergies result in abnormal patterns of posture and movement and interfere with normal recovery and function. Treatment is focused on inhibiting or eliminating these patterns.
- Attempts are made to normalize postural tone:
  - Tone is increased through use of facilitation techniques if tone is too low (hypotonia).
  - Tone is decreased through the use of inhibitory techniques if tone is too high (spasticity).
  - Low effort maximizes performance in the presence of spasticity; high effort and maximal resistance are contraindicated with spasticity.
- Treatment is aimed at promoting active control of movements. Assistance and facilitation are provided as needed:
  - Normal functional activities that are meaningful and goal oriented are promoted (such as rolling over, sitting up, standing, and walking).
  - Use of involved segments and integration of body segments is promoted (forced recovery).
  - Substitution (compensatory) movements are not permitted.
  - Isolated, selective movements (out-of-synergy combinations) are promoted (for example, for the patient with stroke).
  - Automatic balance reactions (righting, equilibrium, and protective reactions) are facilitated.
  - Control of trunk movements is considered critical to postural control and limb function.
  - Gravity-eliminated positions are used initially; progression is made to weight-bearing, antigravity positions.
  - Selective movements in midranges are promoted to establish initial control (placing and holding); progression is made to active control in end ranges, moving into and out of a posture.

- Carryover is promoted through family, caregiver, and staff education. Carryover can be expected only if treatment activities and techniques are consistently applied by all who engage the patient.

Neurodevelopmental Treatment Techniques

NDT techniques of treatment (described in Part 3) include:

Guided movement; active-assistive movement
Handling (key points of control)
Rhythmic rotation (RRo)

Volitional control of movement can be facilitated through the use of:
  ◦ Proprioceptive inputs (weight bearing, stretching, tapping, and other manipulations)
  ◦ Exteroceptive inputs (rubbing and stroking)
  ◦ Verbal commands

The use of proprioceptive facilitation techniques and exteroceptive stimulation techniques is described fully in Part 4.

Movement Therapy in Hemiplegia

Movement Therapy is a treatment approach developed by Signe Brunnstrom, PT, to promote recovery in patients with stroke. Patients relearn movement control through structured activities that promote resumption of normal function. Brunnstrom was the first to describe the stereotypic patterns of recovery and synergistic patterns of movement typically seen in patients recovering from stroke.[4] Recovery progresses in sequence from mass movement patterns (flexion and extension synergies) to movement that involves components of the two patterns and then to isolated joint control.

Basic Principles and Treatment Strategies

- Careful assessment can delineate recovery stages as well as stroke deficits such as tone changes, abnormal synergies, and impaired voluntary movement.
  ◦ The development of an accurate assessment tool is a major contribution of Brunnstrom. Brunnstrom's Hemiplegia Classification and Progress Record[5] forms the basis of the Fugl-Meyer Assessment of Physical Performance currently in use.
  ◦ Variability in recovery can occur between limbs (the lower extremity may recover more than the upper extremity) and within limbs (the shoulder may recover more than the hand). Recovery can also plateau at any stage.
- Training procedures were developed based on the unique sensorimotor difficulties common to patients with stroke.
  ◦ Out-of-synergy combinations needed for everyday function, such as hand function and walking, are promoted.
  ◦ Movement control progresses from small range to large range.
  ◦ Isometric and eccentric contractions progress to isotonic contractions.
- Patients with low-level recovery are encouraged to gain control of basic limb synergies first. Once initial control is achieved, out-of-synergy combinations are promoted. Note: Because repeated use of synergies may make isolated movements difficult to achieve and limit recovery to largely synergistic control, this concept is now viewed as inappropriate. Practice of abnormal synergies is contraindicated.
- Fatigue, pain, and heavy resistance are avoided because they have a detrimental effect on voluntary control.
- Positive reinforcement and repetition are key elements to successful motor learning.

Movement Therapy Techniques of Treatment

Volitional control of movement can be facilitated through the use of:

- Proprioceptive inputs (resistance, weight bearing, stretching, tapping, and other manipulations)
- Exteroceptive inputs (rubbing and stroking)
- Verbal commands
- Use of the sound side to facilitate movement on the involved side (transfer effects)

Sensory Stimulation

Sensory stimulation is a component of all the neurotherapeutic approaches (neurophysiologic approaches), and is based on the work of Rood,[6] Knott and Voss,[2] and the Bobaths.[3] Historically, the techniques are based on the premise that movements can be stimulated by peripheral inputs (using a reflex or stimulus-response theory of motor control). Once movements are initiated through stimulation, they can progress to automatic voluntary control. Problems arise with the inappropriate use or overuse of stimulation techniques. Patients may experience difficulty in the transition to active movement control and fail to develop independent movement patterns needed for function.

Basic Principles and Treatment Strategies

- Indications: Absent or severely disordered motor control; difficulty in initiating or sustaining movement—for example, the patient with traumatic brain injury during an early recovery management program (coma stimulation program).
- Contraindications: Hands-on stimulation is not beneficial in the presence of sufficient voluntary control to initiate and perform active movement, or if the ability to self-correct based on intrinsic feedback mechanisms is intact (for example, in the middle and later stages of motor learning).
- Response to stimulation is dependent on multiple factors, including level of intactness of CNS and initial central set (readiness of postural and movement mechanisms).
  - Sensory stimulation techniques are contraindicated for patients with excess tone, generalized arousal, or autonomic instability (fight-or-flight responses).
  - Excessive stimulation impairs voluntary control of movement.
- Early use of sensory stimulation techniques should be phased out as soon as possible in favor of active movement control.
- Cumulative effects can be achieved with summation of sensory stimulation techniques: this may be necessary to produce the desired response in some patients with very low-level function (for example, the patient with traumatic brain injury who demonstrates low-level recovery and arousal)
  - Spatial summation: simultaneous use of multiple sensory stimulation techniques
  - Temporal summation: repeated use of the same sensory stimulation technique
- The cumulative effects of all environmental influences, together with the effects of sensory stimulation, must be considered in treatment.
  - Overstimulation or bombardment of the central nervous system (CNS) with excessive sensory inputs must be avoided. This is referred to as overload.
  - Overstimulation may prove extremely counterproductive by causing the CNS to shut down (the patient may become unresponsive), or may produce sympathetic fight-or-flight reactions (the patient may become agitated and combative).
- Consideration must be given to the types of stimuli that may yield optimal performance and learning—for example, proprioceptive stimuli are naturally occurring during movement.

COMPENSATORY TRAINING APPROACH

In compensatory training, the focus is on the early resumption of functional independence by using the uninvolved segments for function. For example, a patient with left hemiplegia is taught to dress using the right upper extremity; the patient with a complete T1-level spinal cord lesion is taught to roll using upper extremities and momentum. Central to this approach is the concept of **substitution.** Changes are made in the patient's overall approach to functional tasks.

Basic Principles and Treatment Strategies

- The patient is made aware of movement deficiencies.
- Alternate ways to accomplish a task are considered, simplified, and adopted.
- The patient is taught to use the segments that are intact to compensate for those that have been lost.
- The patient practices and relearns the task; repeated practice results in consistency and habitual use of the new pattern.
- The patient practices the functional skill in environments in which function is expected to occur.
- Energy conservation techniques are taught to ensure that the patient can complete all daily tasks.
- The patient's environment is adapted to facilitate relearning of skills, ease of movement, and optimal performance.
- Assistive devices are incorporated as needed.

General Considerations

- Focusing on the uninvolved segments to accomplish daily tasks may suppress recovery and contribute to learned nonuse of the impaired segments. For example, the patient with stroke may fail to learn to use the involved extremities.
- Focusing on task-specific learning may result in the development of **splinter skills** in patients with brain damage. Splinter skills cannot easily be generalized to other environments or variations of the same task.
- Compensatory training may be the only approach possible when:
  - Very little additional recovery is expected and improved function is the desired outcome (for example, in the patient with a complete spinal cord lesion).
  - Severe sensorimotor deficits and extensive co-morbidities limit the patient's ability to use the affected extremities and to relearn motor skills.

Therapeutic Exercise Techniques

TERMINOLOGY

Approximation. Approximation (joint compression) involves applying a force to joints, typically through gravity acting on body weight; force can be applied through manual contacts or weight belts. Indications for this technique include instability of extensor muscles in weight bearing and holding, poor static postural control, and/or weakness.

Agonist reversals (ARs). AR involves a slow isotonic, shortening contraction through the range followed by an eccentric, lengthening contraction using the same muscle groups. ARs are performed through increments of range; they are typically used in bridging, sit-to-stand transitions, and stepping up and down a step. Indications for this technique include weak postural muscles, inability to control body weight eccentrically during movement transitions, and poor dynamic postural control.

Alternating isometrics (AI). In AI, isometric holding is facilitated first in agonists acting on one side of the joint, followed by holding of the antagonist muscle groups. Resistance may be applied in any direction (anterior/posterior, medial/lateral, or diagonal). Indications for this technique include instability in weight bearing and holding, poor static postural control, and/or weakness.

Contract-relax (CR). CR is a relaxation technique usually performed at a point of limited range of motion (ROM) in the agonist pattern. Isotonic movement in rotation is followed by an isometric hold of the range-limiting muscles in the antagonist pattern against slowly increasing resistance; this is followed by voluntary relaxation and passive movement into the new range of the agonist pattern.

Contract-relax active contraction (CRAC). CRAC is similar to CR except movement into the newly gained range of the agonist pattern is active, not passive. Active contraction serves to maintain the inhibitory effects through reciprocal inhibition. Indications for this contraction include limitations in ROM caused by muscle tightness and spasticity.

Facilitation techniques. Neuromuscular facilitation techniques are a group of techniques used to facilitate or inhibit muscle contraction (see discussion in Part 4).

Guided movement (GM) or active-assistive movement (AAM). In GM, the movements are actively guided or assisted in some way. Guidance reduces errors, promotes early learning during the acquisition phase of motor skill learning, and reduces frustration and movement anxiety.

Manual assists may be maximal, moderate, or minimal. The therapist removes support when the patient is able to take over the movement and resumes guiding as needed. Verbal assists cue the patient through a movement.

Active movement control is the overall goal of GM. Effective problem solving is promoted as the key to independent function. Indications for guided movement include inability to move, impaired tactile and kinesthetic inputs that normally guide movements, and perceptual dysfunction.

Handling. Physical handling techniques are used to inhibit abnormal movements, tone, or reflexes and to facilitate normal tone and patterns of movement. Indications for handling include inability to move because of spasticity and abnormal reflex activity.

- **Key points of control** are parts of the body the therapist chooses as optimal to control tone and movement.
  - *Proximal key points* (trunk, head, shoulders and pelvis) are used to ensure control of trunk and proximal segments before facilitating active limb movements. Proximal key points are also generally effective in influencing tone throughout the entire limb.
  - *Distal key points* (hands and feet) may also be used.
- Tone is normalized before active movements are attempted.
- Examples of key points of control to decrease tone include:
  - **Head and trunk:** Flexion decreases shoulder retraction, trunk and limb extension.
  - **Humerus:** External rotation and flexion to 90 degrees decreases flexion tone of the upper extremity.
  - **Thumb:** Abduction and extension of the thumb with forearm supination decreases flexion tone of the wrist and fingers.
  - **Hip:** Femoral external rotation and abduction decreases extensor adductor tone of the lower extremity.

Hold-relax (HR). HR is a relaxation technique usually performed at the point of limited ROM in the agonist pattern. An isometric contraction of the range-limiting antagonist pattern is performed against slowly increasing resistance, followed by voluntary relaxation and passive movement into the newly gained range of the agonist pattern.

Hold-relax active contraction (HRAC). Active contraction can also be performed in the newly gained range of the agonist pattern. This contraction serves to maintain the inhibitory effects through reciprocal inhibition. Indications for HR and HRAC include limitations in ROM caused by muscle tightness, muscle spasm, and pain.

Hold-relax active motion (HRAM). HRAM is an isometric contraction performed in the middle to shortened range, followed by voluntary relaxation and passive movement into the lengthened range. Tracking resistance is applied to an isotonic contraction as movement occurs from the lengthened to the shortened range. Indications for this contraction include an inability to initiate movement, hypotonia (poor spindle-stretch sensitivity), weakness, and marked imbalances between opposing muscle groups.

Repeated contractions (RCs). RCs are repeated isotonic contractions induced by quick stretches and enhanced by resistance performed through the range or part of the range at a point of weakness. RC is a unidirectional technique; an isometric hold can be added at a point of weakness. Indications for this technique include weakness, incoordination, muscle imbalances, and/or diminished muscular endurance.

Resisted progression (RP). In RP, stretch and tracking resistance are applied to facilitate progression in walking, creeping, kneel-walking, or movement transitions. Indications for RP include impaired timing and control of lower trunk/pelvic segments (pelvic rotation) and lack of endurance.

Rhythmic initiation (RI). RI begins with voluntary relaxation followed by passive movements through increments in range, followed by active-assistive movements progressing to resisted movements using tracking resistance (light, facilitatory resistance) to isotonic contractions. RI may be unidirectional or performed in both directions. Indications for RI include inability to relax, hypertonicity (spasticity, rigidity), inability to initiate movement (apraxia), motor learning deficits, and communication deficits (aphasia).

Rhythmic rotation (RRo). RRo uses voluntary relaxation combined with slow, passive, rhythmic rotation of the body or body part around a longitudinal axis, followed by passive movement into the antagonist range (opposite to the spastic pattern). Rotation may be combined with active movements to promote relaxation and gain new range or hold in the new range. Indications for this technique are hypertonia with limitations in function or ROM.

Rhythmic stabilization (RS). RS is an isometric contraction of the agonist pattern followed by the antagonist pattern. The technique is performed without relaxation using careful grading of resistance; this results in co-contraction of opposing muscle groups. RS emphasizes rotational stability control. Indications for RS include instability in weight bearing and holding, poor static postural control, and weakness as well as limitations in ROM caused by muscle tightness and painful muscle splinting.

Shortened held resisted contraction (SHRC). SHRC uses resistance applied to an isometric contraction of muscle(s) holding in the shortened range. The resistance is typically applied to extensor muscles in modified pivot prone positions such as sidelying or supported sitting. Indications for SHRC include instability in weight bearing and holding, poor static postural control, and weakness.

Slow reversals (SRs). SRs begin with a slow, isotonic contraction in the agonist pattern followed by contraction in the antagonist pattern using careful grading of resistance and optimal facilitation. Then the patterns are reversed (reversal of antagonists) with emphasis on slow, controlled movement and progression through increments of range.

Slow reversal-hold (SRH). In SRH, an isometric hold is added at the end of the range or at a point of weakness. The hold may be added in both directions or only in one direction. Indications for SRs and SRH include inability to reverse directions, muscle imbalances, weakness, incoordination, and lack of endurance.

Tapping. Tapping provides stimulation via a quick stretch to the muscle spindle; the stimulus is applied directly over the muscle belly. **Sweep-tapping** results in widespread activation of the muscle being tapped. Indications for tapping and sweep-tapping include weakness and/or hypotonia.

Timing for emphasis (TE). TE uses maximum resistance to elicit a sequence of contractions of major muscle components of a pattern of motion. This technique allows overflow to occur from strong to weak components; it can be performed within a limb (one muscle group to another) or using overflow from limb to limb or trunk to limb. TE is typically combined with repeated contractions (TE/RCs) to strengthen the weaker components. Indications for TE and TE/RC include weakness and/or incoordination.

Traction. Traction is a distraction force applied to joints; the force is typically applied through manual contacts. Indications for traction include inability of flexor muscles to function in mobilizing patterns and weakness.

Part 4

Neuromuscular Facilitation Techniques

Neuromuscular facilitation techniques are a group of techniques used to facilitate or inhibit muscle contraction or responses.

PROPRIOCEPTIVE FACILITATION TECHNIQUES

Quick Stretch

- The stimulus is a quick stretch applied to a muscle.
  - A quick stretch activates muscle spindles and facilitates Ia endings, making them more sensitive to velocity and length changes.
  - The muscle spindle provides input to spinal neurons (stretch reflex) and higher centers (functional stretch response).
- Quick stretch facilitates or enhances agonist contraction, inhibits antagonists, and facilitates synergists through reciprocal innervation effects.
- Techniques include:
  - Quick stretch
  - Tapping over muscle belly or tendon
- Comments: Quick stretch evokes a low-threshold phasic response that is relatively short-lived. The therapist must add resistance to maintain muscle contraction. Stretch is more effective when applied in the lengthened range to initiate contraction.
- Adverse effects: Quick stretch may increase spasticity.

Prolonged Stretch

- The stimulus is a slowly applied, maintained stretch, especially in lengthened ranges.
  - A prolonged stretch activates muscle spindles (Ia and II endings) and Golgi tendon organs (Ib endings), sensitive to length and tension changes.
  - The muscle spindle provides input to spinal neurons (stretch reflex) and higher centers (functional stretch response).
- The stimulus inhibits or dampens muscle contraction and tone.
- Techniques include:
  - Manual contacts
  - Inhibitory splinting, casting
  - Reflex-inhibiting patterns
  - Mechanical low-load weights
- Comments: Prolonged stretching evokes a higher threshold response. It may be more effective in extensor muscles than flexors due to the added effects of II inhibition. To maintain inhibitory effects, the antagonist muscles should be activated.

Resistance

- The stimulus is a force exerted to muscle.
  - Resistance activates muscle spindles (Ia and II endings) and Golgi tendon organs (Ib endings), making them more sensitive to changes in velocity and length.
  - Muscle spindle provides input to spinal neurons (stretch reflex) and higher centers (functional stretch response).
- The response facilitates or enhances muscle contraction. It facilitates agonist patterns, inhibits antagonists and facilitates synergists and reciprocal innervation effects. Resistance also recruits both alpha and gamma motoneurons and additional motor units. Resistance hypertrophies extrafusal muscle fibers and enhances kinesthetic awareness.
- Techniques include:
  - Manual resistance, adjusted to produce smooth, coordinated movement
  - Use of body weight and gravity
  - Mechanical weights
- Comments: Light, tracking resistance is used to strengthen weak muscles. With weak hypotonic muscles, eccentric and isometric contractions are used before concentric contractions (this enhances muscle spindle support of contraction with less spindle unloading). Maximal resistance may produce overflow to other muscles. Resistance also enhances patient awareness of movement.
- Adverse effects: Too much resistance can easily overpower weak, hypotonic muscles and prevent voluntary movement or encourage substitution. Excessive resistance may increase spasticity. Breath-holding may accompany maximal resistance and should be avoided.

Joint Approximation

- The stimulus is compression of joint surfaces. Approximation activates joint receptors (greatest effects on static, type I receptors).
- The response facilitates postural extensors and stabilizers. Joint compression enhances joint awareness.
- Techniques include:
  - Joint compression, either manual or mechanical using weight cuffs or belts
  - Bouncing while sitting on a Swiss ball
- Comments: Compression is typically applied in extensor patterns, in middle to short-ened ranges while the patient is weight bearing. Resistance must be used to maintain the contraction.
- Adverse effects: Approximation is contraindicated in inflamed joints.

Joint Traction

- The stimulus is distraction of joint surfaces. Traction activates joint receptors (greatest effects on phasic, type II receptors).
- The response facilitates agonists. Traction enhances contraction and joint awareness.
- Technique: Manual distraction is used.
- Comments: Joint traction is used as a facilitatory stimulus in flexor patterns and pulling actions. Slow, sustained traction to joints can be used to improve mobility, re-lieve muscle spasm, and reduce pain with techniques of joint mobilization. Resistance must be used to maintain the contraction.

Inhibitory Pressure

- The stimulus is prolonged pressure applied to long tendons. Inhibitory pressure activates muscle receptors (muscle spindles and Golgi tendon organs) and tactile receptors.
- The response is inhibition; the pressure dampens muscle tone.
- Techniques include:
  - Firm pressure, applied manually or with body weight; positioning at end ranges
  - Mechanical pressure: holding firm objects (cones) in hand
  - Inhibitory splints, casts
- Comments: Weight-bearing postures are used to provide inhibitory pressure; for example, quadruped or kneeling postures can be used to promote inhibition of quadriceps and long finger flexors. Sitting with the hand open and elbow extended, with the arm (UE) supporting body weight, can be used to promote inhibition of long finger flexors.
- Adverse effects: Sustained positioning may dampen muscle contraction and affect functional performance.

EXTEROCEPTIVE STIMULATION TECHNIQUES

Light Touch

- The stimulus is brief, light contact with skin. Light touch activates fast-adapting tactile receptors with input into the central nervous system (CNS) and sympathetic division of the autonomic nervous system.
- The response is increased arousal and withdrawal from the stimulus. Light touch evokes phasic withdrawal responses, including flexion and adduction of the extremities.
- Techniques: Light touch is applied to areas of high tactile receptor density (hands, feet, lips) that are more sensitive to stimulation. Techniques include:
  - A brief, light stroke of the fingertips
  - A brief swipe with an ice cube (quick icing)
  - Light pinching or squeezing
- Comments: Light touch evokes a low-threshold response; the patient accommodates rapidly. Light touch can be effective in initially mobilizing patients with low response levels, for example, the patient with traumatic brain injury during early recovery stages. Resistance must be applied to maintain contraction.
- Adverse effects: Light touch causes increased sympathetic arousal and may produce fight-or-flight responses. It is contraindicated in patients with generalized arousal or autonomic instability (for example, the patient with traumatic brain injury who is agitated and combative).

Maintained Touch

- The stimulus is maintained contact or pressure. Maintained touch activates tactile receptors with input into the CNS and parasympathetic division of the autonomic nervous system.
- The response is a calming effect and generalized inhibition. Maintained touch desensitizes skin receptors.
- Techniques include:
  - Firm manual contacts
  - Firm pressure applied to the midline of the abdomen, the back, lips, palms, and/or the soles of the feet
  - Firm rubbing

- Comments: Maintained touch is useful for patients with high arousal and a hypersensitivity to sensory stimulation. Maintained touch can be applied to hypersensitive areas to normalize responses, for example, in the patient with peripheral nerve injury and paresthesias.
- Adverse effects:
  - Brief touch stimuli should be avoided.
  - Maintained touch can be used in combination with other maintained stimuli.

Slow Stroking

- The stimulus is slow stroking, applied to the paravertebral spinal region over the posterior primary rami. Slow stroking activates tactile receptors in the parasympathetic division of the autonomic nervous system.
- The response is a calming effect and generalized inhibition.
- Techniques
  - The patient is placed in a supported position such as prone, or sitting with the head and arms supported and resting on a table top.
  - The therapist uses a flat hand to apply firm, alternate strokes downward to the paravertebral region for approximately 3 to 5 minutes.
- Comments: Slow stroking is useful with patients who demonstrate high arousal and increased sympathetic (fight-or-flight) responses.

Manual Contacts

- The stimulus is firm, deep pressure of the hands in contact with the body. Manual contacts activate tactile receptors and muscle proprioceptors.
- The response is contraction in the muscle(s) directly under the hands. Manual contacts provide sensory awareness and directional cues to movement. The contacts also provide security and support to unstable body segments.
- Comments: Manual contacts can be used with or without resistance.
- Adverse effects: Manual contacts are contraindicated over spastic muscles and open wounds.

Prolonged Icing

- The stimulus is application of cold water or ice. Prolonged icing activates thermoreceptors.
- The response is decreased neural and muscle spindle firing. Icing inhibits muscle tone and painful muscle spasm. Prolonged icing also decreases the metabolic rate of tissues.
- Techniques include:
  - Immersion in cold water, ice chips
  - Ice towel wraps
  - Ice packs
  - Ice massage
- Comments: Effects should be monitored carefully.
- Adverse effects: Prolonged icing can cause sympathetic nervous system arousal and evoke protective withdrawal responses, including fight-or-flight responses. Prolonged icing is contraindicated in patients with sensory deficits, generalized arousal, autonomic instability, or vascular problems. Exposure to skin should be limited to avoid frostbite.

Neutral Warmth

- The stimulus is retention of body heat. Neutral warmth activates thermoreceptors in the parasympathetic division of the autonomic nervous system.
- The response is generalized inhibition of tone. Neutral warmth produces a calming effect—relaxation; it also can decrease pain.
- Techniques include:
  - Wrapping the body or body parts with Ace wraps or towel wraps
  - Applying snug-fitting clothing (gloves, socks, or tights) or air splints
  - Immersing the body or body part in tepid baths
- Comments: Neutral warmth should be applied for approximately 10 to 20 minutes. It is useful for patients with high arousal or increased sympathetic activity, including spasticity.
- Adverse effects: Overheating should be avoided. Excessive warmth may produce rebound effects (increased arousal or tone).

VESTIBULAR STIMULATION TECHNIQUES

Slow, Maintained Vestibular Stimulation

- The stimulus is low-intensity, slow vestibular stimulation (for example, slow rocking). Low-intensity stimulation primarily activates otolith organs (facilitating tonic receptors); it has less effect on the semicircular canals (phasic receptors).
- The response is generalized inhibition of tone. Slow, maintained vestibular stimulation decreases arousal and has a calming effect.
- Techniques include:
  - Slow, repetitive rocking movements (for example, slow rolling)
  - Assisted rocking with equipment such as a rocking chair, Swiss ball, equilibrium board, hammock, or swing, using slow, rolling movements
- Comments: Low-intensity vestibular stimulation is useful with patients who are hypertonic, hyperactive, or who demonstrate high arousal, or tactile defensiveness. Rocking can be combined with cognitive relaxation techniques.

Fast Vestibular Stimulation

- The stimulus is high-intensity vestibular stimulation (for example, fast spinning, irregular movements with an acceleration and deceleration component). Fast vestibular stimulation activates semicircular canals (phasic receptors); it has less effect on otoliths (tonic receptors).
- The response is generalized facilitation of tone. Fast vestibular stimulation improves motor coordination and retinal image stability; it decreases postrotatory nystagmus.
- Techniques include:
  - Fast spinning (for example, spinning in a chair, mesh net, or hammock)
  - Fast acceleration-deceleration movements (for example, fast rolling movements in prone position on a scooter board)
- Comments: Fast vestibular stimulation is useful in patients with hypotonia (for example, the individual with Down's syndrome) and in patients with sensory integrative dysfunction or coordination problems (for example, patients with stroke or cerebral palsy). It can be helpful in overcoming the effects of akinesia or bradykinesia in patients with Parkinson's disease.
- Adverse effects: Fast vestibular stimulation can cause behavioral changes, seizures, or sleep disturbances. Fast spinning or rolling is contraindicated for patients with recurrent seizures or those who are intolerant to sensory stimulation.

Application of Therapeutic Exercise Techniques to Stages of Motor Control

INITIAL MOBILITY

Strategies/Techniques to Improve Mobility

Initial mobility is characterized by movements that are not well controlled. They subserve a large protective function and therefore have a large reflex base (for example, protective withdrawal). Initial mobility is generally developed in non-weight-bearing postures such as supine, sidelying, or prone positions.

Immobility due to Hypertonicity (High Tone)

Patients who demonstrate problems with decreased mobility may be too stiff (because of spasticity or rigidity) to move. These patients typically exhibit range of motion (ROM) restrictions that prevent or limit movement. Patients may exhibit pain (painful spasm) resulting in decreased mobility and desire to move. The overall goal is to decrease tone or spasm and to promote active movements and ROM.

Emphasis should be placed on:

- Cognitive relaxation (voluntary relaxation)
- Tone-reduction techniques (rhythmic rotation) followed by voluntary movement
- Promotion of normal patterns of movement with inhibition of abnormal muscle tone and primitive reflex patterns
- Low effort with an overall focus on controlled movement
- Use of functional positions and activities to facilitate ease of movement (for example, gravity-assisted movements)
- Promotion of newly acquired movements
  - Focus is placed on active holding or movement in the newly gained range.
  - The utilization of the agonist pattern results in reciprocal inhibition of antagonists.
- Cautious use of resistance
  - Carefully graded resistance (light, tracking resistance) is applied to agonists.
  - Gravity can be an effective form of resistance.
  - Maximal resistance is contraindicated.
- Repetition of newly gained (agonist) movement patterns

Specific neuromuscular facilitation techniques may include:

Rhythmic initiation (RI)
Hold-relax (HR) and contract-relax active contraction (CRAC)
Rhythmic rotation (RRo)
Active-assistive and guided movements, handling techniques

Sensory stimulation inputs may include:

Cold modalities to decrease tone
Neutral warmth
Slow stroking
Slow vestibular stimulation (rocking)
Maintained touch to decrease arousal levels

Immobility due to Hypotonia (Low Tone) and Weakness

Decreased mobility may also result from problems associated with decreased tone (hypotonia), decreased muscle strength, motor programming deficits (dyspraxia), or decreased responsiveness (hyposensitivity) to sensory stimuli. Patients may be too weak to move after prolonged bed rest or inactivity, or they may be too lethargic to respond to their environment after head injury and coma. These patients may benefit from techniques designed to improve motor control by increasing sensory responsiveness, tone, and initiation of movement.

Emphasis should be placed on:

- Sensory experiences and normalization of sensory inputs
- Carefully graded resistance to enhance muscle function (loading of muscle spindles via proprioceptive stimulation)
  - Light, tracking resistance
  - Resistance of gravity in weight-bearing positions
- Isometric holding to develop muscle spindle-stretch sensitivity
- Progression from isometric to eccentric to concentric contractions to facilitate voluntary control
- Repetition of newly gained movements throughout the range

Specific neuromuscular facilitation techniques may include:

Rhythmic initiation (RI)
Hold-relax active movement (HRAM)
Repeated contractions (RCs) using resistance and stretch to tolerance
Active-assistive and guided movement, handling techniques

Sensory stimulation inputs may include carefully graded phasic stimuli such as a quick stretch, tapping, and light touch (including quick icing) to facilitate movement. Prolonged use of sensory inputs should be avoided. Active movement should be promoted and sensory inputs should be phased out as quickly as possible.

STABILITY

Strategies/Techniques to Improve Stability

Stability (static postural control) refers to the ability to maintain a position against gravity. Muscles co-contract to stabilize around a joint and ensure maintenance of upright posture against gravity.

Stability control is developed in weight-bearing postures:

Prone-on-elbows (PoE) posture promotes development of head, upper trunk, and proximal (shoulder) control.
Quadruped (all-fours) posture promotes the additional components of lower trunk, hip, and elbow control.
Sitting promotes upright head and upper trunk control.

Kneeling promotes lower trunk and hip control in addition to upright head and trunk control.

Modified plantigrade position (weight bearing in standing position with extended elbows—upper and lower extremity support) promotes control of the trunk and proximal extremities (upper and lower extremities).

Standing promotes knee, foot, and ankle control in addition to upright head, trunk, and hip control.

Patients who demonstrate problems with stability control may be unable to hold a posture for several reasons including tonal imbalances (hypotonia, hypertonia), impaired voluntary control (decreased strength, lack of stretch sensitivity), hypermobility (athetosis, ataxia), sensory hypersensitivity (tactile-avoidance reactions), and/or increased arousal (high sympathetic tone).

Emphasis should be placed on:

- Isometric contractions in the shortened range (postural extensors), progressing to midrange control (co-contraction)
- Weight bearing and holding in antigravity postures
- Specific motion deficits (for example, patients with hyperkinesia, including ataxia and athetosis) may benefit from gradually decreasing ROM progressing to steady holding

Specific neuromuscular facilitation techniques may include:

Alternating isometrics (AI) or rhythmic stabilization (RS)
Slow reversal-hold (SRH) through decrements of ROM
Placing and holding: hold after positioning

Sensory stimulation inputs may include:

Joint approximation (manual compression and weight bearing or gentle bouncing while sitting on a Swiss ball) to facilitate stabilizing muscles
Weights and Theraband or surgical tubing to increase proprioceptive loading
Pool therapy to provide antigravity support and proprioceptive loading via resistance of water

CONTROLLED MOBILITY

Strategies/Techniques to Improve Controlled Mobility

The ability to move while maintaining a stable upright posture is referred to as **controlled mobility.** It is characterized by the combined function of both mobilizing and stabilizing components with smooth reversal of the antagonists.

Closed-chain activities refer to those functional activities that involve a total body movement with the distal end of the extremity fixed in space while the proximal segments (trunk and proximal joints—shoulders and/or hips) are moving.

Examples of activities in which controlled mobility function is used include rocking, weight shifting, or movement transitions (shifting from one posture to another) while maintaining upright posture. For example, the patient is asked to rock slowly from side to side in sitting or quadruped position, or the patient can be asked to assume a quadruped position from a side-sitting position.

A variation of this level of control is termed **static-dynamic control.** While maintaining a static posture, one limb is freed to move through space (for example, reaching or stepping). From a quadruped position one upper limb is lifted, then one upper limb and the opposite lower limb are lifted simultaneously. This requires dynamic stability because of the reduction in the overall base of support and the shift of the center of mass over the support limbs.

Deficits in controlled mobility are associated with an inability to maintain a posture while moving (dynamic stability). A number of factors can produce deficits in controlled mobility, including tonal imbalances, ROM restrictions, impaired reciprocal actions of the antagonists, or impairment of proximal stabilization.

Emphasis should be placed on:

- Smooth movements and antagonist patterns (changing direction)
- Carefully graded assistance using key movement elements only
- Light, tracking resistance only, or antigravity resistance
- Eccentric control to concentric control
- Gradually increasing ROM
- Functional activities (for example, sitting and reaching and supine-to-sitting transitions)
- Steady holding of a posture while dynamic limb segments are moving (static-dynamic control)
- Repetition of movements

Specific neuromuscular facilitation techniques may include:

Slow reversals (SRs) through increments of range
Slow reversal-hold (SRH)
Timing for emphasis/repeated contractions (TE/RCs)
Agonist reversals (ARs)
Active-assistive to active movements and movement transitions
Swiss ball activities (for example, sitting on the ball and moving the ball while maintaining the sitting position)
Stability techniques to facilitate static segments as needed (AI, RS, and approximation)

SKILL

Strategies/Techniques to Improve Skill

Skill movements are highly coordinated with precise timing and direction. They also are highly consistent and allow attainment of a goal with an economy of effort. The proximal segments (trunk and proximal joints) stabilize the body while the distal segments are free for function. Activities requiring skill function include upper extremity grasp and manipulation (functional tasks of daily living), locomotion, and movement within the environment (reciprocal creeping, walking with a heel-toe gait pattern and a reciprocal arm swing), and oral-motor activities (speech and feeding).

There are many factors that can have a negative impact on the development of motor skills. Performance may be seriously or irreversibly limited with the presentation of any of the problems previously mentioned. In addition, impairments in balance (postural synergies and reactions), motor planning (apraxia, dyspraxia), or motor-control mechanisms (incoordination) may affect skill development. Impairments may also be cognitive and learning based (for example, deficits in attention and memory).

Emphasis should be placed on varying tasks to include:

- Coordination tasks that foster active control of movements. Refinement of sequential and temporal organization of movement is emphasized:
  - Timing can be improved with the use of equipment that allows for speed control (for example, a stationary bicycle with a metronome, a treadmill, or an isokinetic device). Speed can be increased as control improves.
  - Movements can be selected to foster control of multiple body segments, for example, bilateral symmetrical or bilateral asymmetrical PNF patterns, or reciprocal upper extremity and/or lower extremity patterns.

- Dual tasks can be selected to develop control of simultaneous movements (for example, walking and talking or walking and bouncing a ball).
- Training of mechanisms that foster postural control (balance). Activities should include both reactive and proactive activities (for example, Swiss ball activities, balance boards, and functional reach activities).
- Agility tasks that combine both coordination and upright postural control, such as jumping jacks (reciprocal overhead arm movements coupled with jumping and reciprocal leg movements out to the side and together).
- Practice of motor skills in a variety of environmental contexts progressing from closed (fixed) environments such as the physical therapy clinic to open (variable) environments such as the community. Emphasis should be on functional environments (for example, home, work, and community).
- Carefully graded resistance to promote balanced contributions of agonists and antagonists and smooth timing (overall there is limited use of hands-on techniques during skill training).

Specific neuromuscular facilitation techniques may include:

Slow reversals (SRs) and slow reversal-hold (SRH)
Timing for emphasis/repeated contractions (TE/RCs)
Agonist reversals (ARs)
Resisted progression (RP)/normal timing

Motor Learning Approach

TERMINOLOGY AND TREATMENT STRATEGIES

Motor learning is a set of internal processes associated with practice or experience leading to relatively permanent changes in the capability of skill (Schmidt, 1988).[7]

- Feedback and practice are essential for learning; feedback and practice schedules should be organized carefully.
- Overall arousal levels should be carefully assessed; both low arousal and intense arousal yield poor performance and learning.
- The learner (patient) should be involved in goal setting. The task should be desirable to the individual, functionally relevant, and important to learn.
- Active participation and discovery learning should be emphasized. The patient should be encouraged to develop individual solutions for mastery.

Feedback

Feedback is response-produced information acquired during or after performance; information is used to make error corrections. There are two main categories of feedback—*intrinsic* and *augmented*:

Intrinsic feedback is naturally occurring or inherent information derived from the patient's own sensory and perceptual systems, such as visual, auditory, proprioceptive, and tactile feedback.

Augmented feedback is supplemental or added feedback derived from external sources such as verbal cues, electromyogram (EMG) biofeedback, and videotaped performance. Augmented feedback is subdivided into two types—knowledge of results and knowledge of performance:

Knowledge of results (KR) is augmented feedback related to the nature of the result or outcome produced in terms of the environmental goal; for example, the patient with a spinal cord lesion successfully transfers from wheelchair to mat without a transfer board or assistance.

Knowledge of performance (KP) is augmented feedback related to the nature of the movement characteristics produced; for example, the patient with a spinal cord lesion successfully scoots to the edge of the chair, pushes up and lifts the body, and laterally shifts the pelvis over onto the mat using reverse movements of the head and upper trunk.

- Precise and accurate feedback should be used. The patient should be assisted in recognizing and pairing intrinsic feedback with movement responses. Consideration should be given to videotaping and analyzing performance.
- Feedback given after every trial improves *performance*; feedback given after several trials improves *learning and retention*. Consideration should be given to use of different timing for feedback:
  - **Summed feedback** is given after a set number of trials (for example, every third trial).

- ○ **Fading feedback** is given after every trial, then every third trial, every fifth trial, and so forth.
  - ○ **Bandwidth feedback** is given only if performance exceeds an expected error range.
- Early training should focus on visual feedback (the cognitive phase of learning); later training should emphasize proprioceptive feedback—the "feel of the movement" (the associated phase of learning).
- Augmented feedback should be provided about knowledge of results and knowledge of performance. The therapist should emphasize different aspects at different stages:
  - ○ During early learning, it is important to emphasize the correct aspects of performance.
  - ○ During the middle and later stages of learning, errors should be emphasized only as they become consistent.
- Use of feedback should be carefully monitored. Feedback dependency should be avoided with attention focused on reducing augmented feedback as soon as possible and allowing the patient active introspection and decision making (participation improves learning and retention).
- Extraneous environmental stimuli must be reduced early in learning; practice should occur in a closed environment. During later learning the focus can be shifted to adapting performance to varying environmental demands; practice should now occur in an open environment.
- Supportive feedback can be used to motivate the patient and shape (reinforce) behavior.

Practice

Constant practice is practice of a single motor skill repeatedly; repetitive practice.

Variable practice is practice of a motor skill in a context in which the patient is required to make rapid modifications of the skill in order to match the demands of the situation.

Mass practice is practice in which the amount of rest time is small; rest time is less than the total practice time. Mass practice may lead to decreased performance and fatigue.

Distributed practice is practice in which the rest time is relatively large; practice time is less than the total rest time.

Mental practice is cognitive rehearsal of a motor skill without making overt physical movements.

Practice order is the order in which practice of tasks is organized:

Blocked practice order is practice of the same task within the practice session; for example, task A can be practiced repeatedly, in a block—AAAAAA. Blocked practice order results in improved acquisition of a skill and performance.

Serial practice order is practice of a group or class of motor skills in a predictable order within a series (for example, ABCABC).

Random practice order is practice of a group or class of motor skills in a random, unpredictable order (for example, ACBBAC). Random practice order represents higher contextual interference, resulting in improved retention of the skill.

A practice schedule should be established. *Distributed practice* is used when the task is complex, long, or energy costly; when superior performance is desired; when motivation is low; or when the patient has a short attention span, poor concentration, or fatigues easily. *Mass practice* is used when the task is highly meaningful and the patient has an adequate attention span, concentration, high motivation, and endurance.

Practicing tasks within a class of different but related skills provides contextual interference and increases the depth of cognitive processing; for example, a serial or random practice order results in improved retention of the skill. Variable practice will promote generalizability of skills to different environments.

Mental practice can be used to improve learning; the patient verbalizes task components and critical task elements required for performance.

- Mental practice is effective when the task has a large cognitive component and cognition is intact.
- Mental practice can help to decrease anxiety or fear.

Transfer refers to the effect (gain or loss) of previous practice of a skill on learning a new skill, or on the performance in a new context. Transfer may be either positive (assisting learning) or negative (hindering learning).

- **Part-whole transfer** is a learning technique in which the motor task is broken down into its component parts for separate practice before practice of the integrated whole.
- **Bilateral transfer** occurs when improvement in movement skill performance with one limb results from practice with the opposite limb.

Practice of *parts to whole* is used when the task is complex, with highly independent parts (for example, a transfer). Part-whole transfer should also be used when the patient has limited memory or attention or difficulty with a particular component of a task. The practice session should always include both the parts and the integrated whole; practice of the whole should not be delayed. Practice of parts to whole is not as effective when the task has highly integrated, dependent components such as gait.

Practice of bilateral movements *(bilateral transfer)* should stress identical movements from one side to the other and the similarity of task components. Practice of tasks should occur in similar performance situations.

MOTOR RELEARNING PROGRAMME FOR STROKE

Janet Carr and Roberta Shepherd,[8] both physiotherapists, developed a Motor Relearning Programme (MRP) for stroke. The emphasis of this approach is on retraining motor control using everyday functional activities. Facilitation techniques are deemphasized in favor of motor learning strategies. The patient must demonstrate intact cognition and concentration in order to relearn control of movements.

Basic Principles and Strategies

In the MRP for stroke, focus is on using motor learning strategies to retrain the patient to perform functional activities (skills). Muscles are retrained with an emphasis on the control and timing needed for specific tasks.

- Feedback and practice are essential for learning.
- Facilitation techniques are not emphasized.

MRP uses a problem-solving approach for evaluation and treatment:

1. Analysis of the task involves careful observation of the patient's motor performance with identification of missing components.
2. Each missing component is practiced before the entire activity is attempted:
   - Therapy is goal directed.
   - Instruction and demonstration are used carefully.
   - Verbal, visual feedback, and manual guidance are provided as needed.
   - Progression is made from passive to active to resistive movement.

  ◦ The environment is structured to optimize learning.
  ◦ Positive reinforcement is stressed to motivate the patient.
3. The entire activity is practiced; training is task specific:
  ◦ Goals are reinforced.
  ◦ Cues and guidance are provided as needed.
  ◦ Learned errors and learned nonuse are avoided.
  ◦ The effects of physical and mental fatigue are eliminated or reduced.
  ◦ Flexibility is encouraged.
4. Transference of learning is the ultimate goal:
  ◦ The task is practiced in varying environmental contexts.
  ◦ Self-monitoring by the patient to ensure independent practice is stressed.
  ◦ The family and caregivers are taught supportive techniques.
  ◦ Continued practice shifts learning from cognitive to associative and automatic phases.

Facilitating Skill Development: Functional Mobility Training

This portion of the manual focuses on activities and techniques that can be used to promote development of functional mobility skills. A description of the general characteristics of each skill is provided along with general comments, treatment strategies, and considerations. Patient outcomes are organized by specific motor control goals: acquisition of initial mobility, stability, controlled mobility, and skill level of function. Appropriate suggestions for lead-up and follow-up skills are given.

Part
7

Initial Activities in Supine or Sidelying Position

ROLLING

General Characteristics

- The base of support (BOS) in supine is large.
- The center of mass (COM) is low.
- This posture is very stable; rolling does not require upright postural control.
- Weight bearing occurs through large segments of body.
- Minimal antigravity postural control is required:
  - Transitions from supine to sidelying movements are resisted by gravity acting on the trunk and extremities.
  - Transitions from sidelying to prone movements are assisted by gravity.
- Normal rolling is typically accomplished with a segmental trunk pattern; either the shoulder/upper trunk or pelvis/lower trunk leads first. A log-rolling pattern (rolling with the trunk as a whole) is less common with adult patients.
- Head/neck motions are combined with upper trunk rotation (UTR) as normal components of movement:
  - Head/neck flexion and rotation with UTR assist in transitions from supine to sidelying movement.
  - Head/neck extension and rotation with UTR assist in transitions from prone to sidelying movement.
- During normal rolling, the hands are not used to pull the body over; the hands or feet do not push the body up from the supporting surface.
- Normal postural reactions contribute to rolling:
  - Body-on-body righting reactions
  - Neck righting reactions
- Hyperactive tonic reflexes coupled with excess tone can interfere with rolling movements and segmental trunk patterns:
  - Symmetrical Tonic Labyrinthine Reflex (STLR): Excess extension or flexion tone impedes motion. Consider sidelying training to eliminate reflex influences.
  - Asymmetrical Tonic Neck Reflex (ATNR): Upper extremity (UE) position impedes motion. Normal head/neck alignment should be maintained.
- Dependent positions (full supine or prone) may be difficult or contraindicated for patients with cardiopulmonary problems such as chronic obstructive pulmonary disease or congestive heart failure or with recent surgical interventions involving the trunk.

Treatment Strategies and Considerations

- Begin working in sidelying position and progress from small ranges to larger ranges, and finally to full range of motion—for example, rolling from supine to prone.
- Limb movements and momentum can assist rolling:
  - Upper extremities (UEs) or lower extremities (LEs) or both can flex up and across the body to facilitate rolling from supine to sidelying position.

- The addition of weights (wrist cuffs) can assist in momentum and functional training (for example, training the patient with quadriplegia to roll).
- Limbs should be pre-positioned before rolling begins:
  - UEs: The lowermost arm should be flexed overhead to avoid getting it "trapped" under the body.
  - LEs: The uppermost limb can be positioned in hip and knee flexion with the foot flat on the supporting surface (a modified hooklying position).
- The therapist should be positioned in front of the patient to assist individuals with communication deficits (aphasia) or those who depend heavily on visual cueing.

Rolling: Therapeutic Activities and Techniques

Position/Activity: Rolling from Supine to Sidelying Position

The patient is in supine position. The therapist is standing next to the treatment table or half-kneeling next to the platform mat. The therapist assists the motion of the patient's trunk and/or limbs.

The patient is instructed to lift the LE (or UE) off the mat and swing it up and across the body. The trunk and remaining extremity follow. The therapist gives maximum assistance at the beginning of the range (when the maximum effects of gravity are felt) and reduces assistance from midrange on as the patient can move more easily.

Comments

The patient's movements are timed with the therapist's verbal commands (VCs): "On three, I want you to lift your arm and leg up and toward me and roll onto your side. One, two, and three . . ."

The therapist gives only as much assistance as necessary to accomplish the motion.

Active-assistive movements (AAM) should progress toward active movements (AM)— to promote voluntary control as soon as possible.

The therapist's position and movements should not restrict or limit the patient's ease of movement.

Speed influences the amount of effort required: the slower the movement, the greater the effort required to roll.

Patients recovering from stroke need to practice rolling over onto the affected side and over onto the sound side (a more difficult activity). The UE affected by the stroke can be effectively supported using a prayer position (hands clasped together with both elbows extended and shoulders flexed) to keep the shoulder forward and the elbow extended.

Position/Activity: Rolling into Sidelying-on-Elbow Position

From supine, the patient turns and lifts the trunk up into the sidelying-on-elbow position. The therapist assists rotation of the upper trunk by lifting the trunk with both hands on patient's sides under the axillae (Fig. 7–1A and B).

Comments

The patient's lowermost UE is pre-positioned with the elbow in 90 degrees of flexion.

The patient's uppermost UE is pre-positioned with the elbow extended and the hand placed on the therapist's shoulder for support. (This minimizes the effect of gravity dragging the shoulder back.)

The patient is gently placed into the sidelying-on-elbow position; the elbow should not be "slammed" into the support surface.

The left leg can be crossed over the right to facilitate the roll or the leg can be flexed with foot flat.

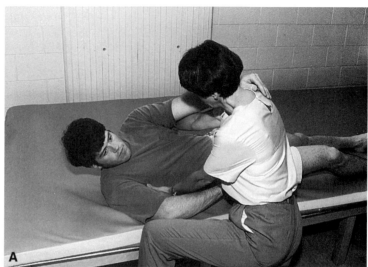

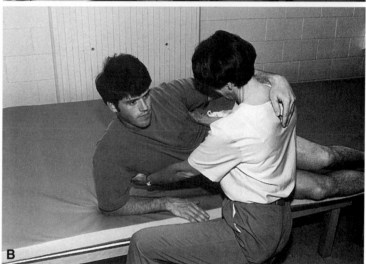

Figure 7–1*A* and *B*. Rolling into sidelying-on-elbow position.

For patients recovering from stroke, this is an excellent exercise to promote early weight bearing on the affected shoulder with elongation of the affected side. (This is important for inhibition of spastic trunk side muscles).

Motor control goals. Mobility (active-assistive movement—AAM), progressing to controlled mobility (active movement—AM).

Indications. Dependent function due to weakness, disordered motor control.

Functional outcome. The patient is able to roll independently from supine to prone, a lead-up skill to independent transfers from supine to sitting and dressing in bed.

Position/Activity: Sidelying, Log Rolling

The patient is positioned in sidelying with the LEs extended in midposition or in slight flexion; the UEs are positioned with the lowermost arm flexed overhead. The patient's uppermost arm can be positioned overhead or at the side, with the hand resting on the pelvis or in a pants pocket if shoulder range-of-motion (ROM) limitations exist.

The therapist heel-sits or kneels in front of or behind the patient. The therapist places one hand on the side of the trunk, under the axilla or over the top of the shoulder, and one hand on the pelvis. (Manual contacts should *not* be on the arm or waist).

TECHNIQUES

Rhythmic Initiation

The upper trunk/shoulder moves together as one unit with the lower trunk/pelvis, hence the term "log roll." In rhythmic initiation (RI) movements are first passive, then active-assistive, then lightly resisted with **tracking resistance**. Progression to the next phase of movement is dependent upon the patient's ability to relax and participate in each phase of the movements (Fig. 7–2).

The therapist's manual contacts are fixed during the first two phases of RI. During the final resistive phase, the therapist's hands slide forward or backward on the patient's trunk to resist the movement. **Verbal commands** (VCs) for RI: "Relax—let me move you back and forth" (timed with passive movements). "Now move with me, back and forth" (timed with active movements). "Now pull forward, and push backward" (timed with resisted movements).

Comments

Movements should be slow and rhythmic (moving the patient too fast may increase tone).
Verbal commands should be soothing, slow, and rhythmic—well timed with movements.
Light, tracking resistance during the resistive phase is used to facilitate muscle contraction through loading of the muscle spindle. A facilatory quick stretch can also be used to initiate the movement and should be well timed with VCs.
Repetition is important for relaxation and motor learning.
Rocking movements (slow vestibular stimulation) may facilitate a decrease in hypertonia.

Motor control goal. Mobility.

Indications. Dependent function due to muscle hypertonia (for example, spasticity or rigidity); impaired ability to initiate rolling (dyspraxia), impaired cognition and motor learning.

Functional outcome. The patient is able to roll independently from supine to prone position.

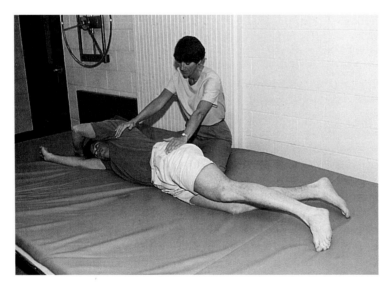

Figure 7–2. Sidelying: log rolling—rhythmic initiation.

Once the patient is relaxed and can actively move in the log-rolling pattern, the technique can be altered to promote **controlled mobility** function using **slow reversal (SR)** and **slow reversal-hold (SRH).**

Slow Reversals

In slow reversals (SRs), the therapist places both hands first on the anterior trunk (shoulder and pelvis) to resist flexion, then slides both hands to the posterior to resist extension.

Slow Reversal-Hold

A hold (SRH) may be added if the patient demonstrates difficulty in completing the contraction in the shortened range.

Comments

The hold is a momentary pause (held to one count); the antagonist movement is then facilitated.

The hold can be added in one direction only or in both directions.

Movements begin with small-range control (one-quarter turn forward to one-quarter turn backward) and progress to full-range control (from full prone to full supine position).

Position/Activity: Sidelying, Rolling

The patient is in sidelying position. The therapist heel-sits or kneels behind the patient to activate abdominals or in front of the patient to focus on extensor muscles. The therapist's hands are positioned on the patient's upper trunk and pelvis.

TECHNIQUES

Hold-Relax Active Motion

Hold-relax active motion (HRAM) is beneficial for weak abdominals. The patient is tipped forward one-quarter of the range (shortened range for abdominals) and holds, followed by active relaxation. The therapist then moves the trunk backwards quickly one-quarter of the range past neutral and asks the patient to contract actively through the range back to the original position (Fig. 7–3). **Verbal commands** for HRAM: "Hold this position; don't let me pull you backward. Hold, hold; now relax. Now pull forward."

Comments

Resistance of the isometric hold recruits muscle-spindle support of contraction and should be built up gradually.

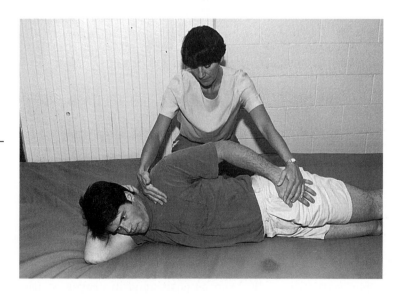

Figure 7–3. Sidelying: rolling— hold-relax active motion.

The active relaxation is important; the patient should not be moved backward until the contraction is completely released.

Resistance of the isotonic movement is light (tracking).

VCs are dynamic and should reflect a buildup of effort.

A quick stretch can be applied in the lengthened range to facilitate the return movement.

HRAM is a unidirectional technique, emphasizing movement only in one direction. Active extension is not permitted because reciprocal inhibition effects might further weaken the abdominals.

The hold is built up slowly. The patient is quickly moved back through the range once relaxation is achieved; isotonic movement from the lengthened to shortened range is slow.

The technique is repeated until patient fatigue is evident.

Midrange control is achieved first; then progression is to full-range control.

Motor control goal. Mobility.

Indications. Dependent function due to muscle weakness, hypotonia, inability to initiate or sustain contraction (lack of muscle spindle-stretch sensitivity).

Functional outcome. The patient is able to roll independently from supine to prone position.

Position/Activity: Rolling from Supine to Sidelying Using PNF D1F Extremity Patterns

Upper extremity D1F pattern with roll assumes function of upper extremity (UE) with overflow of limb movements to weaker trunk muscles. The patient is positioned in supine, or one-quarter turn toward sidelying using a pillow for support. The lower extremity (LE) is positioned in modified hooklying position, with one foot flat on the mat.

The therapist kneels or heel-sits at one side of the patient. One of the therapist's hands assists (or resists) the UE or LE pattern; the other hand (on the trunk) helps the patient roll onto the sidelying position (Fig. 7–4A and B).

TECHNIQUES

Rhythmic Initiation

In rhythmic initiation (RI), the patient's arm (UE) is brought up and across the body in D1F pattern and back down through the D1E pattern. Movement is first passive (PM), then active-assistive (AAM), then resistive (RM). AAM and RM are unidirectional, emphasizing D1F. Movements in D1E are passive (the patient is not allowed to push back down to the side). **Verbal commands** (VCs): "Relax; let me move your arm up and across your face. Turn your head. Now move with me, up and across your face. Now pull up and across your face. Now pull up and roll onto your side."

Comments

The movement and momentum of the UE is used to facilitate rolling into the sidelying position.

The patient should be instructed to turn the head and follow the hand with the eyes. (This prevents the limb from smothering the mouth and nose when it comes up and across the face).

Rhythmic initiation (RI) is ideal for motor learning. Once the patient achieves control, a progression is made to slow reversals (SRs) or active movement (AM).

Rolling with Lower Extremity D1F Pattern

The patient's lower extremity is positioned in slight flexion over the therapist's knee. Manual contacts are on the dorsal/medial foot and the thigh; resistance is applied to both the thigh and the foot as the (LE) moves up and across the body (Fig. 7–5A and B). The upper extremities (UEs) can be positioned in prayer position with the hands clasped together in front of the body.

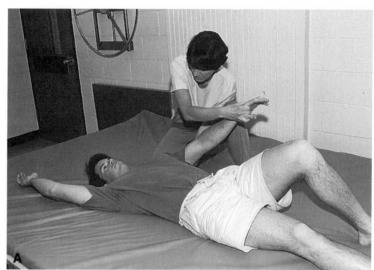

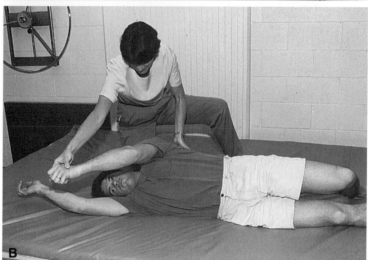

Figure 7–4 *A* and *B*. Rolling: supine to sidelying using PNF UE D1 flexion pattern.

Rolling with Simultaneous Upper Extremity and Lower Extremity D1F Patterns
In simultaneous D1F patterns both the UE and the LE move together up and across the body. The therapist can assist or resist one extremity while the other extremity moves actively.

Motor control goals. Mobility (AAM), progressing to controlled mobility (AM).

Indications. Dependent function due to weak trunk muscles. The simultaneous UE and LE patterns use overflow of strong limb movements to weaker trunk muscles, a compensatory technique in the absence of trunk muscle function (for example, in patients with spinal cord lesions).

Functional outcome. The patient is able to roll independently from supine to prone position.

Position/Activity: Rolling from Supine to Sidelying Using PNF Reverse Chop or PNF Lift Patterns

The **reverse chop pattern** combines upper trunk extension (UTE) with rotation. The lead UE moves in D1F; the patient holds one hand on top of the wrist of the lead limb.

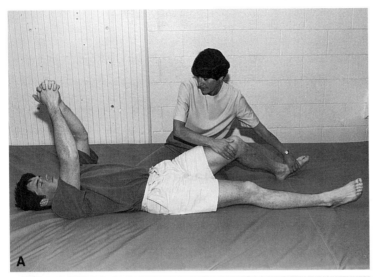

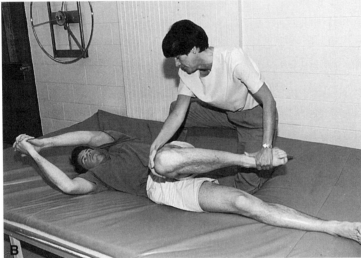

Figure 7–5A and B. Rolling: supine to sidelying using PNF LE D1 flexion pattern.

The **lift pattern** combines upper trunk extension (UTE) with rotation. The lead arm (UE) moves in D2F; the patient holds one hand underneath the wrist of the lead limb.

TECHNIQUES

Rolling Using Reverse Chop to the Right
The patient is positioned in supine. The left LE is flexed at the hip and the knee is flexed with one foot flat on the mat (modified hooklying position).

The therapist kneels or heel-sits next to the patient on the left side. Manual contacts are on the lead UE: the therapist holds the forearm (left UE) as it moves up and across the body in D1F; the therapist's other hand helps the patient roll to the right by supporting the trunk in the scapular region. The patient rolls to the right sidelying position (Fig. 7–6A and B). **Verbal commands** (VCs): "Relax; let me move your arms up and across your face. Now move with me, up and across your face. Now turn your head, lift your arms up and across your face, and roll onto your right side."

Rolling Using Lift to the Right
The patient is supine, with the right LE flexed at the hip and knee with one foot flat on the mat (modified hooklying position).

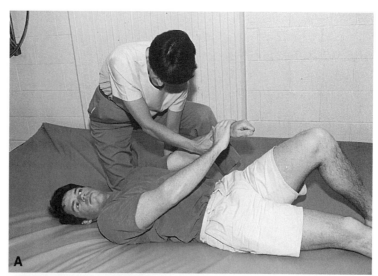

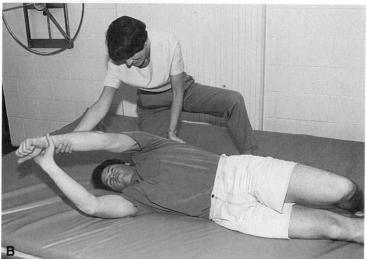

Figure 7–6*A* and *B*. Rolling: supine to sidelying using PNF reverse chop pattern.

The therapist kneels or heel-sits next to the patient on the left side. Manual contacts are on the left (lead) UE: the therapist holds the forearm of the lead UE as it moves up and out (Fig. 7–7*A* and *B*). **Verbal commands** (VCs): "Relax; let me move your arms up and toward me. Now move with me, up and toward me. Now turn your head, lift your arms up and toward me, and roll onto your left side."

Comments

The therapist should use an open hand (not a tight grasp) on the lead UE to allow rotation and movement through the pattern.

In the reverse chop or lift, active-assistive movements occur in only one direction; movements in the opposite direction are passive.

The LE can be flexed at the hip and the knee, with one foot flat, or can actively move in D1F pattern.

Rhythmic initiation (RI) is ideal for promoting motor learning; once the patient achieves control, a progression to slow reversals (SRs) or active movement (AM) can be made.

Chop or lift patterns increase the amount of upper trunk rotation (UTR) that occurs with rolling (as compared to unilateral limb patterns); this results from closing of the kinematic chain.

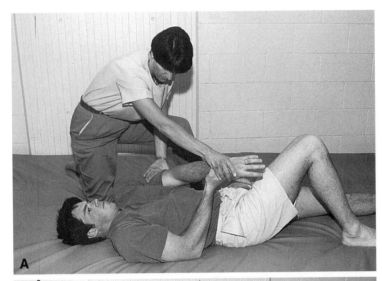

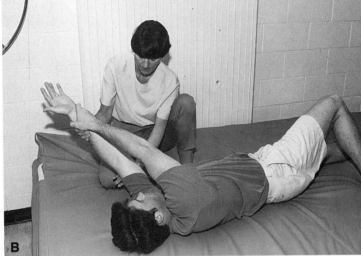

Figure 7–7A and B. Rolling: supine to sidelying using PNF lift pattern.

Motor control goals. Mobility (AAM), progressing to controlled mobility (AM).

Indications. Dependent function due to weak trunk muscles. Chop or lift patterns use overflow of strong limb movements to weaker trunk muscles, which encourages increased upper trunk rotation.

Functional outcome. The patient is able to roll independently from supine to prone position.

SIDELYING

General Characteristics

- The base of support (BOS) in sidelying is large.
- The center of mass (COM) is low.
- This posture is very stable; sidelying does not require upright postural control.
- Tonic reflex activity is reduced in sidelying.

Treatment Strategies and Considerations

- The posture can be used to work on trunk extension and trunk rotation patterns in patients who lack upright (antigravity) control.
- During any isometric contractions, the patient should be encouraged to breathe regularly. Breath holding increases intrathoracic pressures, producing a Valsalva effect.
- Good body mechanics for the therapist are important: The back should be kept straight, with the elbows relatively extended; avoid bending over the patient; and avoid hyperextension of the wrists.

Sidelying: Therapeutic Activities and Techniques

Position/Activity: Sidelying, Holding in Extension

The patient is positioned in sidelying. The patient's head is extended slightly with the trunk and LEs in midline; the uppermost shoulder is extended with the elbow flexed (a modified pivot prone position). The lowermost LE can be flexed slightly; the lowermost UE can also be flexed, supporting the head.

The therapist heel-sits behind the patient. Manual contacts are variable: To assist patients who have poor head control, the therapist can use one hand to support the head and apply resistance to the neck extensors through the base of the hand. The therapist's other hand should be positioned on the patient's upper trunk or elbow to resist shoulder extension and scapular adduction. For patients with trunk extensor weakness the therapist can place one hand on the upper trunk or arm and one hand on the pelvis/lower trunk or thigh.

TECHNIQUES

Shortened Held Resisted Contraction
In shortened held resisted contraction (SHRC) resistance to extension is applied at multiple points (the head, upper trunk, arm, and pelvis). An isometric hold is built up gradually to achieve and maintain a maximum contraction. Overflow to other extensor muscles throughout the trunk is expected (Fig. 7–8A and B). **Verbal commands** for SHRC: "Hold—don't let me push you forward. Hold, hold."

Comments
The focus is on developing initial extensor control.
SHRC in sidelying position (modified pivot prone) is a lead-up activity to stability control in sitting position (sitting in modified pivot prone position with SHRC or sitting and holding).

Motor control goals. Stability, static postural control.

Indications. Weak postural extensors, inability to sustain a contraction, poor sitting control and posture (for example, the patient with kyphosis who slouches forward).

Functional outcome. The patient is able to stabilize the trunk in postural extension.

Position/Activity: Sidelying, Holding

The patient is in sidelying position with the trunk in midrange. The lowermost extremities are flexed slightly to increase the base of support (BOS). The uppermost LE is in extension; the uppermost UE is flexed overhead. Patients who do not have sufficient shoulder ROM to position the UE overhead can hold the UE on the side of the trunk, with one hand on the pelvis or one hand in a pants pocket.

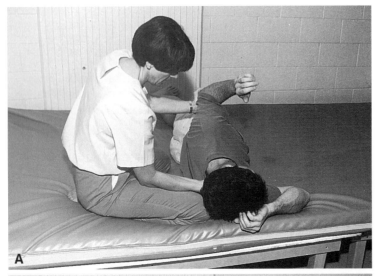

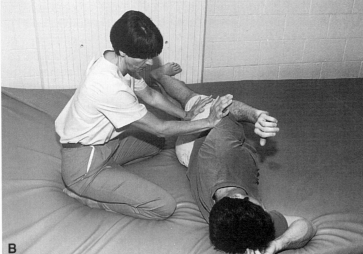

Figure 7–8*A* **and** *B*. Side-lying: holding—shortened held resisted contraction.

The therapist heel-sits behind or in front of the patient. Manual contacts are on the upper trunk, either under the axilla or over the top of the shoulder, and on the pelvis. The therapist's hands are slid over the top of the trunk from anterior to posterior surfaces; flat open hands (a lumbrical grip, using metacarpophalangeal flexion with interphalangeal extension) are used to apply resistance, not tightly grasped fingers.

TECHNIQUES

Alternating Isometrics
In alternating isometrics (AI) the patient is asked to hold the sidelying position while the therapist applies resistance alternately, first to the trunk extensors, then to the flexors. Resistance is built up gradually from very light resistance to the patient's maximum. The isometric contraction is maintained for several counts (Fig. 7–9).

Verbal commands for AI: "Hold—don't let me push you forward. Hold, hold. Now don't let me pull you backward. Hold, hold." The therapist must give the transitional command ("Now don't let me pull you the other way") before sliding the hands to the opposite surface. (This allows the patient to make preparatory postural adjustments.)

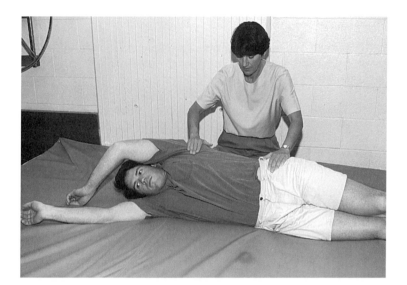

Figure 7–9. Sidelying: holding—alternating isometrics.

Comments

A quick stretch can be used to facilitate muscles or segments that are not responding.
The patient is not allowed to relax between contractions.
Steady holding of the posture is the goal, not jerky movements forward or backward.

Rhythmic Stabilization

In rhythmic stabilization (RS) the patient is asked to hold the position while the therapist applies resistance: one hand resists the upper trunk flexors while the other hand resists the lower trunk extensors. Resistance is then reversed: one hand resists upper trunk extensors while the other hand resists the lower trunk flexors (Fig. 7–10). **Verbal commands** for RS: "Hold—don't let me twist you. Hold, hold. Now don't let me twist you the other way. Hold, hold."

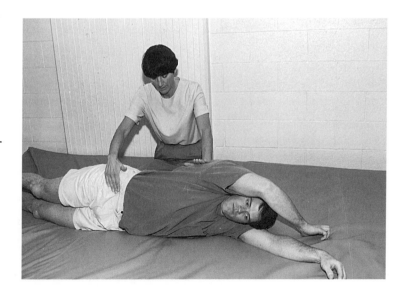

Figure 7–10. Sidelying: holding—rhythmic stabilization.

Motor control goal. Stability, static control.

Indications. Weakness of trunk muscles. Rhythmic stabilization (RS) increases emphasis on the stabilizing action of the trunk rotators.

Functional outcome. The patient is able to stabilize the trunk in postural extension.

Position/Activity: Sidelying, Trunk Rotation

Upper and Lower Trunk Rotation

The patient is in sidelying position. In **upper trunk rotation** (UTR) the patient moves the upper trunk/shoulder forward and backward while keeping the lower trunk/pelvis stationary. The sequence is reversed for **lower trunk rotation** (LTR): The pelvis/lower trunk moves forward and back while the upper trunk/shoulder remains stationary. The therapist heel-sits behind or in front of the patient. Manual contracts are on the upper trunk and pelvis.

TECHNIQUES

Slow Reversal

In slow reversal (SR), the therapist keeps one hand on the stationary segment being stabilized while the other hand resists the movement, first on the anterior trunk; then the hand slides to the posterior to resist the opposite movement. Verbal commands for SRs: "Keep your pelvis still and pull your shoulder forward. Now push back; pull forward; now push back."

Comments

Movements begin with small range control and progress to larger ranges.

Light, tracking resistance is used to promote smooth reversal of antagonists.

A facilitatory quick stretch can be used to initiate the movement and should be timed to coincide with VCs.

Patients may find it easier to move one segment more than the other. Lower trunk rotation (LTR) is usually more problematic.

Slow reversals (SRs) can be combined with PNF scapular patterns to promote scapula/shoulder movements.

Patients with a retracted pelvic position (commonly seen in stroke) will benefit from LTR with an emphasis on forward rotation. (The reverse motion can be passive or assisted, not resisted.)

Slow Reversal-Hold

A hold (SRH) may be added if the patient demonstrates difficulty in completing the movement into the shortened range. (The isometric hold adds additional muscle spindle support.)

Comments

The hold is a momentary pause, held for one count.

The antagonist movement is then facilitated.

The hold can be added in one direction only or in both directions.

Motor control goals. Controlled mobility, static-dynamic control of trunk.

Indications. Impairment of segmental trunk patterns; an important lead-up skill for independent rolling, assumption of supine to sit, and trunk counterrotation and reciprocal upper extremity/trunk movements in gait.

Functional outcome. Patient is able to perform segmental trunk patterns (isolated upper trunk and lower trunk rotation).

Position/Activity: Sidelying, Trunk Counterrotation

Patient is positioned in sidelying. The upper trunk/shoulder moves forward while the lower trunk/pelvis move backward in the opposite direction. The movements are then reversed.

The therapist heel-sits behind or in front of the patient.

Manual contacts are on the upper trunk under the axilla and on the pelvis (Fig. 7–11*A* and *B*).

TECHNIQUES

Rhythmic Initiation

The patient is instructed to relax while the therapist passively moves each trunk segment in opposite directions (the lower trunk/pelvis moves forward while the upper trunk/shoulder moves backward). The movements are reversed and continued until patient moves easily. The patient is then asked to participate actively in the movements.

Verbal commands for RI: "Relax—let me move you; let me twist you. Now let me twist you the other way. Now move with me; twist; now twist the other way."

Figure 7–11*A* and *B*. Sidelying: trunk counterrotation—rhythmic initiation.

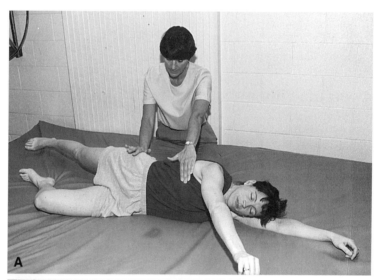

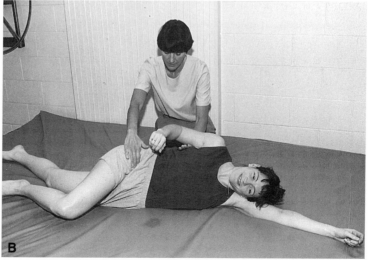

Comments

Trunk counterrotation is a very difficult movement to achieve. RI is the technique of choice to assist in motor learning of difficult tasks.

Movements are assisted passively at first, slowly progressing to active-assistive and then resisted movements.

The resisted movement is usually very difficult and may not be attempted during early practice attempts.

If the resistive phase is used, the therapist's hands must slide forward and backward on the trunk to resist the movements.

Once learning occurs, RI can progress to slow reversals (SRs).

Active reciprocal extremity movements simulating arm swing and stepping movements in gait can be requested (this allows the complete motor program to be called up).

Smooth reversal of antagonists is the goal. The movements should look coordinated, the movement sequence continuous; the therapist and patient must be in rhythm together.

Motor control goal. Skill-level control for the trunk.

Indications. Impaired reciprocal trunk movements during gait (trunk counterrotation).

Functional outcome. The patient is able to perform reciprocal trunk patterns and coordinated reciprocal trunk/UE movements during gait.

Part

8

Prone Activities

PRONE EXTENSION (PIVOT PRONE)

General Characteristics

- The base of support (BOS) in prone position is large.
- The center of mass (COM) is low.
- This posture is very stable.
- The patient lies prone and lifts the head, upper extremities (UEs), upper trunk, and lower extremities (LEs) off the mat in a total extension pattern.
- The shoulders may be externally rotated, abducted, and extended with the elbows flexed to 90 degrees or extended; the LEs are extended through the hips and knees.

Treatment Strategies and Considerations

- The pattern of extremity lifts can be varied: (1) one or both UEs can lift off the support surface; (2) one or both LEs can lift off the support surface; and (3) the opposite UE and LE can lift off the support surface.
- Prone activities are generally performed as active movements. The resistance of gravity provides enough challenge for most adults; it requires at least fair muscle strength.
- Weight cuffs can be added to the wrists or ankles to increase resistance.
- Hip flexor tightness may limit position and range.
- Prone positions may be contraindicated in patients with cardiopulmonary impairments (for example, cardiovascular disease or respiratory insufficiency).
- The presence of strong flexor tone, strong tonic labyrinthine prone reflexes, and the absence of righting reflexes may prevent any active lifting.

Movement Transitions into Prone-on-Elbows Position

Prone Lying to Prone-on-Elbows Position
The patient is lying in prone position with the shoulders pre-positioned at approximately 120 degrees of abduction and the elbows flexed to 90 degrees. The patient actively lifts the head and upper trunk, pulling both elbows under the shoulders.

The therapist is half-kneeling over the patient. Both hands are on the patient's anterior trunk; the hands are cupped over the clavicles to relieve any bony pressure. The therapist lifts the patient on a count of three, and assists the patient gently onto the elbows (Fig. 8–1A and B). **Verbal commands** (VCs): "On the count of three I want you to lift your head up. I will help you lift up your upper trunk to come onto your elbows. One, two; now lift."

Comments
The therapist must lift the patient high enough—approximately 1 inch (2.5 cm) off the mat—so gravity will allow the elbows to fall under the shoulders.

Once the patient is prone on elbows, approximation can be applied directly over the shoulders to facilitate stabilizing muscles.

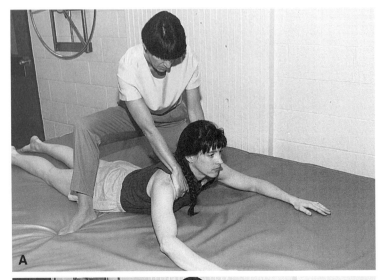

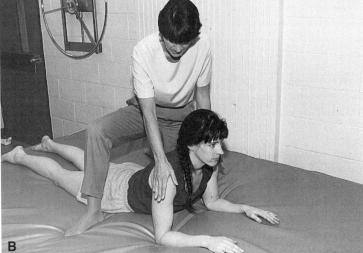

Figure 8–1A and B. Prone to prone-on-elbows position—active-assistive movement.

If the elbows are not directly lined up under the shoulders (too abducted), the patient can be unweighted to one side. Gravity will pull the opposite arm in under the shoulder; this can be repeated to align the other side.

As control increases, the patient learns to lift the trunk actively and pull both elbows under the shoulders.

Sidelying-on-Elbow to Prone-on-Elbows Position

The patient is in sidelying-on-elbow position. The patient rotates the upper trunk and moves into the prone-on-elbows position.

The therapist is half-kneeling over the patient with both hands on the sides of the patient's upper trunk, under the axillae. The patient is assisted into the position by rotating (twisting) the trunk until both elbows are resting on the mat (Fig. 8–2A and B). **Verbal commands** (VCs): "On the count of three I want you to turn (rotate) your upper body and come down onto both elbows. One, two, three."

Comments

This transition is useful for the patient with strong UE and trunk spasticity or strong tonic labyrinthine reflex in prone position.

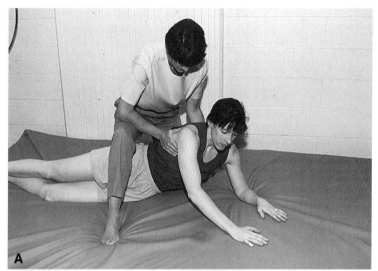

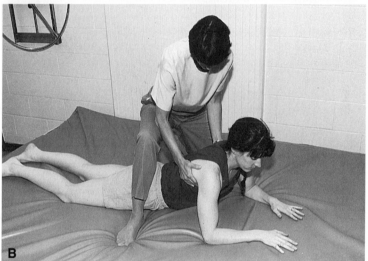

Figure 8–2A and B. Side-lying-on-elbow to prone-on-elbows position—active-assistive movement.

For the patient with UE spasticity (for example, the patient with hemiplegia), the affected UE is positioned with the hand open and flat on the mat with neutral rotation of the shoulder.

Motor control goals. Mobility (active-assistive movements), progressing to controlled mobility (active movements).

Indications. Dependent function due to weakness, disordered motor control. These activities are important lead-up skills for independence in bed mobility.

Functional outcome. The patient is able to assume prone-on-elbows (PoE) position independently.

PRONE-ON-ELBOWS

General Characteristics

- The base of support (BOS) in prone-on-elbows (PoE) position is large.
- The center of mass (COM) is low.

- This posture is very stable.
- The head and upper trunk are elevated with weight supported on the elbows and forearms. The elbows are flexed to 90 degrees and are positioned directly under the shoulders.
- This position involves primarily head, upper trunk, and shoulder control. Active holding of the PoE posture requires scapular and shoulder stability. (The serratus anterior stabilizes the scapula on the thorax; the rotator cuff muscles and pectoralis major stabilize the humerus under the body). Active holding of PoE also requires midrange control of neck extensors.
- Normal righting reactions—optical righting reactions (ORR) and labyrinthine righting reactions (LRR) along with body on head (BOH)—contribute to maintenance of head position.

Treatment Strategies and Considerations

- Shoulder/scapular weakness (for example, weakness in the serratus anterior or shoulder stabilizers) may limit the patient's ability to assume or hold in this posture. Shoulder pain or passive ROM (PROM) limitations may also limit tolerance of the position and the amount of weight borne.
  - A wedge cushion can be used to reduce loading in PoE.
  - The patient can be positioned in sitting with the elbows bearing weight on a table top (modified PoE).
  - The patient can be positioned in sitting, with one arm at the side. Unilateral weight bearing can occur through the elbow positioned on a stool at the side of the patient.
- Upper extremity spasticity (typically flexion-adduction-internal rotation pattern) may pull the UE into an abnormal position, adducting and internally rotating the arm; the hand is usually fisted.
  - Gentle rocking from side to side may relax tone.
  - Rounding the thoracic spine by raising the chest can relax tone through active protraction movements.
  - Inhibitory handling can be used to promote relaxation: The hand is opened by grasping the thumb and gradually supinating the forearm; the hand should then be positioned open and flat on the surface with the shoulder in neutral rotation; gentle stroking on top of the fingers can assist in relaxation.
  - Active holding is the goal of treatment; resistive techniques may be contraindicated.
- Abnormal reflex activity may interfere with the patient's ability to assume or hold the posture.
  - An abnormal STNR (head-up position) may increase extension in the upper extremities.
  - An abnormal STLR (head-down position) may prevent head and trunk extension.
  - An abnormal ATNR may cause one UE to collapse.
- Active holding in the PoE posture may be indicated to improve prone extension in lumbar spine dysfunction. When the patient is pain free in this position, he or she can progress to a prone-on-hands position with elbows extended (the McKenzie approach).[9]
- Prone-on-elbows position may be contraindicated for patients with cardiovascular impairments or respiratory insufficiency.
- Tightness in the trunk or hip flexors may limit extension into this posture. A pillow under the abdomen can be used to assist initial positioning.

Prone-on-Elbows: Therapeutic Activities/Techniques

Position/Activity: Prone-on-Elbows, Holding

The patient is in prone-on-elbows (PoE) position, with the head in midposition. Both scapulae should be flat on the thorax. Scapular winging (when the vertebral border of the scapula is more than 1 inch off the thorax) indicates weakness of the serratus anterior muscle and is a contraindication for use of the PoE posture. Modified PoE postures that limit weight bearing (for example, resting on a wedge, or sitting with the elbows on a table top) should be considered. With slight winging, the therapist can place a hand in the mid-scapular region and ask the patient to flatten the back into the hand. The patient is then instructed to maintain this position (flat back) at all times.

TECHNIQUES

Alternating Isometrics: Medial/Lateral Resistance

The therapist heel-sits at the patient's side, at the level of the shoulder. One hand is positioned on the contralateral side of the trunk, pushing on the vertebral border of the scapula or pulling on the axillary border of the scapula. The other hand is positioned on the near side of the upper trunk, pushing on the axillary border of the scapula or cupping the scapula and pulling on the vertebral border of the scapula (Fig. 8–3). **Verbal commands** for alternating isometrics (AI): "Hold this position—don't let me push you away. Hold, hold. Now don't let me pull you toward me. Hold, hold."

Alternating Isometrics: Anterior/Posterior Resistance

The therapist straddles the patient in half-kneeling position. The therapist's hands are positioned on the inferior border of the scapula, pushing forward and upward or over the top of the shoulders on the anterior trunk (hands cupped over the clavicle), pulling backward. **Verbal commands** for AI: "Hold—don't let me push you up and away. Hold, hold. Now don't let me pull you back. Hold, hold."

Rhythmic Stabilization

The therapist straddles the patient in half-kneeling position. The hands are positioned on the upper trunk: one hand is on the lateral border of the scapula (posterior trunk), the other hand on the contralateral anterior trunk. Resistance is applied in a twisting motion,

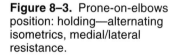

Figure 8–3. Prone-on-elbows position: holding—alternating isometrics, medial/lateral resistance.

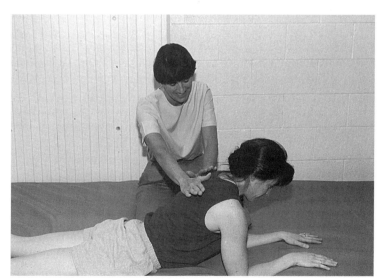

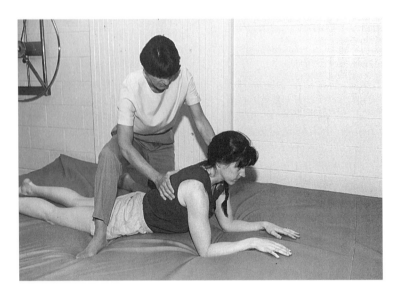

Figure 8–4. Prone-on-elbows position: holding—rhythmic stabilization.

trying to rotate the upper trunk; the patient resists the movement (Fig. 8–4). **Verbal commands** for rhythmic stabilization (RS): "Hold—don't let me twist you. Hold, hold. Now don't let me twist you the other way. Hold, hold."

Comments

Isometric control is the goal. Resistance should build up gradually; the hold should be steady, not jerky, with no visible movement of the trunk.

The therapist's hands should slide quickly during transitions. The patient is not allowed to relax at any time.

The therapist should give the transitional command ("Now don't let me . .") just before the hands change position. This allows the patient to adjust to the expected resistance through feed-forward mechanisms.

Isometric holds (reversals) are repeated three or four times or until patient fatigue becomes evident.

Rhythmic breathing should be encouraged; breath holding should be avoided during all isometric work.

Good body mechanics for the therapist are important: the back should be kept straight, and wrist hyperextension should be avoided.

Manual contacts can include the head along with the upper trunk to increase stabilizing responses of the neck muscles. All resistance to head motion should be light; flat open hands should be used.

Theraband tubing can be tied around the forearms; the patient is instructed to keep the forearms apart, holding against the tubing. This will increase the proprioceptive loading of the shoulder stabilizers, especially the rotator cuff muscles.

Motor control goal. Stability, static control of the head, upper trunk, and shoulders.

Indications. Dependent function due to weakness; disordered control of head, upper trunk, and shoulder muscles. These activities are important lead-up skills for head control in upright antigravity postures (sitting and standing).

Functional outcomes. The patient is able to stabilize in PoE.

Position/Activity: Prone-on-Elbows, Weight Shifting

The patient is positioned in prone-on-elbows (PoE), with the head in midposition. The patient shifts weight from side to side or down (out of the posture) to up (into the posture). This activity requires dynamic stability: the posture must be stabilized while moving. Slow, rhythmic active movements can be used to relax hypertonicity in the UEs.

TECHNIQUES

Slow Reversals: Medial/Lateral Shifts

The therapist applies light, tracking resistance to the upper trunk during weight shifts. Resistance during slow reversals (SRs) is facilitatory, to assist proprioceptive loading (Fig. 8–5A and B). The therapist heel-sits at the patient's side, at shoulder level. As the patient moves toward the therapist, one hand is positioned on the contralateral side of the trunk, resisting the motion from the vertebral border of the scapula; the other hand is positioned on the near side of upper trunk, resisting from the axillary border. As the patient moves away from the therapist, the hands stay on the same sides of the trunk but reverse their position on the scapular borders to resist the opposite direction. **Verbal commands** for SRs: "Push toward me; now pull away. Push toward me; now pull away."

Slow Reversals: Anterior/Posterior Shifts

The patient is initially positioned with the elbows slightly lateral and posterior, to allow movement down to the mat and back up into the PoE position. The therapist straddles the patient in half-kneeling position and applies resistance to the movement, first on the anterior chest (with hands cupped over the clavicles) to resist the downward anterior movement, then on the posterior trunk (the inferior border of the scapula) to resist the return movement to PoE. **Verbal commands** for the shifts: "Pull down to the mat. Now push up to the on-elbows position. Pull down; now push up."

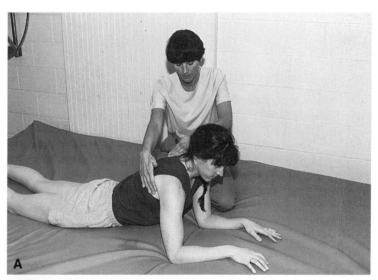

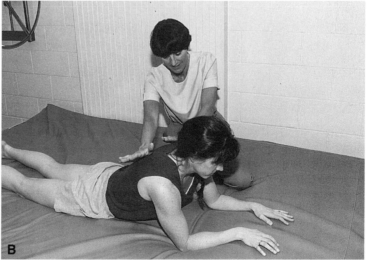

Figure 8–5A and B. Prone-on-elbows position: weight shifting—slow reversals, medial/lateral shifts.

Comments

The emphasis is on smooth reversal of antagonists; movement does not stop in either position.

The therapist's hands move in advance of the verbal command (VC) to ensure smooth reversals of the antagonist movement.

A facilitatory stretch can be used to initiate the antagonist movement and should be well timed to coincide with the VCs.

Small-range control is used initially and progresses to full-range control (through increments of ROM).

Movements are continued until patient fatigue sets in or control is diminished.

A hold (slow reversal-hold) can be added in the on-elbows position to improve stability control.

Agonist Reversals: Anterior/Posterior Shifts

In agonist reversals (ARs), the therapist applies resistance to both the eccentric contraction (controlled lowering out of the posture) and the concentric contraction (return to the PoE posture). The manual contacts remain on the posterior trunk and the inferior border of the scapula throughout both motions (Fig. 8–6A and B). Verbal commands for ARs: "Make me work at pushing you down (or go down slowly). Now push up into prone-on-elbows."

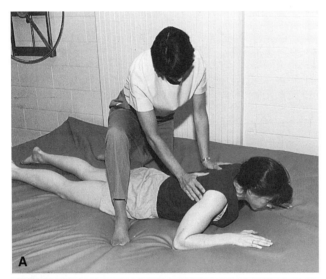

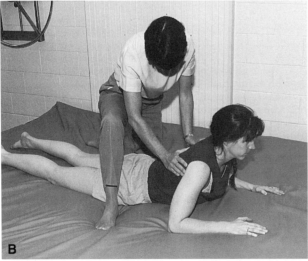

Figure 8–6A and B. Prone-on-elbows position: agonist reversals—anterior/posterior shifts.

Motor control goals. Controlled mobility function of head, upper trunk, and shoulders.

Indications. Dependent function due to weakness; disoredered control of head, upper trunk, and shoulder muscles. These activities are important lead-up skills for dynamic balance control in PoE.

Functional outcomes. The patient is independent in bed mobility and assumption of PoE posture.

Position/Activity: Prone-on-Elbows, Limb Movements

The patient is positioned in PoE, with the head in midposition. For all static-dynamic activities, the center of mass (COM) must shift toward the weight-bearing limb in order to free the dynamic limb for movement. Active reaching or a cone-stacking task can be used. The therapist holds the target cone and asks the patient to place a cone on it. The cone position can be varied with each trial: initially, the target cone should be across from and in front of the patient to facilitate weight transfer to the static limb. As control increases the target cone can be shifted to other locations to challenge control. This task requires eye-hand coordination.

TECHNIQUES

Upper Extremity D1 Thrust Pattern, Slow Reversals
The therapist is positioned in half-kneeling or heel-sitting at the patient's shoulder, positioned diagonally opposite from the dynamic limb (UE). The patient is instructed to shift weight onto the static UE. The dynamic UE is unweighted and passively taken through the range once or twice before resistance is applied. The dynamic UE begins in shoulder hyperextension and scapular retraction, supination, then elbow, wrist, and finger flexion. The UE moves forward and upward across the patient's face, moving into scapular protraction, shoulder flexion and adduction, elbow extension, pronation, wrist and finger extension (D1 thrust). This pattern is a protective pattern for the face. The patient then reverses direction and brings the UE back down to the start position (withdrawal or reverse thrust). The dynamic UE is non-weight-bearing at all times.

   The therapist resists the motion of the dynamic UE with one hand grasping the patient's wrist or forearm. As the patient moves into the thrust pattern the therapist must also move from supination to pronation. The therapist's other hand is positioned lightly on or near the top of the shoulder of the static limb. The therapist applies light, tracking resistance to the dynamic upper limb. The amount of resistance applied to the dynamic limb is determined by the patient's ability to hold the static limb and trunk steady. Approximation can be applied to increase stabilizing responses as needed (Fig. 8–7A and B). **Verbal commands** for slow reversals (SRs) in this pattern: "Shift your weight over onto your left elbow. Now lift your right arm up and across your face. Now pull the arm down and back to your side."

Comments
The therapist may actually block movement in the thrust pattern if positioned in midline
   directly in front of the patient.
Contact with the static shoulder should be minimal; the patient should not be supported
   by the therapist's hand.
A hold (slow reversal-hold) can be added in either direction; the hold is most commonly
   applied to the D1 thrust pattern.

Motor control goals. Controlled mobility and static-dynamic control of the upper trunk and upper extremity. This activity is an important lead-up skill for UE function in PoE.

Indications. Impairments in static-dynamic control in PoE.

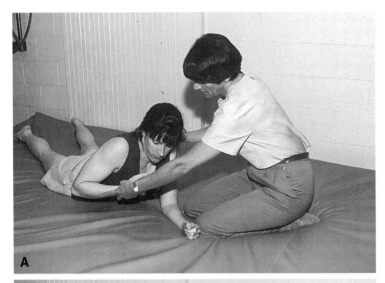

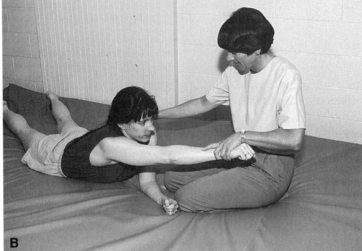

Figure 8–7A and B. Prone-on-elbows position: PNF UE thrust/reverse thrust pattern—slow reversals.

Functional outcomes. The patient is independent in prone-on-elbows position and can perform UE reach and grasp activities.

Position/Activity: Prone-on-Elbows, Balance Training Activities

Balance training begins with static holding (static postural control) and progresses to weight shifts in all directions (dynamic postural control). The patient learns how far to shift in any one direction before losing balance and falling out of the PoE position. Re-education of the limits of stability (LOS) is one of the first activities in a balance training sequence.

Additional activities that challenge anticipatory balance control in PoE include UE reaching and elevation activities (cone stacking) and look-arounds: the head and upper trunk rotate first to one side, then the other.

Activities that can be used to challenge reactive balance control include side-to-side tilts on an equilibrium board (self-initiated or therapist-initiated). Lateral curvature of head and upper trunk is a normal response: the head and trunk rotate toward the raised or elevated side.

Motor control goals. Static and dynamic balance control.

Indications. Severely disordered balance control. Balance training in PoE promotes balance control in a stable posture with a large base of support (BOS).

Functional outcomes. The patient demonstrates appropriate functional balance in the PoE posture.

Movement Transitions into Quadruped (All-Fours) Position

Prone-on-Elbows into Quadruped Posture

Starting in the PoE position, the patient walks backward on the elbows until the knees are directly under the hips. The patient then extends both elbows, lifting the upper trunk into a hands-and-knees position.

The therapist initially is squatting behind the patient with both hands on the patient's hips. The therapist pulls backward and upward, first on one hip then the other, walking the patient back into quadruped. Movement of the pelvis facilitates shoulder extension by stretching the latissimus dorsi on the same side. Once the patient's knees are positioned directly under the hips, the therapist straddles the patient, keeping both knees in contact with the patient's hips to stabilize the hip position (Fig. 8–8A and B). The therapist's

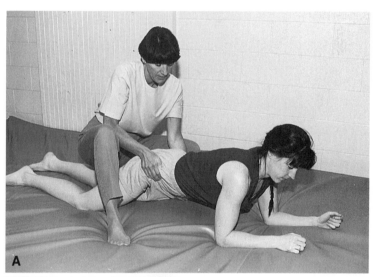

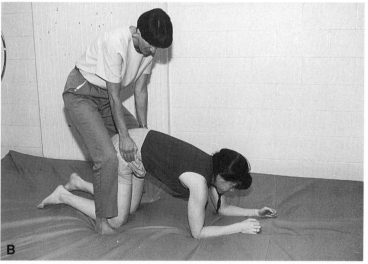

Figure 8–8A and B. Prone-on-elbows to quadruped—active-assistive movement.

hands then shift to the upper trunk to assist upper trunk/UE movement into quadruped. **Verbal commands** (VCs): "On three, I want you to walk back on your elbows until your hips are over your knees. One, two, three; step, step, step. Now push up with your hands and arms, and come up onto your hands and knees."

Comments
If the knees are too far apart in quadruped, weight can be shifted onto one knee; the opposite unweighted knee will adduct into its proper alignment.

Side-sitting to Quadruped
The patient is in side-sitting position with the upper trunk rotated and the elbows extended; both hands are weight bearing (the hands should be shoulder-width apart). The hips and knees are pre-positioned to 90 degrees of flexion. The patient twists (rotates) the lower trunk from side-sitting into quadruped.

The therapist is half-kneeling near the patient's hips or squatting over both legs. Manual contacts are on both hips. The therapist assists the movement of the hips (lower trunk rotation) into quadruped (Fig. 8–9*A* and *B*). **Verbal commands** for the transition: "On three, I want you to twist your hips around, coming up onto your hands and knees. One, two, three."

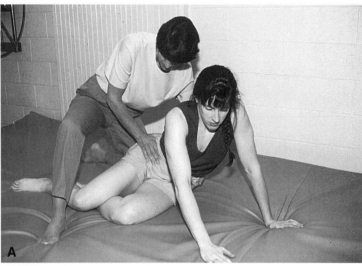

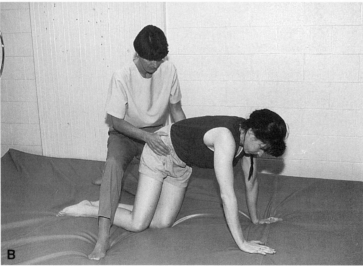

Figure 8–9*A* and *B*. Side-sitting to quadruped—active-assistive movement.

Comments

Maximum assistance is required in the beginning of the movement; as the hips move closer to the final position, less assistance is given.

Pre-positioning of the limbs is key to achieving the correct final position.

A Swiss ball can be used to assist the movement of the hips while providing support for the trunk during early quadruped activities. The ball size is important: it should be large enough to support the trunk in quadruped but not too large to interfere with assumption of the posture or postural alignment in the position.

Motor control goals. Mobility (active-assistive movements), progressing to controlled mobility (active movements).

Indications. Dependent function due to weakness, disordered motor control. These activities are important lead-up skills for floor-to-standing transfers.

Functional outcome. The patient is able to assume quadruped position independently.

QUADRUPED (PRONE KNEELING)

General Characteristics

- The base of support (BOS) in quadruped is large.
- The center of mass (COM) is higher than in PoE but still low.
- Quadruped (kneeling on all fours) is a stable, four-limb posture.
- The shoulders are flexed to 90 degrees, with the elbows extended and the hands positioned directly under the shoulders. The hips are flexed to 90 degrees, with the knees positioned directly under the hips; the back is straight (flat).
- Assuming and maintaining quadruped posture requires head/neck, upper trunk, upper extremity (shoulder/elbow), and lower trunk/hip control.
- Normal righting reactions (ORR, LRR, BOH) contribute to the maintenance of head position.
- Quadruped posture involves increased demands for balance, especially with dynamic shifting activities.
- Abnormal reflexes may interfere with the patient's ability to assume and maintain this position:
  - Asymmetrical tonic neck reflex (ATNR) may cause one UE to flex if the head turns to the opposite side.
  - Symmetrical tonic neck reflex (STNR) may cause the UEs to flex with head/neck flexion or the hips to flex with head/neck extension.

Treatment Strategies and Considerations

- Ability to hold in this posture may be limited due to inhibitory pressure on quadriceps and wrist/finger flexors. The hand can be positioned over a sandbag or the end of a platform mat, or weight bearing can occur on a fisted hand to reduce UE inhibitory effects.
- Patients with LE extensor or finger flexor hypertonicity may benefit from the effects of inhibitory pressure inherent in this posture. Quadruped can be a useful lead-up activity to relax tone before standing and walking or hand activities.
- Patients with UE spasticity secondary to retracted scapula with shoulder internal rotation and adduction and elbow flexion (for example, the patient with stroke) may benefit from rounding the back, then hollowing; this requires active scapular protraction movements. The UE should be positioned in elbow extension, forearm supination, and shoulder flexion and external rotation.

- Patients with knee pain (for example, older adults with osteoarthritis) may find quadruped and kneeling activities uncomfortable. A folded towel or small pillow placed under the knees can be used to increase comfort levels.
- Patients with shoulder pain and limited ROM (for example, the patient with hemiplegia who has a painful, subluxed shoulder) may find this posture too stressful. For these patients a modified plantigrade posture or sitting with weight bearing on elbows or extended upper extremities may be used to achieve the benefits of early weight bearing.
- Quadruped posture may be contraindicated in patients with LE flexor spasticity.

Quadruped: Therapeutic Activities/Techniques

Position/Activity: Quadruped, Holding

The patient is positioned in quadruped, with the head in midposition and the back flat. The patient actively holds in the all-fours posture. If scapular winging is present, the therapist can place a hand over the midscapular region and ask the patient to flatten the back into the hand. If increased lumbar lordosis (sway back) is present, the therapist can place a hand over the lumbar region and ask the patient to flatten the back into the hand and hold the back level (flat). Modified holding in quadruped with limited weight bearing can be achieved by positioning the patient over a Swiss ball.

TECHNIQUES

Alternating Isometrics: Medial/Lateral Resistance
The therapist is half-kneeling at the patient's side. Resistance is given in medial/lateral (M/L) directions. One hand is positioned on the contralateral side of upper trunk, and resists either on the vertebral or axillary borders of the scapula; the other hand is positioned on the ipsilateral lower trunk, and resists either on the lateral border of pelvis or is cupped and pulls on the midpelvic region (Fig. 8–10). Alternately, both hands can resist on the sides of the trunk, switching from ipsilateral to contralateral. This may be problematic in large patients with a broad trunk. **Verbal commands** for alternating isometrics (AI): "Hold this position—don't let me push you away. Hold, hold. Now don't let me pull you toward me. Hold, hold."

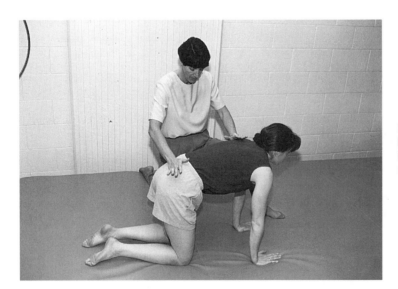

Figure 8–10. Quadruped: holding—alternating isometrics, medial/lateral resistance.

Alternating Isometrics: Anterior/Posterior Resistance

The therapist is kneeling directly behind the patient. Resistance is given in anterior/posterior (A/P) directions. Both hands are positioned on the pelvis, pushing forward (sliding the hands down over the lower pelvis/ischium) or pulling backward (sliding the hands up over the top of the iliac crest). Alternately, one hand can be on the upper trunk and one hand on the pelvis (Fig. 8–11). This may be problematic in very tall patients with a long trunk. **Verbal commands** for AI: "Hold—don't let me push you up and away. Hold, hold. Now don't let me pull you back. Hold, hold."

Alternating Isometrics: Diagonal Resistance

The therapist is half-kneeling next to the patient, positioned on the diagonal. Resistance is given in diagonal directions. **Verbal commands** for AI: "Hold—don't let me push you up and over your right arm. Hold, hold. Now don't let me pull back and over your left hip. Hold, hold."

Rhythmic Stabilization

The therapist is half-kneeling next to the patient or standing with both knees flexed. One hand is positioned on the upper trunk, either on the lateral border of the scapula (posterior trunk) or on the anterior trunk/shoulder. The other hand is positioned either on the posterior or anterior pelvis. The therapist applies resistance to trunk rotation, pushing forward and downward on the upper trunk while pulling upward and backward on the pelvis (twisting the trunk). The hands are then reversed, maintaining their respective positions on the pelvis and upper trunk. The patient resists the movement, holding steady (Fig. 8–12). **Verbal commands** for rhythmic stabilization (RS): "Hold—don't let me twist you. Hold, hold. Now don't let me twist you the other way. Hold, hold."

Comments

Isometric control is the goal. Resistance should build up gradually. The hold should be steady, not jerky, with no visible movement of the trunk.

The therapist's hands are slid quickly during transitions; the patient should not be allowed to relax at any time.

The therapist should give the transitional command ("Now don't let me . .") just before the hands change position. This allows the patient to adjust to the expected resistance through feed-forward mechanisms.

The isometric holds (reversals) are repeated three or four times or until patient fatigue becomes evident.

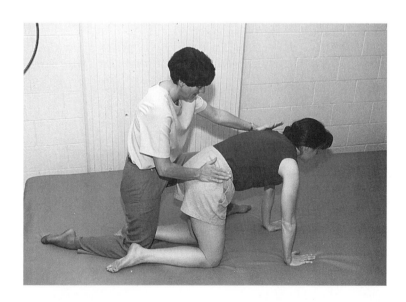

Figure 8–11. Quadruped: holding—alternating isometrics, anterior/posterior resistance.

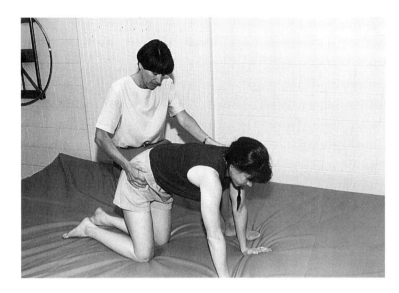

Figure 8–12. Quadruped: holding—rhythmic stabilization.

Rhythmic breathing should be encouraged. Breath holding should be avoided by the patient during all isometric work.

Good body mechanics for the therapist are important: the back should be straight (not stooped or flexed), and wrist hyperextension should be avoided.

Theraband tubing can be placed around the patient's UEs (to increase lateral stabilization of the shoulders) or around the patient's thighs (to increase lateral stabilization of the hips). The patient is instructed to keep the limbs apart, holding against the tubing.

Motor control goal. Stability, static control of head, upper and lower trunk, shoulders, and hips.

Indications. Dependent function due to weakness, disordered motor control. Kneeling on all fours is an intermediate posture and lead-up skill for independent assumption of floor-to-standing transfers

Functional outcomes. The patient is able to stabilize in the quadruped posture independently.

Position/Activity: Quadruped, Weight Shifting

The patient is in quadruped (all-fours) position, with the head in midposition and the back flat. The patient shifts weight from side to side (in M/L shifts), forward and backward (in A/P shifts), or diagonally. This activity requires dynamic stability: the patient must maintain the posture while moving. Movement begins with small-range control and progresses to full-range control (through increments of ROM).

TECHNIQUES

Slow Reversals: Medial/Lateral Shifts
In slow reversals (SRs), the therapist applies light, tracking resistance to the trunk during weight shifts. Resistance is facilitatory (proprioceptive loading). The emphasis is on a smooth reversal of antagonists; the patient does not stop in either position. The therapist's hands move in advance of the verbal command to ensure smooth reversals to the antagonist movement. A facilitatory stretch can be used to initiate the antagonist movement and should be well timed to coincide with the verbal commands. A hold (slow reversal-hold) can be added if shortened range control is lacking in any direction.

The patient shifts weight first onto the ipsilateral UE and LE, then shifts weight onto the contralateral limbs. The therapist is half-kneeling at the patient's side. Both hands resist at the side of the trunk: one hand is on the upper trunk, the other hand is on the pelvis. As the patient pushes toward the therapist, both hands resist the movement on the ipsilateral side of the trunk. As the patient pulls away, both hands resist the movement on the contralateral side of the trunk. Using an alternate hand position, the therapist keeps one hand positioned on the contralateral side of the upper trunk, resisting first the vertebral border of the scapula, then the axillary border; the other hand is positioned on the ipsilateral pelvis, resisting first on the lateral pelvis, then on the midpelvis. **Verbal commands** for the SRs: "Push toward me. Now pull away. Push toward me. Now pull away."

Slow Reversals: Anterior/Posterior Shifts
The patient shifts weight forward onto both UEs, then backward onto both LEs. The therapist is half-kneeling directly behind the patient. Resistance is given to the movement, first on the upper pelvis (iliac crest), then on the lower pelvis (ischium) (Fig. 8–13).

Slow Reversals from Quadruped to Heel-sitting Position
The patient can move from the quadruped position down into heel-sitting. The shoulders are flexed and the hands remain on the mat. The patient then moves back up into quadruped position (Fig. 8–14). Weight shifts from quadruped down into heel-sitting can be used to improve shoulder ROM; this may be useful in unsuspecting patients who may be otherwise anxious about passive range of motion (PROM). Repeated movements can be effective in inhibiting spasticity in the UEs. A prayer seat (small wooden bench) may be used to decrease the range of the movements down into heel-sitting. A small wooden bench seat allows the patient to sit with knees flexed under the seat. The prayer seat is useful for patients who find it difficult to get up from the full heel-sitting position. **Verbal commands** for the SRs: "Pull forward. Now push backward."

Slow Reversals: Diagonal Shifts
The patient shifts weight diagonally forward and over onto one UE, then backward and diagonally over the opposite knee. The therapist is half-kneeling, positioned on the diagonal. The movements are resisted, using one hand on the contralateral upper trunk and one hand on the ipsilateral pelvis.

Quadruped to Heel-sitting on One Side
The patient diagonally shifts down from quadruped into heel-sitting on one side (Fig. 8–15). This activity can be used to elongate the trunk and reduce spasticity (for example, in the patient with hemiplegia who demonstrates spasticity in the lateral trunk flexors). A side seat or sandbags can be used to decrease the range of movements down into side-sitting. This is useful for patients who find it difficult to get up from the full side-sitting position.

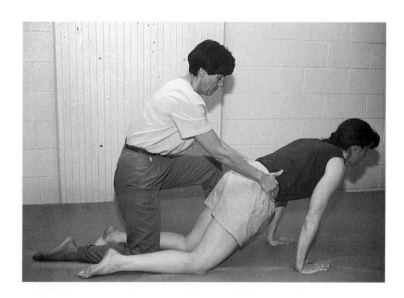

Figure 8–13. Quadruped: weight shifting—slow reversals anterior/posterior shifts.

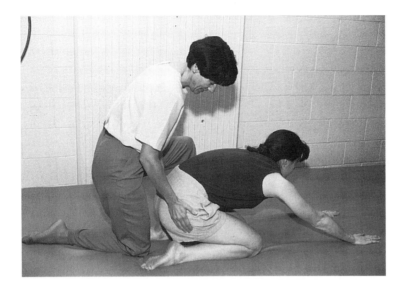

Figure 8–14. Quadruped to heel-sitting—slow reversals.

Quadruped to Side-sitting

The patient moves from quadruped to the side-sitting position using lower trunk rotation; the hands remain on the mat. This activity requires considerable flexibility through the lower trunk and pelvis. Patients with limited ROM can be instructed to move through the available ranges only. A Swiss ball can be used to support the trunk and assist the motion from side to side (Fig. 8–16). The therapist first guides the motion, then verbally cues the patient's active movements. Patients who have difficulty getting up from the full side-sitting position can be assisted into the range by tapping.

Motor control goals. Controlled mobility function of the upper/lower trunk and shoulders/hips.

Indications. Dependent function due to weakness, disordered motor control. These activities are important lead-up skills for dynamic balance control in quadruped position and creeping (progression on hands and knees).

Functional outcomes. The patient is able to assume and weight-shift in quadruped posture.

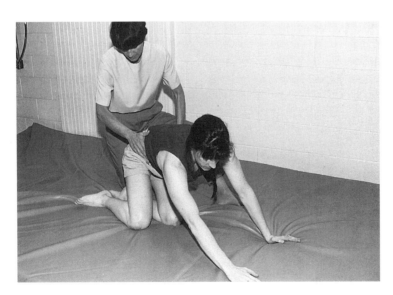

Figure 8–15. Quadruped to heel-sitting on one side—slow reversals.

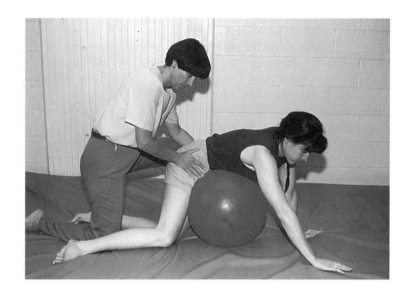

Figure 8–16. Quadruped to side-sitting using a Swiss ball—active-assistive movement.

Position/Activity: Quadruped, Limb Movements

The patient is in quadruped (all-fours) position, with the head in midposition and the trunk stable (back flat). For all static-dynamic activities, the center of mass (COM) must shift toward the weight-bearing limbs in order to free the dynamic limb for movement.

Upper Extremity Reaching

The patient is asked to weight-shift onto one side and lift the opposite limb off the mat. The therapist can provide a target by holding a hand in space (within the patient's reach) and asking the patient to touch it. The therapist can also hold a cone and ask the patient to place a second cone on it—a cone-stacking task (Fig. 8–17). The position can be varied with each trial: the initial location of the target should facilitate weight transfer onto the static limbs. As control increases the target can be shifted to other locations to challenge control. UE reaching requires eye-hand coordination.

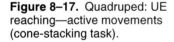

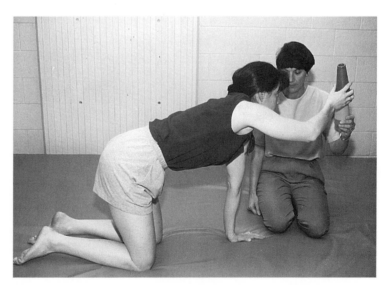

Figure 8–17. Quadruped: UE reaching—active movements (cone-stacking task).

Lower Extremity Lifting

The patient is asked to weight-shift to one side and extend the LE back and up behind the body. Various combinations can be used: alternate lifting of one UE, then the other; one LE, then the other; or the opposite UE and LE (Fig. 8–18).

TECHNIQUES

The therapist applies light, tracking resistance to the dynamic limb. The amount of resistance applied to the dynamic limb is determined by the patient's ability to hold the static limb and trunk steady.

Slow Reversals: Upper Extremity PNF D2 Flexion and Extension

The patient is instructed to weight-shift toward the static UE. The dynamic UE is unweighted and passively taken through the range once or twice before resistance is applied. The dynamic UE begins in shoulder extension, adduction and internal rotation with pronation, wrist and finger flexion; the fisted hand is placed on opposite pelvis, anterior superior iliac spine, ASIS. The hand opens, turns, and lifts up and out moving the arm into shoulder flexion, abduction, and external rotation with supination, wrist, and finger extension. The patient then reverses direction and brings the UE back down to the start position. The dynamic UE is non-weight-bearing at all times.

The therapist is half-kneeling at the patient's shoulder, diagonally opposite the dynamic limb. The therapist resists the motion of the dynamic UE with one hand resting on top of the patient's forearm with a loose grasp. The therapist's other hand is positioned lightly on or near the top of the shoulder of the static limb. Approximation can then be applied to the static limb if needed to increase stabilizing responses (Fig. 8–19A and B). **Verbal commands** (VCs): "Shift your weight over onto your right arm. Now open your hand, turn, and lift your left hand up and out toward me. Now pull that hand down and across to your hip."

Comments

The therapist may actually block the movement of the arm if he or she is positioned too far in front of the patient.

Contact with the static shoulder should be minimal—the patient should not be supported by the therapist's hand.

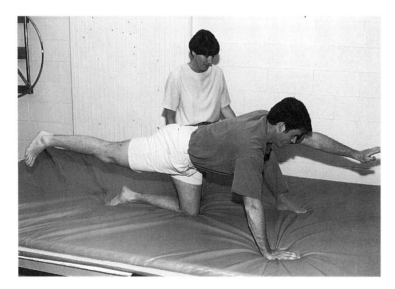

Figure 8–18. Quadruped: UE and LE reaching—active movements.

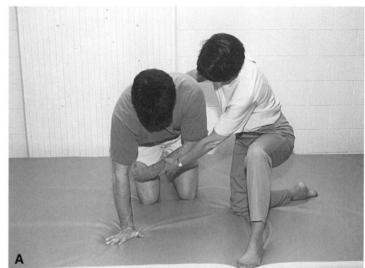

Figure 8–19*A* and *B*.
Quadruped: PNF UE D2 flexion and extension patterns—slow reversals.

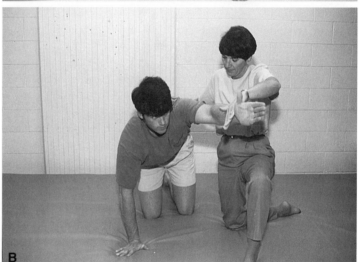

Slow Reversals: Lower Extremity PNF D1 Flexion with Knee Flexed and D1 Extension with Knee Extended

The patient is instructed to weight-shift toward the static LE. The dynamic LE is unweighted and passively taken through the range once or twice before resistance is applied. The dynamic LE begins in hip flexion and adduction with the knee flexed toward the opposite hand. The knee moves backward and upward, moving the hip into extension and abduction. The knee extends upward and behind the patient. The patient then reverses direction and brings the knee back down and across toward the opposite hand. The dynamic LE is non-weight-bearing at all times.

The therapist is half-kneeling behind the patient. The therapist resists the motion of the dynamic LE with one hand on the anterior or posterior lower leg. The therapist's other hand is positioned lightly on or near the top of the pelvis of the static limb. Approximation can be applied to the static lower limb to increase stabilizing responses as needed (Fig. 8–20*A* and *B*).

Slow Reversal-Hold

A hold (slow reversal-hold) can be added to increase the degree of difficulty and postural challenge to the trunk and static limbs. Typically the hold is added when the dynamic limb is lifted up (either UE D2F or LE D1E).

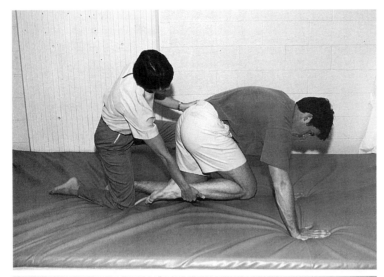

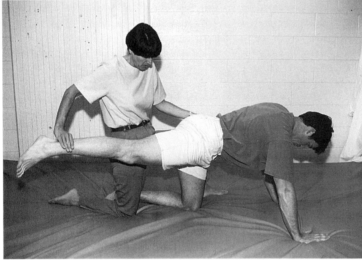

Figure 8–20A and B. Quadruped: PNF LE D1 flexion and extension patterns—slow reversals.

Motor control goals. Controlled mobility/static-dynamic control of the trunk and extremities.

Indications. Impairments in static-dynamic control in quadruped. These activities are important lead-up skills for skill level function in the posture, creeping.

Functional outcomes. The patient is independent in quadruped position and can perform UE reaching and LE movements.

Position/Activity: Quadruped, Creeping

The patient is in quadruped, with the head in midposition and the back flat. The patient moves forward or backward using the limbs (hands and knees) for locomotion.

A **four-point creeping pattern** can be used initially for maximum stability. The patient advances only one limb at a time: first one hand, then the opposite knee. The patient then shifts weight to advance the opposite hand, then the contralateral knee. The sequence is repeated for continued progression.

In a **two-point creeping pattern** the patient advances one hand and the opposite knee simultaneously. Weight is then shifted onto these limbs and the opposite hand and knee are advanced together. The sequence is repeated for continued progression. A two-point pattern allows for a more continuous movement sequence. Some patients may adopt an ipsilateral pattern in which the hand and the knee on the same side move together. This pattern should be discouraged in favor of a contralateral pattern, with the opposite hand and knee moving together. This activity can be an important lead-up activity for skilled gait, which requires trunk counterrotation and contralateral limb movements.

TECHNIQUES

Resisted Progression
Therapist applies light, tracking resistance to the pelvis, resisting both the forward progression as well as the pelvic rotation that accompanies the advancement of the LEs. A light stretch can be used to facilitate initiation of pelvic and LE movements. In resisted progression (RP), the therapist must move when the patient does (Fig. 8–21).

As an alternative, the therapist's hands can be placed on the patient's ankles to resist forward progression. The therapist is in a full squatting position and must move forward each time the patient moves. Ankle cuffs attached to a wall-pulley system can also be used to resist the forward progression. Movements must be well timed with appropriate commands. **Verbal commands** for RP: "On three, I want you to move your right arm and left leg together. One, two, and step, step, step."

Comments
Some patients may be resistant to creeping as a training activity, feeling it is too childish. The therapist needs to stress the clinical relevance of this activity to other functional activities. For example, the counterrotation pattern is important for gait; patients may need this skill if they fall and have to get to the nearest chair or support to pull themselves up.

Motor control goals. Skill.

Indications. Development of skilled locomotion pattern, trunk counterrotation with contralateral UE and LE movements.

Functional outcomes. The patient is able to move independently in quadruped using a reciprocal trunk and limb pattern.

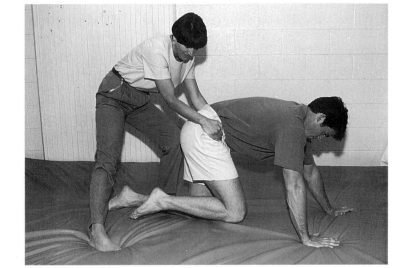

Figure 8–21. Quadruped: creeping—resisted progression.

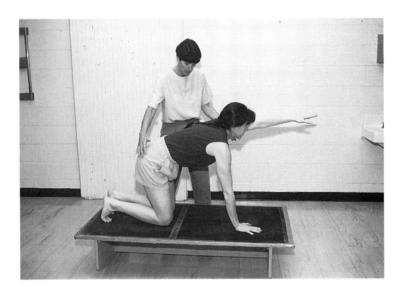

Figure 8–22. Quadruped: balancing using three-limb support on a balance board—active movements.

Position/Activity: Quadruped, Balance Training Activities

Balance training begins with static holding (static postural control) and progresses to weight shifts in all directions (dynamic postural control). The patient learns how far to shift in any one direction before losing balance and falling out of the quadruped position Re-education of the limits of stability (LOS) is one of the first activities in a balance training sequence.

Additional activities that challenge anticipatory balance control in quadruped posture include arm lifts, leg lifts, and combined arm and leg lifts as well as look-arounds (the head and upper trunk rotate first to one side, then the other) and transitions from quadruped to side-sitting to quadruped using pelvic/lower trunk rotation.

Activities that can be used to challenge reactive balance control include side-to-side tilts on the equilibrium board (self-initiated or therapist-initiated). Lateral curvature of the head and upper trunk is a normal response; the head and trunk rotate toward the raised or elevated side. Progression is from four-limb support to three-limb to two-limb support while balancing on the equilibrium board (Fig. 8–22). Self-initiated tilts challenge both anticipatory and reactive balance control.

Motor control goals. Static and dynamic balance control.

Indications. Disordered balance control, impairments in strength and coordination of postural muscles; these activities promote dynamic balance control in a stable, four-limb posture.

Functional outcomes. The patient demonstrates appropriate functional balance in quadruped position.

Lower Trunk Activities

HOOKLYING (CROOKLYING)

General Characteristics

- The base of support (BOS) in hooklying is large.
- The center of mass (COM) is low.
- This posture is very stable.
- Hooklying primarily involves lower trunk, hip, and knee control:
  - Activation of the lower trunk rotators and hip abductors/adductors allows the patient to actively move the knees from side to side away from midline.
  - Activation of the hamstrings allows the patient to keep the knees flexed in the hooklying position.

Treatment Strategies and Considerations

- Hooklying activities are important lead-up activities for controlled bridging, kneeling, and bipedal gait.
- Abnormal reflex activity may interfere with assumption or maintenance of the posture.
  - In supine, the symmetrical tonic labyrinthine reflex (STLR) may cause the lower extremities (LEs) to extend.
  - A positive support reaction (applying pressure to the ball of the foot) may also cause the LE to extend; a heel-down position minimizing contact of the ball of the foot may need to be adopted.
- Active movements of the knees from side to side involve crossing the midline and can be an important treatment activity for patients with unilateral neglect (for example, the patient with left hemiplegia).
- Patients with gluteus medius weakness (for example, the patient with a Trendelenburg gait pattern) may benefit from hooklying activities to activate the abductors in a less stressful, non-weight-bearing position.
- Lower trunk rotation (LTR) should occur without accompanying upper trunk rotation (UTR) or log rolling.
  - The upper extremities (UEs) can be positioned in extension and abduction on the mat.
  - A prayer position (hands clasped together with both elbows extended and shoulders flexed to 90 degrees) may be used with the patient recovering from stroke who demonstrates excess flexor tone in the UE.

Hooklying: Therapeutic Activities and Techniques

Position/Activity: Hooklying, Lower Trunk Rotation

The patient is in hooklying position.

TECHNIQUES

Rhythmic Rotation

Rhythmic rotation (RRo) is a passive technique designed to promote relaxation in the patient with LE hypertonicity. Rhythmic rotation is repeated until relaxation occurs, generally for several minutes.

The patient is in hooklying position with both feet placed flat on the mat or on the therapist's knees. The therapist is in heel-sitting position at the base of the patient's feet. The therapist instructs the patient to relax and let the therapist move the legs. The therapist places both hands on top of the patient's knees and slowly rocks the knees side to side. Range of motion in lower trunk rotation (LTR) is gradually increased as tone decreases.

An alternate approach involves positioning the patient's legs on a Swiss ball (hips and knees are flexed to approximately 90 degrees). The therapist is half-kneeling, holding onto the patient's legs. The therapist slowly rocks the ball from side to side (Fig. 9–1). This technique eliminates tactile input to the bottom of the feet, thereby reducing the possible negative effects of a hyperactive positive support reflex. The ball also allows the patient to move from side to side easily and may be a more effective intervention for patients with high levels of spasticity (for example, the patient with multiple sclerosis and strong LE extensor tone).

Rhythmic Initiation

In rhythmic initiation (RI) the lower trunk is rotated as the knees are moved slowly from side to side. As the patient relaxes, range is gradually increased until the knees move laterally down to the mat on each side. The movements are first passive (as in rhythmic rotation), then active-assistive, then lightly resisted with **tracking resistance.** Progression to next phase is dependent upon the patient's ability to relax and participate in the active and resistive phases.

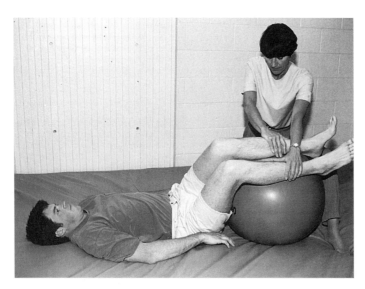

Figure 9–1. Hooklying: lower trunk rotation (LEs on a Swiss ball)—rhythmic rotation.

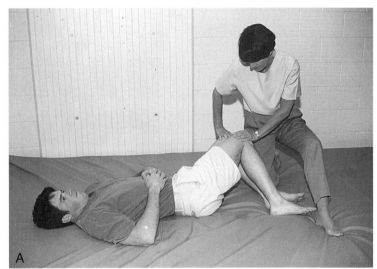

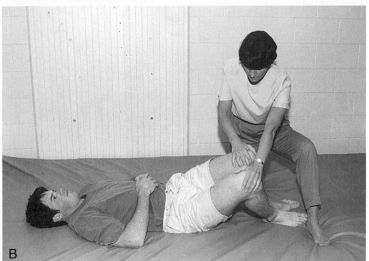

Figure 9–2A and B. Hook-lying: lower trunk rotation—rhythmic initiation.

The patient is positioned in hooklying. The therapist is at the patient's side in a half-kneeling position. Manual contacts are fixed on top of the knees during the first two phases. During the final (resistive) phase the therapist's hands slide to the side (the medial side of one knee and the lateral side of the opposite knee) to resist both knees as they pull away and then slide to the opposite sides of the knees to resist the return movement. The therapist's hands pivot in order to resist the complete return movement of the knees down to the mat (Fig. 9–2A and B).

Motor control goals (RRo and RI).   Mobility.

Indications.   Impaired function due to hypertonia (LE extensor spasticity, rigidity) and decreased LTR.

Functional outcomes.   The patient performs independent bed-mat mobility.

Hold-Relax Active Motion
In hold-relax active motion (HRAM), the patient's knees are moved toward one side (away from the therapist) one-quarter range. The patient is asked to hold this position, slowly building up the isometric contraction. The patient is then asked to actively relax. The therapist then moves the knees quickly in the opposite direction past midline and

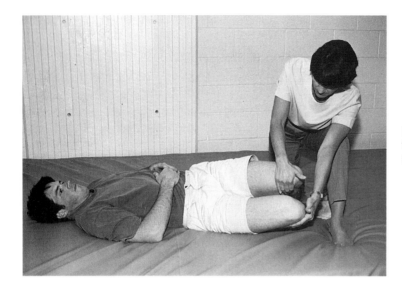

Figure 9–3. Hooklying: lower trunk rotation—hold-relax active motion.

asks the patient to actively contract through the range back to the original position (Fig. 9–3).

The sequence is an isometric hold followed by active relaxation, then passive movement into the lengthened range followed by a resisted isotonic contraction back into the shortened range. The active relaxation is important; return movement should not be initiated until the isometric contraction is completely released.

The patient is positioned in hooklying. The therapist is half-kneeling at the patient's side. The therapist's hands are positioned on top of the patient's knees. The therapist applies greater resistance to the weaker LE, which typically has weak hip abductors on one side. The isometric contraction is built up slowly; resistance of the isotonic movement is light (tracking). **Verbal commands** are dynamic and should reflect the buildup of effort. A quick stretch can be applied in the lengthened range to facilitate the return movement.

HRAM emphasizes movement in one direction only. Midrange control is achieved first; progression is to full-range control.

Motor control goals (HRAM). Mobility.

Indications. Weak, hypotonic muscles (lower trunk rotators, hip abductors).

Functional outcomes. The patient performs independent bed-mat mobility.

Position/Activity: Hooklying, Holding

In hooklying, the patient actively holds both knees stable and apart, in midline position. Active holding (maintaining the hooklying position with feet in contact with mat surface) is a useful activity for the patient recovering from stroke. The ability to hold the foot flat while in hooklying position on the mat is an out-of-synergy combination that avoids the influence of the mass movement synergies. In synergy, the patient will flex the hip and the knee off the mat with accompanying hip abduction and external rotation. With the LE in this out-of-synergy combination, the patient is asked to actively hold the foot flat.

As control increases, the position of the foot can be varied, progressing to various degrees of knee extension. This promotes the development of selective knee control. Progression can also be achieved by altering the activity from bilateral to unilateral. Theraband tubing can be placed around the patient's thighs to increase the proprioceptive loading of the hip abductors.

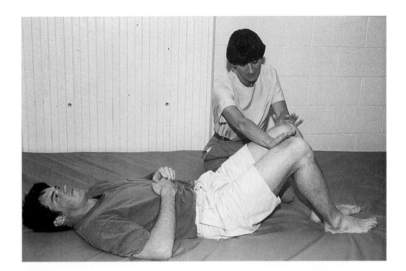

Figure 9–4. Hooklying: holding—alternating isometrics.

TECHNIQUES

Alternating Isometrics

The patient is asked to hold the hooklying position while the therapist applies resistance to the knees. Side-to-side resistance is applied with one hand on the medial side of the knee and the opposite hand on the lateral side of the other knee. The hand placements are then reversed to resist holding in the other direction (Fig. 9–4).

The resistance is built up gradually from very light resistance to the patient's maximum. The isometric contraction is maintained for several counts. The therapist must give a transitional command ("Now don't let me pull you the other way") before sliding the hands to resist the opposite muscles; this allows the patient the opportunity to make appropriate preparatory postural adjustments.

In alternating isometrics (AI) resistance can be applied side to side, or diagonally. The position of the therapist will vary according to the line of force that needs to be applied. Resistance applied to both hip abductors may be used to gain overflow from strong to weak muscles (for example, in the patient recovering from stroke). In this situation, resistance to abductors is typically maximized while resistance to adductors in minimal. Resistance can also be applied to the ankles. This variation shifts the focus more distally, recruiting more activity of the knee muscles, especially the hamstrings.

Motor control goals. Stability.

Indications. Weakness and instability of the lower trunk (for example, in the patient with low back dysfunction); weakness and instability of the hip muscles (for example, in the patient with abductor weakness and a Trendelenburg gait pattern). These activities are important lead-up skills for lower trunk/pelvic stabilization during bipedal gait.

Functional outcomes. The patient is able to stabilize the lower trunk/pelvis during bed-mat activities.

Position/Activity: Hooklying, Lower Trunk Rotation

In hooklying, the patient moves both knees together in side-to-side movements. Depending on the range of motion available, the knees can move all the way down to the mat on one side, then the other.

TECHNIQUES

Slow Reversals

The knees are moved passively from side to side for a few repetitions to ensure that the patient knows the movements expected. The movements are then resisted. The therapist

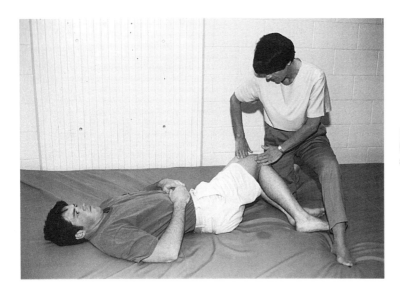

Figure 9–5. Hooklying: lower trunk rotation—slow reversals.

alternates hand placement, first on one side to resist the knees pulling away from midline, then on the other side to resist the return movement (Fig. 9–5).

Smooth reversals of antagonists are facilitated by well-timed verbal commands ("Pull away" or "Push back") and a quick stretch to initiate the reverse movement (SR). Progression is from partial-range to full-range control.

Slow Reversal-Hold

A hold (SRH) may be added in one or both directions if the patient demonstrates difficulty in maintaining the contraction into the shortened range. The resisted hold is a momentary pause (held for one count); the antagonist contraction is then facilitated.

Slow Reversal-Hold with Repeated Contractions

Repeated contractions (RCs) can be added if weakness exists—typically the hip abductors are weak on one side. When weakness is detected, the isotonic contractions to one side are repeated. The patient's knees are repeatedly pulled back toward the mat surface (repeated stretches) and verbal commands ("Pull away," "And again pull away") are given to facilitate the movement. The contractions may be applied through partial range and progress to full range.

Motor control goals.   Controlled mobility.

Indications.   Weakness and instability of the lower trunk and hip muscles. Lower trunk rotation in hooklying is an important lead-up skill for upright antigravity control in kneeling, standing, and gait.

Functional outcomes.   The patient performs independent bed-mat mobility and can ambulate with adequate control of lower trunk/pelvic movements.

BRIDGING

General Characteristics

- The base of support (BOS) in bridging is large.
- The center of mass (COM) is low.
- This posture is very stable.
- Bridging is similar to hooklying in that it primarily involves the **lower trunk, hip, and knee muscles.**

○ The lower trunk muscles and hip abductors and adductors stabilize the hip and lower trunk.
○ The low-back and hip extensors elevate the pelvis.
○ The hamstrings keep the knees flexed and the feet under the knees.

Treatment Strategies and Considerations

• Bridging allows early weight bearing through the foot and ankle without the body weight constraints of a fully upright posture. It is an appropriate early posture for patients recovering from ankle injury.
• Bridging activities are important lead-up activities for later functional activities such as moving in bed and scooting to the edge of the bed, sit-to-stand transitions, and stair climbing.
• Precautions:
○ Breath holding is common during bridging activities; this may present problems for the patient with hypertension and cardiac disability and should be closely monitored. Patients should be encouraged to breathe rhythmically during all bridging activities.
○ Elevating the hips higher than the head (the head-down position in bridging) may be contraindicated for patients with uncontrolled hypertension or elevated intracranial pressures (for example, the patient with acute traumatic brain injury).
• Abnormal reflex activity may interfere with assumption or maintenance of the bridging posture (as in hooklying).
• Bridging promotes selective control (hip extension with knee flexion) and may be indicated for patients recovering from stroke who demonstrate influence of the mass movement synergies (when hip and knee extension are firmly linked together with hip adduction and ankle plantarflexion).
• Initially the patient can be allowed to stabilize the upper trunk by extending and abducting the upper extremities (UEs) on the mat. Reducing this stabilization can increase difficulty; the UEs can be gradually adducted and brought closer to the trunk, flexed across the chest, or the hands can be clasped together in a prayer position.

Bridging: Therapeutic Activities/Techniques

Position/Activity: Bridging, Pelvic Elevation

The patient is supine with the hips and knees flexed and the feet flat on the mat (in hooklying position). The therapist instructs the patient to raise the hips from the mat until the hips are fully extended and the pelvis is elevated and level. The patient then lowers the pelvis down to the mat slowly, rather than "plopping" or collapsing down.

The therapist can facilitate pelvic elevation by placing both hands on the patient's lower thighs and pushing down on the knees, pulling the distal thighs toward the feet. Tapping over the gluteus maximus can also be used to stimulate muscle contraction.

Patients with a unilateral weakness of the gluteal muscles (for example, the patient who is recovering from a hip fracture) will not be able to hold the pelvis level—the pelvis will drop down on the weaker side. The therapist can hold a wand across the pelvis to demonstrate this problem visually to the patient. As control increases, difficulty can be increased by progressing from bilateral to unilateral LE support.

TECHNIQUES

Slow Reversals

The therapist is half-kneeling at the side of the patient. The hips are assisted up and down for a few repetitions to ensure the patient knows the movements expected. The movements are then lightly resisted. The therapist alternates hand placement, first on

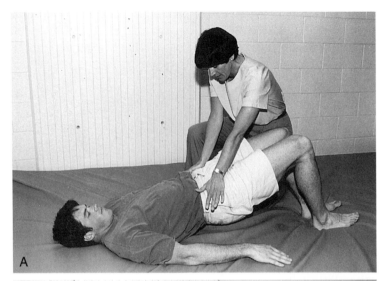

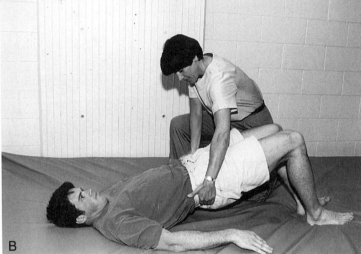

Figure 9–6A and B. Bridging: pelvic elevation—slow reversals.

the top of the pelvis to resist the hips as they rise up, then on the buttocks to give a directional cue for the return (SR) to the mat. Resistance is minimal in the return motion (Fig. 9–6A and B). Smooth motions of opposing muscle groups (reversals of antagonists) are facilitated by well-timed verbal commands ("Push up" or "Pull down").

Slow Reversal-Hold

A hold (SRH) may be added in the direction of pelvic elevation if difficulty is experienced in maintaining the contraction in the shortened range. The hold is a momentary pause (held for one count); the antagonist contraction is then facilitated.

Agonist Reversals

Agonist reversals (ARs) provide resistance to the lower back and hip extensors during both concentric (shortening) contractions and eccentric (lengthening) contractions. This is an important lead-up activity for the patient with poor eccentric control who has difficulty sitting down slowly.

The therapist is half-kneeling at the patient's side with both hands positioned on the anterior pelvis during the elevation and lowering phases of bridging (Fig. 9–7). **Verbal commands** for ARs include "Push up" and "Now go down slowly."

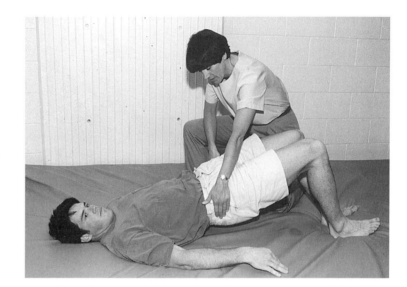

Figure 9–7. Bridging: pelvic elevation—agonist reversals.

Motor control goal. Controlled mobility.

Indications. Weakness of the low-back extensors, gluteals, and hamstring muscles. Bridging helps break up mass movement synergies by combining hip extension with knee flexion (for example, in the patient recovering from stroke). These activities are important lead-up skills for sit-to-stand and stand-to-sit transfers, and for ambulation up and down stairs.

Functional outcomes. The patient performs independent bed-mat mobility.

Position/Activity: Bridging, Holding

Maintenance of the bridge position can be difficult for many patients. Partial-range control may need to be established before full-range control is achieved. It is important for the patient to avoid breath holding during all isometric work and bridging activities.

TECHNIQUES

Alternating Isometrics
In alternating isometrics (AI), the patient is asked to hold the bridge position while medial/lateral resistance is applied to the pelvis, first on one side pushing the pelvis away from the therapist, then pulling the pelvis toward the therapist. The resistance is built up gradually from very light resistance to the patient's maximum. The isometric contraction is maintained for several counts. The therapist must give a transitional command ("Now don't let me pull you the other way") before sliding the hands to resist the opposite muscles; this allows the patient the opportunity to make appropriate preparatory postural adjustments.

Resistance can also be applied at the pelvis in anterior/posterior directions or diagonally. Resistance applied at the knees increases the length of the lever and recruits more lower-limb muscles, especially foot and ankle muscles. The position of the therapist will vary according to the line of force required.

Theraband tubing placed around the distal thighs increases the proprioceptive loading and contraction of the lateral hip muscles (gluteus medius). Thus, simultaneous contraction of gluteal muscles (maximus and medius) is achieved.

Rhythmic Stabilization
The patient is asked to hold the bridge position while the therapist applies rotational resistance to the pelvis. One hand is placed on the posterior pelvis on one side, pulling up at

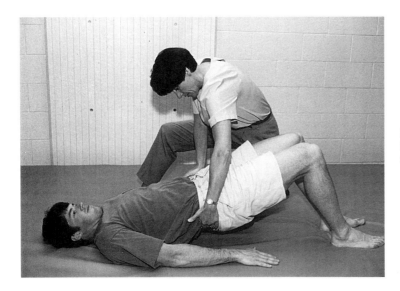

Figure 9–8. Bridging: holding—rhythmic stabilization.

the hip while the other hand is on the opposite side, pushing down on the anterior pelvis (Fig. 9–8). **Verbal commands** for rhythmic stabilization (RS) include "Don't let me twist you; now don't let me twist you the other way."

Motor control goal. Stability.

Indications. Weakness of the low-back extensors, gluteals, and hamstring muscles; instability of the pelvis at midstance (a Trendelenburg gait pattern). These activities are important lead-up skills for stabilization needed during upright antigravity activities (kneeling, standing, bipedal gait).

Functional outcomes. The patient is able to the stabilize the lower trunk, pelvis, and hip during bed-mat activities.

Position/Activity: Bridging, Weight Shifting

The patient actively shifts the pelvis from side to side (in medial/lateral shifts). Small-range shifts are stressed and can be an important lead-up activity for the pelvic lateral control required for gait.

Bridge and Place
The patient is instructed to move up into the bridge position, shift the pelvis laterally to one side, and lower the pelvis down to the new side position. The therapist manually assists the lateral motion for the first few repetitions; tactile cueing (tapping on the side of the pelvis) and verbal cueing are used to assist the patient (Fig. 9–9A and B).

Motor control goal. Controlled mobility.

Indications. Bridge and place is a valuable treatment activity for the patient in the early stages of recovery from stroke. Movement of the pelvis toward the sound side stretches and elongates the upper trunk on the affected side. This counteracts a common problem of shortening of the trunk side flexors on the stroke side. The hands can be clasped together with the elbows extended in a prayer position to counteract the common flexor and adductor posturing of the UEs (see Fig. 9–9).

Functional outcomes. The patient is independent in bed-mat mobility (scooting side to side and scooting to the edge of the bed prior to sitting up).

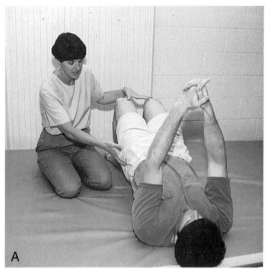

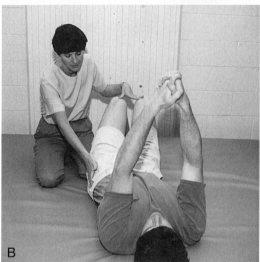

Figure 9–9A and B. Bridge and place to left side—active movements.

TECHNIQUES

Slow Reversals
The therapist is kneeling at the side of the patient. The movement of the hips is assisted for a few repetitions to ensure that the patient knows the movements expected. Side-to-side movements are then lightly resisted. The therapist alternates hand placement, first on one side of the pelvis resisting the pelvis as it pulls away, then on the opposite side as the pelvis pushes back. Smooth reversals of antagonists are facilitated by well-timed **verbal commands** ("Pull away" or "Push back"). Manual contacts at the knees increase the length of the lever and recruit medial and lateral ankle and foot muscles to shift the body from side to side.

Motor control goal. Controlled mobility.

Indications. Weakness of the low-back extensors and gluteals, the hamstring muscles, and the foot/ankle invertors and evertors; instability of the pelvis at midstance (Trendelenburg gait); and instability of medial/lateral foot/ankle muscles. This is an important lead-up activity to upright stance and balance training for patients recovering from ankle injury.

Functional outcomes. Patient ambulates independently with normal control of pelvic excursion and LE control.

Position/Activity: Bridging, Advanced Stabilization Activities

Bridging, Leg Lifts

The patient is asked to lift one leg up while maintaining the bridge position using single-limb support. Lifts can include knee extension (Fig. 9–10) or marching in place (hip and knee flexion). The patient is asked to alternate limbs, lifting first one leg, then the other. Patients with instability will demonstrate a pelvic drop on the side of the dynamic, non-weight-bearing limb. A wand can be placed across the pelvis to provide a visual reminder to keep the pelvis level.

Movements can be assisted with tactile or verbal cueing. UE stabilization (arms abducted and extended with hands on mat) is essential during initial training; as control progresses, difficulty can be increased by reducing the UE support (by increasing shoulder adduction or crossing the UEs over the chest or holding the hands in a prayer position). The speed and range of movements can be varied to increase the difficulty of the activities. Patients can work up to marching, then running in place or running side to side.

Bridging Using a Swiss Ball

A medium-size Swiss ball can be placed under the patient's legs. The patient is then instructed to elevate the pelvis, extending the hips while keeping the knees straight and the legs on the ball (Fig. 9–11). This activity significantly increases the postural challenge of pelvic elevation because the base of support is not fixed. The patient must stabilize the legs on the ball and maintain the ball position in addition to elevating the pelvis. The more distally the ball is placed under the legs, the more difficult the activity. The hamstrings participate more fully in stabilization with the legs extended. UE stabilization (with hands on mat) should be encouraged initially and reduced as control increases.

Sit-to-Bridge Transitions Using a Swiss Ball

A more difficult variation involves sit-to-bridge transitions on the ball. The patient begins by sitting on an appropriately sized ball. The hips and knees should be flexed to 90 degrees. The patient is instructed to walk both feet away from the ball. The ball will roll under the trunk until the head and shoulders are resting on the ball (Fig. 9–12A and B). The patient is instructed to maintain the hips in the fully extended bridge position with the

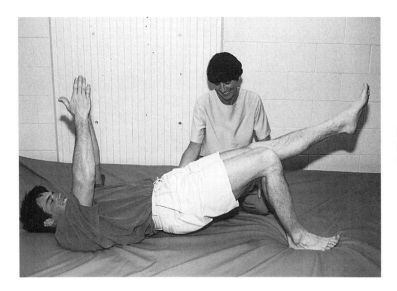

Figure 9–10. Bridging: leg lifts—active movements.

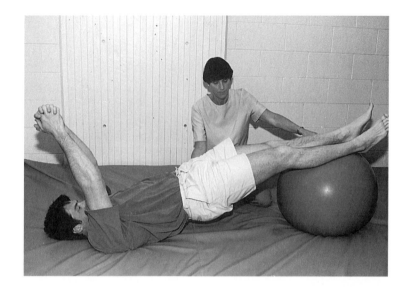

Figure 9–11. Bridging using a Swiss ball—active movements.

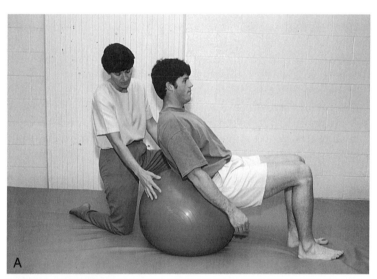

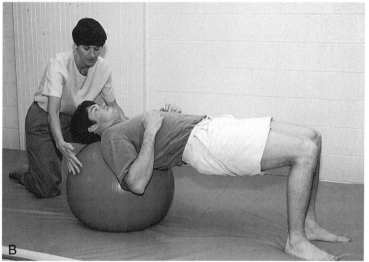

Figure 9–12*A* **and** *B*. Sitting-to-bridging transitions using a Swiss ball—active movements.

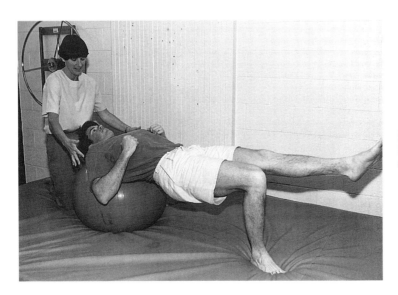

Figure 9–13. Bridging using a Swiss ball: leg lifts—active movements.

pelvis level. Initially, hand touch-down support may be necessary; as control develops, hand contact is removed. The UEs can be hooked on the ball (elbows flexed with shoulders extended and arms adducted around ball) at first; then the patient can progress to the more difficult prayer position.

Static-dynamic challenges to postural control while bridging on the ball provide the highest level of difficulty and should be reserved for late-stage rehabilitation. These challenges can include lifting one lower limb (the dynamic limb can move in hip flexion or knee extension) while the static limb stabilizes the body and maintains the bridge position (Fig. 9–13). Alternate LE lifts (stepping) can then be performed. An additional activity that can be attempted while maintaining a single-limb bridge position on the ball is writing alphabet letters with the foot of the dynamic limb.

Motor control goal. Controlled mobility, static-dynamic control.

Indications. Bridging is advanced postural control work for the lower trunk/pelvis and LEs; it stimulates proprioceptive responses necessary for stabilization and balance.

Functional outcomes. The patient stabilizes the pelvis/hip during upright antigravity activities (kneeling, standing, gait).

Sitting Activities

SITTING

General Characteristics

- The base of support (BOS) in sitting is moderate.
- The center of mass (COM) is higher than in supine or prone positions.
- This posture is relatively stable.
- Sitting involves the head, trunk, and lower extremity (LE) muscles for upright postural control. The extensor muscles of the pelvis and lumbar spine are the primary muscles for antigravity control.
- The head and trunk are maintained on the vertical in midline orientation (upright sitting). Deficits in postural alignment may include a forward head position or a rounded thoracic spine with absent lumbar curve (slumped sitting).
- The pelvis is maintained in midline orientation:
  - Excessive posterior tilting results in extension of the hips, flattening or reversal of the lumbar curve, and sacral sitting.
  - Excessive anterior tilting results in increased lateral rotation and abduction of the hips.
- Effects of tonic reflex activity are minimal if the head is maintained in a neutral position.
- Righting reactions contribute to upright head position (face vertical, mouth horizontal).
- Static postural control is necessary for maintenance of upright posture. Dynamic postural control is necessary for movements in the posture (for example, weight shifting or reaching).
- Reactive balance control is needed for adjustments in responses to changes in COM (perturbation) or changes in the support surface (tilting).
- Anticipatory balance control is needed for preparatory postural adjustments that accompany voluntary movements.

Treatment Strategies and Considerations

- BOS can be varied to alter postural stabilization requirements and difficulty. For example, greater challenges can be incorporated into sitting activities by progressing from:
  - long-sitting to short-sitting
  - bilateral upper extremity (UE) support to single UE support to no UE support
  - feet flat on floor to no floor contact using a high seat or plinth
  - feet flat on a stationary surface to feet on a roller or small ball
  - stationary sitting on a fixed support surface to sitting on an equilibrium board or Swiss ball
- The type of chair used in supported sitting can influence postural alignment:
  - A firm chair (dining room chair) promotes upright alignment.
  - A soft, low chair (upholstered living room chair) or a chair with a seat that is too deep (for example, an improperly fitting wheelchair) encourages slumped sitting (sacral sitting).

○ Firm support for the UEs using a table top or lap tray allows some of the weight to be taken on the upper limbs and increases the overall BOS. Requirements for postural stability are reduced.
- A mirror can be used to assist the patient in perceptual awareness of a symmetrical and vertical sitting posture. Training with mirrors is contraindicated for patients with visual-perceptual spatial deficits such as vertical disorientation or position-in-space deficits.
- Therapist position and level of support for unsupported sitting can vary with the patient's level of control and anxiety.
  ○ A patient with poor sitting control and high anxiety may benefit from having the therapist positioned in front of the patient. This position blocks the patient's vision of the floor and reduces the patient's anxiety about falling forward.
  ○ An anterior sitting position will also allow the therapist to lock his or her knees around the outside of the patient's knees and firmly grasp them. This reduces anxiety and assists the patient by extending the BOS.
  ○ As sitting control progresses, the therapist's position can be varied (to the side or behind) and support reduced.

Movement Transitions: Supine-to-Sit Transfers

Variations in the method used are based on the patient's medical status and functional impairments.

Transitions from Supine to Sidelying to Sitting
From the supine position the patient rolls onto the side (see rolling sequence, supine to sidelying). The hips and knees are flexed and the legs are moved off the bed or mat. The pelvis acts as a fulcrum with the legs as counterweights as they are lowered off the bed or mat to rotate the patient up into sitting position. The patient simultaneously uses both UEs to push up into sitting position.

The therapist can assist the initial rolling sequence into the sidelying position, the lowering of the legs off the mat or bed, or the lifting of the upper trunk. This method is frequently used for the patient with low back pain when trunk rotation is contraindicated due to pain.

Transitions from Supine to Sidelying-on-Elbow to Sitting
From the supine position the patient rotates the head and upper trunk up and rolls onto the flexed elbow of the upper limb nearest the edge of the mat or bed (see rolling sequence, onto sidelying-on-elbow). Once the patient is in the sidelying-on-elbow position with the knees flexed and the legs moved off the mat or bed, the patient pushes up into sitting using both UEs. Individuals with increased control can move from lying to sitting in one smooth motion without using the UEs to push up.

The therapist can assist movement into the sidelying-on-elbow position by holding onto the sides of the patient's trunk and rotating and lifting the upper trunk (Fig. 10–1*A* and *B*). The therapist can also assist the patient by pulling down on the iliac crest, providing an anchoring point for the trunk side flexors. If the patient requires additional assistance the therapist's opposite hand can be placed on the side of the upper trunk on the weight-bearing side to lift the patient into sitting position. Speed influences the amount of effort required: the slower the movement, the greater the effort.

Motor control goals. Mobility (active-assistive movements), progressing to controlled mobility (active movements).

Indications. This is a useful functional activity for the patient recovering from stroke. Rolling onto the hemiplegic side enhances functional recovery and use of the involved extremities. This activity requires the patient to use head and upper trunk rotation and look toward the hemiplegic side (often a problem in patients with unilateral neglect). It also elongates the trunk side flexors (shortening of the trunk side flexors is a common prob-

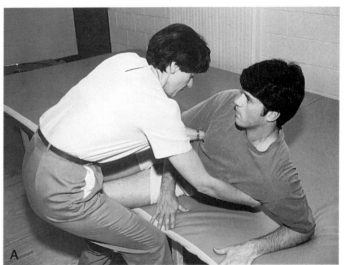

Figure 10–1A and B. Transitions: supine to sidelying-on-elbow to sitting—active-assistive movement.

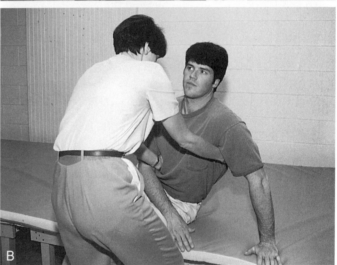

lem). Finally, weight bearing on the affected elbow and extended UE provides joint compression and proprioceptive stimulation and is useful for problems of shoulder instability and subluxation.

Functional outcomes. The patient is able to independently perform supine-to-sit transfers, an important element of independent bed mobility.

Transitions from Supine to Long-sitting Position

From the supine position the patient flexes the head and upper trunk, coming up into the supine-on-elbows position. The patient then rotates to one side, unweighting the opposite UE, and moves the opposite shoulder back into extension and abduction with elbow extension and weight bearing on the hand. This motion is repeated to the other side. The patient then walks up into long-sitting using extended UEs for support.

The therapist can assist the initial head and upper trunk flexion, or the rotation movements to the side. A trapeze bar can also be used to assist the patient with generalized trunk weakness. The patient pulls up into the long-sitting position primarily using the elbow flexors.

Motor control goals. Mobility (active-assistive movements) progressing to controlled mobility (active movements).

Indications. This is a useful functional activity for the patient with quadriplegia. Patients with innervated triceps (C7 and below) will have an easier time than patients with no triceps function who have to use shoulder movements (extension, abduction, external rotation) to position the UEs behind the trunk and lock the elbows for weight bearing. These activities are important lead-up skills for independent bed mobility, dressing in bed, and transfers.

Functional outcomes. The patient is able to perform supine-to-sit transfers independently.

Sitting: Therapeutic Activities/Techniques

Position/Activity: Sitting, Holding

The patient is sitting with the head and trunk vertical, both hips and knees flexed to 90 degrees, and the feet flat on the floor. Posture is symmetrical with equal weight bearing over both LEs. The patient's UEs can be used for support (shoulder and elbows extended with the hands at the side) or the UEs can rest on the LEs.

If additional support is needed during early sitting, the therapist can sit behind the patient on a Swiss ball. The ball is used to support the lumbar spine and maintain the lumbar curve. The patient's arms rest on the therapist's knees for support.

Sitting, Holding with Weight Bearing on an Extended UE
The UE is positioned in shoulder and elbow extension, external rotation with the hand open and flat on the support surface (Fig. 10–2). This is a useful position to counteract UE flexor-adductor spasticity (for example, in the patient recovering from stroke or traumatic brain injury).

Rhythmic rotation (RRo) may be required to move the UE into the extended position initially. Additional stimulation (tapping or stroking) over the triceps and deltoid can be used to assist the patient in maintaining the extended position. The dorsum of the hand can also be stroked to keep the hand open with the fingers extended.

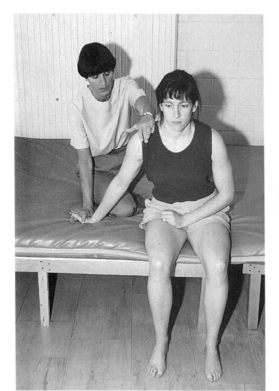

Figure 10–2. Sitting: holding with weight bearing on an extended arm—active-assistive movement.

The patient with shoulder instability (for example, the patient recovering from stroke who has a flaccid, subluxed shoulder) also benefits from weight bearing and compression through an extended UE. The proprioceptive loading that occurs increases the action of stabilizing muscles around the shoulder. The therapist can add additional stimulation by lightly compressing the top of the shoulder downward while stabilizing the elbow as needed. (See discussion of prone progression, UE weight bearing.)

The patient with elbow instability (for example, the patient with C6 quadriplegia who has no triceps function) can be assisted to maintain an extended position using external rotation and extension of the shoulder, locking the elbow into extension. It is important to remember that this patient will need to keep the fingers flexed (interphalangeal flexion) during weight bearing in order to allow for the development of effective tenodesis grasp.

Sitting, Holding in Long-sitting Position

Long-sitting is an important posture for developing initial sitting control in patients with spinal cord lesions. Initially, the hands are positioned behind the patient to maximize the BOS. As control develops the position of the hands can be varied by placing them in front and finally at the sides of the hips. Sitting training then progresses to short-sitting activities, with the knees flexed over the side of a mat. Adequate range of the hamstrings (90 to 110 degrees) is essential to prevent sacral sitting.

Sitting, Holding in Side-sitting Position

In the side-sitting position, the patient sits on one hip with the LEs flexed and tucked to the opposite side. Since this posture elongates the trunk on the weight-bearing side, this is a useful activity for the patient recovering from stroke because it provides inhibition to spastic lateral trunk muscles. The affected UE can be extended and weight bearing or both UEs can be held in front in a prayer position with hands clasped.

TECHNIQUES

Sitting, Holding in Modified Pivot Prone Position (Shortened Held Resisted Contraction)

The patient is sitting on the edge of a mat. The therapist is sitting on a Swiss ball behind the patient. The ball is used to support the patient's lumbar spine and maintain the lumbar curve. The patient's UEs are supported on the therapist's knees; the shoulders are extended, abducted, and externally rotated and the elbows are flexed, a modified pivot prone position.

This is a good initial posture to work on head control in patients with decreased head control. In modified pivot prone position gravity is minimized, as opposed to prone-on-elbows position, where maximum influences of gravity are acting on the head. If needed, the therapist can support the head under the chin and assist it into the extended position. A hold (SHRC) is then asked for; additional proprioceptive stimulation can be provided by gently resisting head extension with the other hand on the back of the head (occiput). As control increases, assistance is gradually removed and the patient actively holds the head up. This is an important lead-up activity for prone-on-elbows stabilization activities for the head and neck.

Upper extremity (UE) and upper trunk extensors can be additionally recruited by resisting first at the posterior shoulder, then on the UEs (posterior elbows, or more distally at the dorsum of the wrists). The therapist's hands are moved progressively from head to trunk to UEs to recruit muscles needed to hold in this posture. Extension throughout the head and upper trunk is facilitated. As control improves, the therapist can remove knee support from the patient's UEs and ball support from the lumbar spine by rolling the ball back and away from the patient (Fig. 10–3).

Light approximation (joint compression) through the head and spine can be used to stimulate postural stabilizers; the therapist clasps both hands together on top of the patient's head and gently compresses downward. Approximation is contraindicated in

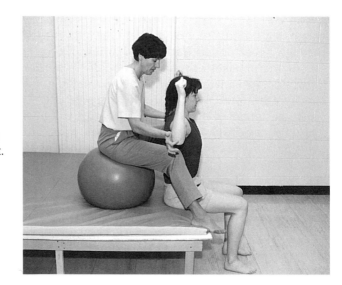

Figure 10–3. Sitting: holding in modified pivot prone position—resisted movement.

patients with spinal deformity or an inability to assume an upright position (for example, the patient with osteoporosis and kyphosis) and in patients with acute pain (for example, disc pathology or arthritis).

Alternating Isometrics

In alternating isometrics (AI), the patient is asked to hold the sitting position while the therapist applies medial/lateral (M/L) resistance to the upper trunk, first on one side pushing the upper trunk away from the therapist, then pulling the upper trunk toward the therapist. Manual contacts are on the lateral aspect of one side of the trunk and the medial portion (vertebral border of the scapula) of the other side; the hands are then reversed. The resistance is built up gradually, starting from very light resistance and progressing to the patient's maximum. The isometric contraction is maintained for several counts.

The therapist must give a transitional command ("Now don't let me pull you the other way") before sliding the hands to resist the opposite muscles. This allows the patient the opportunity to make appropriate preparatory postural adjustments. Resistance can also be applied in anterior/posterior (A/P) directions or diagonally. The position of the therapist will vary according to the line of force that needs to be applied.

Rhythmic Stabilization

In rhythmic stabilization (RS), the patient is asked to hold the sitting position while the therapist applies rotational resistance to the upper trunk. One hand is placed on the posterior trunk of one side (axillary border of the scapula) pushing forward while the other hand is on the opposite side, anterior upper trunk, pulling back (Fig. 10–4). The therapist's hands are then reversed for the opposite movement (each hand remains positioned on the same side of the trunk). **Verbal commands** for RS include "Don't let me twist you, now don't let me twist you the other way."

Motor control goal. Stability, static postural control.

Indications. Instability of the head, upper trunk, shoulder girdle, and upper extremity; impaired static balance control. These activities are important lead-up skills for many activities of daily living (dressing, grooming, toileting, and feeding) as well as later transfer training.

Functional outcomes. The patient is able to maintain sitting position independently.

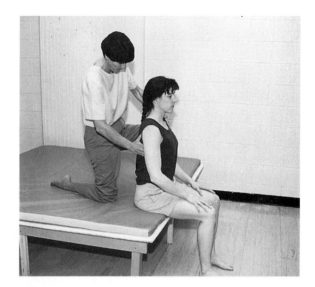

Figure 10–4. Sitting: holding—rhythmic stabilization.

Position/Activity: Sitting, Weight Shifting

The patient is encouraged to shift weight from side to side, forward and backward and diagonally. Re-education of limits of stability (LOS) is one of the first activities in a balance training sequence. The patient is encouraged to shift as far as possible without losing balance and then to return to the midline position. Initially, weight shifts may begin with bilateral or unilateral UE support and progress to no UE support (UEs crossed or cradled).

Active reaching activities can be used to promote weight shifting in all directions, or in the direction of an instability (for example, in the patient with hemiplegia). The therapist can provide a target ("reach out and touch my hand"); a functional task like cone stacking can also be used to promote reaching in any direction. The patient can be instructed to reach down and touch the floor or pick up objects from the floor.

Sitting and crossing one lower limb over the other requires an initial weight shift to unweight and free up the dynamic limb for movement. The therapist can facilitate the action of crossing one limb over the other by appropriate verbal cues (ensuring the initial weight shift) and by manual cues or guided movement of the dynamic limb. This is a useful activity for the patient with stroke, since crossing the affected leg over the sound limb represents out-of-synergy, isolated control.

Sitting, Weight Shifts with Extended Arm Support

Patients with excess UE flexor tone (for example, the patient with stroke or traumatic brain injury) may benefit from weight shifting forward and back with the elbow extended and the hand weight bearing. The rocking provides slow vestibular stimulation and additional inhibition to the spastic muscles. Rhythmic rotation, inhibitory positioning, and stroking to antagonist muscles also provide inhibitory influences.

Sitting, Weight Shifts with a Large Ball

The patient is sitting with both UEs forward, elbows extended, and hands resting on a large ball. The patient is instructed to move the ball slowly forward and backward and side to side (Fig. 10–5). Initially, the therapist can stand on the opposite side of the ball to assist in controlling range and speed of movements.

This activity has a number of benefits. The ball can provide UE support and inhibitory positioning for the patient with a spastic UE. It also reduces anxiety that may occur with weight shifting, since the patient does not feel threatened with falling forward to the floor. Movements can be easily assisted using the ball. Rocking activities that involve moving the ball forward and backward in sitting can be used to promote shoulder ROM in unsuspecting patients who may be otherwise anxious about passive range of motion (PROM).

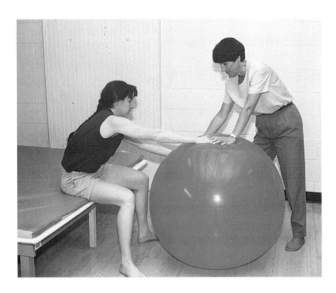

Figure 10–5. Sitting: weight shifts, hands moving a large Swiss ball—active-assistive movements.

Sitting, Weight Shifts with Upper Trunk Rotation

Upper trunk rotation (UTR) with flexion or extension is a difficult movement combination for many patients (for example, the patient with Parkinson's disease who has difficulty with all rotation activities). Holding the UEs in a cradled position, the patient is instructed to bend down with a twist, bringing the shoulder toward the opposite knee, then lift back up and twist. The patient should be instructed to turn the head to follow the movement. The therapist is positioned diagonally in front of the patient to either assist or resist the movements (Fig. 10–6).

TECHNIQUES

Slow Reversals

The patient is moved passively from side to side (in medial/lateral shifts) for a few repetitions to ensure the patient knows the movements expected. The movements are then lightly resisted.

The therapist alternates hand placement, first on one side to resist the upper body pulling away, then on the other side to resist the return movement. Manual contacts are

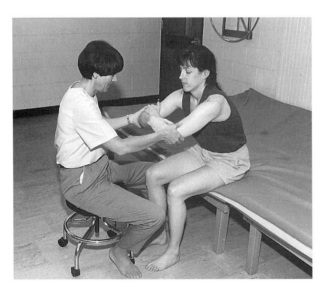

Figure 10–6. Sitting: weight shifts with upper trunk rotation—active-assistive movements.

on the trunk to effectively resist the trunk muscles, not on the lateral shoulders. Typically one hand is on the side of the trunk and the other hand is on the vertebral border of the scapula. The hands are then reversed to the opposite side of trunk and opposite scapula for the return movement (SR). Smooth reversals of antagonists are facilitated by well-timed verbal commands ("Pull away" or "Push back") and a quick stretch to initiate the reverse movement.

Progression is from partial-range to full-range control. Shifts may be resisted in all directions: medial/lateral, anterior/posterior, diagonal, and diagonal with rotation.

Slow Reversal-Hold
A hold (SRH) may be added in one or both directions if the patient demonstrates difficulty in maintaining the contraction into the shortened range. The hold is a momentary pause (held for one count); the antagonist contraction is then facilitated.

Motor control goal.   Controlled mobility, dynamic postural control.

Indications.   Impaired dynamic balance control, instability of the upper trunk with movement.

Functional outcomes.   The patient is able to perform weight shifts, pressure relief, and transfers.

Position/Activity: Sitting, PNF Patterns

PNF patterns can be used to provide a dynamic challenge to postural control and stabilization. The patient can be instructed to actively move in the pattern(s) or the pattern(s) can be resisted. Resistance can be manual, or the patient can use free weights, Theraband tubing, or pulleys that are appropriately positioned.

The benefits of using PNF patterns are many. They promote muscle activity in naturally occurring synergistic combinations. They encourage diagonal and rotational movements and represent advanced control work for many patients. They also promote crossing the midline, an important activity for patients with unilateral neglect of one side (for example, the patient with stroke). The patient's full attention is focused on the correct limb movements and not on the movements of the trunk. Therefore, the PNF pattern assists in promoting automatic postural control of the head and trunk.

The therapist chooses which pattern(s) to use based on the patient's level of control. Unilateral patterns are often used initially when patients are unfamiliar with PNF patterns, or when one extremity is needed for weight bearing and support. As control develops, the therapist can progress to the more difficult bilateral or upper trunk patterns. UE D2 patterns are contraindicated for patients recovering from stroke who are firmly locked into abnormal synergies.

PNF UNILATERAL UE D1 PATTERNS

D1F, Flexion-Adduction-External Rotation
The hand of the dynamic limb is positioned near the side of the ipsilateral hip with hand open and thumb facing down. The patient is instructed to close the hand, turn, and pull the hand up and across the face (Fig. 10–7A and B).

D1E, Extension-Abduction-Internal Rotation
The patient opens the hand, turns, and pushes the hand down and out to the side.

PNF UNILATERAL UE D2 PATTERNS

D2F, Flexion-Abduction-External Rotation
The hand of the dynamic limb is positioned across the body on the opposite hip with hand closed and thumb facing down. The patient is instructed to open the hand, turn, and lift the hand up and out.

Position/Activity: Sitting, Scooting

Scooting, in the Long-sitting Position

The patient is in long-sitting position with the hands held off the mat. Clasping the hands together in a prayer position and holding them straight ahead can help restrict upper trunk movements and isolate the motion to the lower trunk and pelvis. The patient is instructed to weight-shift over onto one hip and, using a forward pelvic thrust, to move the opposite hip forward. The sequence is then repeated to the other side and the body is advanced forward in small increments (Fig. 10–12).

Initially the therapist is positioned at the patient's feet and holds both feet off the mat. This reduces friction effects of the mat on the LEs and allows for easy forward progression. The movements can also be reversed by instructing the patient to move backward.

This is a useful activity for patients who lack lower trunk and pelvic control (for example, the patient recovering from stroke who has a retracted and fixed pelvis). Scooting is also a functional activity for patients with spinal cord lesions and can be a useful lead-up activity to a reciprocal gait pattern. Adequate range of the hamstrings (90 to 110 degrees) is essential to prevent sacral sitting.

Scooting, in the Short-sitting Position

The patient is sitting on a mat, with both feet flat on the floor. The patient is instructed to weight-shift onto one hip and, using a forward pelvic thrust, to move the opposite hip forward. The sequence is then repeated to the other side and the body scoots forward to the edge of the seat (Fig. 10–13).

The therapist assists the motion by lifting and unweighting the thigh to allow for easy forward movement. Scooting in the short-sitting position is an important lead-up activity for sit-to-stand transitions, which require that the patient must initially come forward to the edge of the chair before standing up.

Scooting, onto and off a High Plinth

The patient is sitting on a high plinth with both feet off the floor. The patient is instructed to weight-shift onto one hip and move the opposite hip forward. The sequence is then repeated to the other side until the patient reaches the edge of the plinth. The patient then extends one LE and places that foot on the floor, keeping the other LE flexed and on the plinthe (Fig. 10–14).

Scooting onto and off of a high plinth promotes lower trunk and pelvic control. It also challenges the patient to come down into weight bearing on one limb before the other (uni-

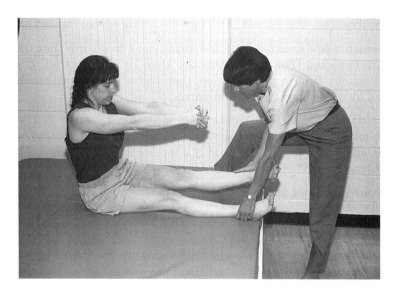

Figure 10–12. Long-sitting: scooting—active-assistive movements.

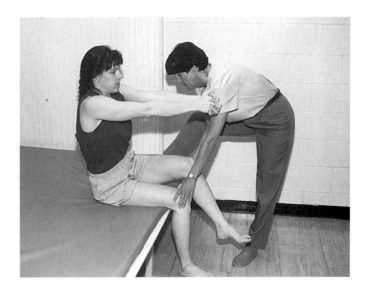

Figure 10–13. Short-sitting: scooting—active-assistive movements.

lateral weight bearing). This is a useful activity for patients who do not demonstrate symmetrical weight bearing in standing position (for example, the patient recovering from stroke who favors the sound side). Because one hip is still on the plinth while the opposite hip and knee are extended, it provides a partial weight-bearing situation and is a good initial training activity. The height of the plinth is important to facilitate proper standing (an adjustable-height treatment table is ideal for this activity).

Motor control goals. Controlled mobility, static-dynamic control.

Indications. Impaired dynamic balance control; impaired control of the lower trunk and LE. Scooting is an important lead-up activity for sit-to-stand transfers and bipedal gait.

Functional outcomes. The patient is able to perform weight shifts and transfers independently.

Figure 10–14. Sitting: scooting off and on a high plinth—active-assistive movements.

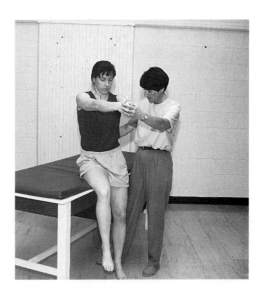

Position/Activity: Sitting, Balance Activities

Balance training begins with static holding (static postural control) and progresses to weight-shifting or reaching activities in all directions (dynamic postural control). The range and speed of the movements can be increased to increase the challenge to postural control.

Additional activities that can be used to challenge anticipatory balance control in sitting position include look-arounds (trunk and head rotation); pushing a large Swiss ball forward and backward and side to side; passing, catching, and throwing a ball (increasing the weight of the ball or decreasing its size increases the challenge); supine-to-sitting/sitting-to-supine transfers; and bending forward and touching the floor, or picking up objects off floor.

Activities that can be used to challenge reactive balance control include manual perturbances (disturbances of the patient's center of mass) in sitting and sitting on an equilibrium board (disturbances of the patient's base of support).

Sitting, Manual Perturbations

The patient is sitting on a stationary surface (mat) with the feet flat on the floor. The therapist provides a displacing force (manual perturbation) to the trunk. Varied, asymmetrical manual contacts (such as tapping the patient out of position) should be used. It is important to ensure appropriate compensatory responses. With backward displacements, hip and trunk flexor activity is required. With forward displacements, hip and trunk extensor activity is required. Lateral displacements (twisting and displacing the trunk) are also important to include and may provide the most difficult challenges for many patients. Protective extension reactions can be initiated with the UEs if the displacements move the center of mass (COM) near the limits of stability or outside of the base of support. If patient responses are lacking, the therapist may need to guide the initial attempts either verbally or manually. The patient can then progress to active movements.

Perturbations should be appropriate for the patient's range and speed of control. It is important to use gentle disturbances; violent perturbations (pushes or shoves) are not necessary to stimulate balance responses. The therapist can vary the base of support (BOS) to increase or decrease difficulty. For example, the patient's feet can be in contact with the floor, or without contact (sitting on a high plinth). The feet can also be positioned apart, together, or LEs can be crossed.

Sitting on an Equilibrium Board, Balance Training

Activities on equilibrium boards (wobble boards) can be used to disturb the patient's base of support. The boards are constructed to allow varying motion; the type and amount of motion is determined by the design of the board: A curved-bottom board allows motion in two directions; a dome-bottom board allows motion in all directions. The degree of curve or size of the dome determines the amount of motion in any direction; motion is increased in boards with large curves or high domes. Selection of the type of board used is dependent upon the patient's dynamic balance control and the type and range of movements permitted.

The patient is sitting on the equilibrium board with the feet flat on the floor. Initial activities include having the patient maintain a balanced (centered) sitting position (Fig. 10–15). The patient can then progress to active weight shifts, tilting the board in varying directions to stimulate balance responses. These patient-initiated challenges stimulate balance using both feed-forward (anticipatory) and feedback-driven adjustments—and reactive balance control.

The therapist can also manually tilt the board to stimulate balance responses (evoking feedback-driven responses). The therapist varies the speed and range of displacements depending on the control exhibited by the patient. The direction of the displacements should

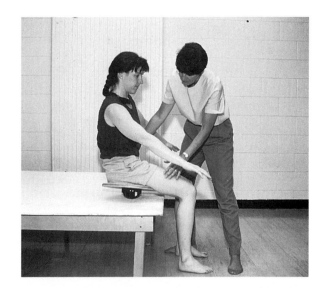

Figure 10–15. Sitting: balancing on a balance board—active-assistive movements.

be varied and unpredictable. It is important to observe the patient's responses carefully and use appropriate safety precautions.

Sitting, Swiss Ball Activities

Activities performed while sitting on a Swiss ball are useful for patients with impaired balance control. Sitting on the ball facilitates intrinsic feedback using visual, proprioceptive, and vestibular inputs; it also challenges CNS sensory integration mechanisms. The use of the ball adds novelty to rehabilitation programs and can be adapted to group classes.

Sitting, Holding

Initially, the patient is assisted into sitting on a Swiss ball by placing the ball directly in front of the patient, who is sitting on a platform mat. The patient scoots forward and sits on the ball. Hips and knees are flexed to 90 degrees with the knees aligned directly over the feet. The therapist sits directly behind the patient on the mat with one knee on either side of the ball, providing lateral support and stabilization to the ball (Fig. 10–16).

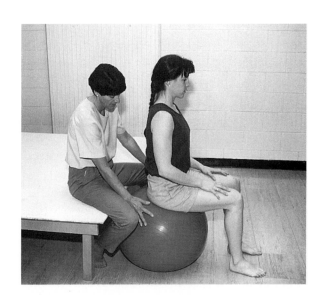

Figure 10–16. Sitting on a Swiss ball: holding—active-assistive movements.

The patient is instructed to maintain a steady position and not let the ball roll in any direction. Sitting off to one side will result in instability and movement of the ball. Approximation can be easily given during this activity by having the patient sit and gently bounce up and down. An immediate and automatic improvement in posture (that is, the patient sits up straight) can be expected with this stimulation.

Static control work on the ball should only be attempted after static control is achieved on a stationary surface (the patient should be able to hold steady while sitting on a mat).

Sitting on a Swiss Ball, Pelvic Shifts

The patient sits on the Swiss ball and shifts the hips forward and backward in anterior/posterior pelvic tilts, or from side to side in medial/lateral shifts (Fig. 10–17). The patient is instructed to roll the ball using his or her hips in the desired direction. The patient starts out with small-range shifts and progresses to larger ranges. The patient can then progress to rotating the hips around in a full circle (pelvic circles or pelvic clock).

The therapist sits behind the patient (either on the mat or on another ball). Initially manual contacts can be used to assist the patient in the correct movements through tapping in the direction of the movement. As control develops, independent practice (a hands-off approach) is desired.

Additional Swiss Ball Activities

Additional activities that can be used to challenge dynamic postural control while sitting on the ball include:

Sitting, unilateral shoulder flexion: One arm is raised overhead; this activity can progress to bilateral symmetrical or alternate arm lifts (Fig. 10–18).

Arm circles: The arms are held out to the sides and rotated first forwards, then backwards.

Sitting, leg lifts (unilateral hip flexion): The patient lifts one leg, then repeats with the other leg; this activity can progress to marching in place (alternate leg lifts) and marching combined with alternate arm lifts.

Sitting, knee extension: The knee is extended; this activity can progress to alternate knee extensions and writing letters of the alphabet in space with one foot.

Sitting, side-steps: The hip is abducted with the knee extended out to the side.

Sitting, alternate leg crosses: One LE is crossed over the other, then the activity is repeated with other LE.

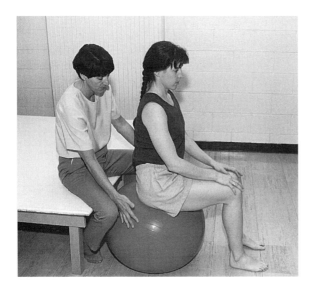

Figure 10–17. Sitting on a Swiss ball: pelvic shifts—active movements.

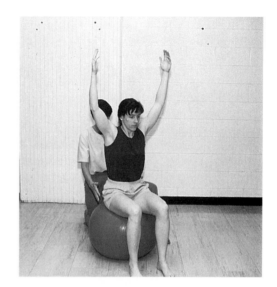

Figure 10–18. Sitting on a Swiss ball: bilateral arm lifts—active movements.

Sitting, jumping jacks: The arms are raised overhead and returned to the sides; arm movements are combined with bouncing movements on the ball.

Sitting, Mexican hat dance: The patient bounces on ball with reciprocal elbow flexion-extension and knee extension-flexion movements.

Sitting, head and trunk rotation: Look-arounds can be combined with arm swings from side to side.

Sitting, with the feet on a roller or small ball: Difficulty can be increased by using a mobile foot support.

Sitting, passing, catching, and throwing a ball: Difficulty can be increased by altering the size or weight of the ball used for throwing or catching.

Motor control goals. Static and dynamic balance control.

Indications. Impairments in balance control; impairments in sensory/kinesthetic awareness.

Functional outcomes. The patient demonstrates appropriate functional balance in sitting.

Movement Transitions: Sit-to-Stand Transfers

Variations in the method used are based on the patient's condition and functional impairments. The goal of these activities is independent assumption of standing.

Sit-to-Stand Transfers, Push-up Assist

The patient scoots to the front of the chair, and positions the feet under the hips (center of mass over the base of support). The patient is instructed to lean forward and push up into standing using both UEs for support. Important lead-up skills for this activity include scooting in short-sitting, sitting forward weight shifts, and sitting push-ups. Adequate height of the armrest is necessary to assist the UEs as they push up into standing.

The therapist can assist the transfer by counting ("On three I want you to shift forward and stand up—one, two, three") and initiating a rocking motion in time to the counts. This enables the patient to use momentum to stand up. The slower the movements, the greater the difficulty. If momentum is too great, the patient may continue forward once standing up, resulting in a loss of balance or fall.

During initial training, the height of the armrests can be varied (a wheelchair with adjustable-height armrests can be used) to increase or decrease the level of assistance. For patients with bilateral amputations, these armrests are essential to ensure independent sit-to-stand transfers.

Sit-to-Stand Transfers without Upper Limb Support

The sit-to-stand transfer is similiar to the above sequence with the exception that the upper limbs are not used to push up. Requirements for this type of transfer to standing include adequate forward weight transfer and lower extremity (LE) strength.

The therapist can facilitate the initial weight transfer forward by placing a stool or low table in front of the patient. The patient then practices partial stand-ups with the hands weight bearing (sit-to-plantigrade transfers). These transfers can also be done using a large ball with the therapist stabilizing the ball from the opposite side. As control develops, anterior support is removed.

A rocking chair can also be used to facilitate forward weight transfer and momentum. This is a useful training device for the patient with Parkinson's disease who has to overcome the effects of akinesia and rigidity.

The height of the seat can be varied (increased or decreased) depending on the strength of the LE muscles to assume the upright position. A higher seat decreases the total range of excursion and facilitates early independent standing. The seat can then be progressively lowered as the patient develops control. The support surface should be firm (such as a mat) as opposed to a soft bed to facilitate ease of transfer.

Upper limb position is an important consideration in facilitating forward weight transfer. The patient's hands can be clasped together in a prayer position with the shoulders flexed and elbows extended (Fig. 10–19). This position is useful for the patient with UE flexor spasticity, such as the patient recovering from stroke or traumatic brain injury. The patient's UEs are positioned over one of the therapist's shoulders (in the patient with stroke, the shoulder opposite the affected side is preferable since it helps maintain a

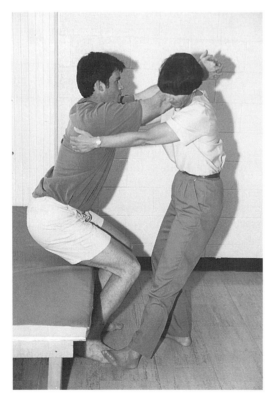

Figure 10–19. Sit-to-stand transfers: UEs in prayer position—active-assistive movements.

stretch to the trunk side flexors). Hands should never be positioned around the therapist's neck since this may result in an inadvertent choke hold. A variation useful for shorter patients involves having the patient hold the extended UEs against the therapist's sides (Fig. 10–20). The therapist maintains manual contacts on the patient's upper trunk and assists in the forward weight shift of the trunk.

Important lead-up activities to independent sit-to-stand transfers include bridging with pelvic elevation and standing, partial wall squats (see Fig. 13–7).

Sit-to-Stand Transfers, Agonist Reversals

This technique provides resistance to hip and knee extensors during both standing up (concentric or shortening contractions) and sitting down (eccentric or lengthening contractions). The therapist sits directly in front of the patient with both hands positioned on the anterior pelvis (Fig. 10–21).

Verbal commands include "Push up into standing" and "Now go down slowly." Resistance is offered at the end range (last 20 degrees) of standing up to ensure complete hip extension and during the first part of sitting down. During the rest of the transfer maximum resistance of gravity is in effect and manual resistance is not helpful.

Sit-to-Stand-to-Sit Transfers, Placing to One Side

During this activity the patient practices standing up, laterally moving the hips to one side, and sitting down adjacent to the original start position (Fig. 10–22). The feet are then repositioned directly in front. The patient can move completely around the mat in one direction by repeating this sequence.

This is an important training activity for the patient with stroke. It elongates the trunk side flexors on the affected side as the patient sits down toward the sound side. Arms should be clasped together in a prayer position and held directly in front to promote lower trunk rotation.

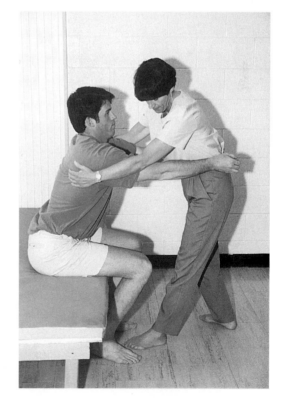

Figure 10–20. Sit-to-stand transfers: UEs extended—active-assistive movements.

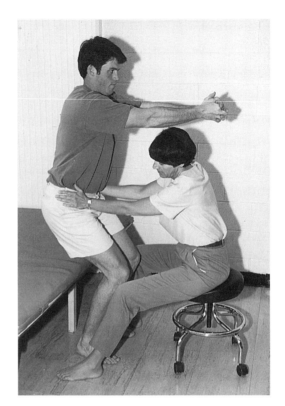

Figure 10–21. Sit-to-stand transfers—agonist reversals.

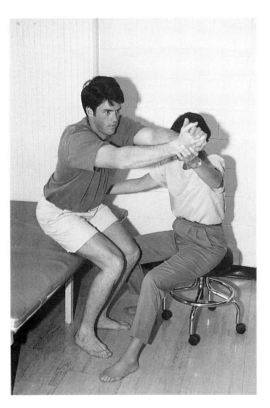

Figure 10–22. Sit-to-stand-to-sit transfers, placing to left side—active-assistive movements.

Motor control goals. Controlled mobility, static-dynamic control.

Indications. Weakness of the lower trunk/lower extremity muscles. These activities promote dynamic balance control and are important lead-up skills for independent gait and stair climbing.

Functional outcomes. The patient is able to perform sit-to-stand transfers independently.

Kneeling Activities

KNEELING (KNEEL-STANDING)

Movement Transitions: Quadruped (Prone Kneeling) to Kneel-Standing

The patient is in quadruped position and pushes the hips back over the heels while extending the hips and lifting the trunk into the upright position. Patients can also be instructed to use a chair or other support to climb up into kneeling using the UEs.

The therapist can assist the transition into kneeling by standing slightly behind and to the side of the patient and placing both hands on the trunk under the axillae. First one shoulder then the other is lifted back. If assistance with hip extension is needed, the therapist can place one foot between the patient's knees and use the side of the knee to gently push the patient's hips into extension.

Motor control goals. Controlled mobility (active-assistive movements progressing to active movements).

Indications. Weakness of trunk and hip muscles; impaired balance, frequent falls. Kneeling activities are important lead-up skills for independent floor-to-standing transfers.

Functional outcomes. The patient is able to assume kneeling independently.

General Characteristics

- The base of support (BOS) compared to quadruped (prone kneeling) is decreased; BOS is limited to the length of the leg and foot and is positioned largely posterior to COM. Thus this posture is more stable to the posterior than the anterior.
- The center of mass (COM) is intermediate; it is higher than in supine or prone positions and lower than in standing position.
- Kneeling involves head, trunk, and hip muscles for upright postural control.
- The head and trunk are maintained vertical in midline orientation, with normal spinal lumbar and thoracic curves.
- The pelvis is maintained in midline orientation with the hips fully extended and the knees flexed (as in bridging but with the trunk vertical).
  - Righting reactions contribute to upright head position (face vertical, mouth horizontal).
  - Static postural control is necessary for maintenance of upright posture. Dynamic postural control is necessary for control of movements in the posture (for example, weight shifting and reaching).
- Reactive balance control is needed for adjustments in response to changes in the COM (perturbation) or changes in the support surface (tilting).
- Anticipatory balance control is needed for preparatory postural adjustments that accompany voluntary movements.
- Effects of tonic reflex activity are minimal if the head is maintained in a neutral position.

- Patients may experience knee discomfort and knee pain from prolonged kneeling; a small pillow can be used to decrease discomfort.

Treatment Strategies and Considerations

- The lower COM and wider BOS (compared to standing) make kneeling an ideal safe posture for initial training of upright trunk and hip control.
  - If the patient loses control, the distance to the mat is small and a fall would be unlikely to result in injury.
  - The degrees of freedom problem is reduced; the patient does not need to demonstrate control of the knee or foot/ankle to maintain upright trunk and hip control.
- Prolonged positioning in kneeling provides strong inhibitory influences (inhibitory pressure) acting on the quadriceps.
  - It is therefore a useful treatment activity to dampen extensor hypertonicity in patients with lower extremity (LE) spasticity.
  - Kneeling may be an important lead-up activity to immediately precede ambulation for the patient with LE extensor spasticity and a scissoring gait pattern.
- Patients with strong abnormal flexor synergy influence (for example, the patient with stroke) will have difficulty maintaining the hip in extension; the tendency will be to recruit hip flexors with knee flexors.
  - The therapist may need to assist the patient with hip extension by using gentle pressure from behind.
  - A patient whose foot pulls strongly into dorsiflexion may require a pillow under the foot to relieve pressure on the toes.
- Kneeling may be contraindicated in some patients such as individuals with osteoarthritis of the knee or patients recovering from recent knee surgery.

Therapeutic Activities and Techniques

Position/Activity: Kneeling, Holding

The patient is kneeling, weight bearing on both knees and legs with the head and trunk upright and hips extended. During initial training in kneeling, the patient with instability may benefit from using a chair or stool placed in front for UE support. Alternate positions include placing the UEs forward with the patient's hands placed on the therapist's shoulders or placed on a wall. Since weight bearing occurs on both hands and knees, these positions are modified plantigrade positions. As control develops the patient can progress from bilateral to unilateral UE support to free kneeling.

TECHNIQUES

Alternating Isometrics
In alternating isometrics (AI), the patient is asked to hold the kneeling position while therapist applies medial/lateral resistance to the pelvis, first on one side pushing the pelvis away from the therapist, then pulling the pelvis toward the therapist. The resistance is built up gradually from very light resistance to the patient's maximum. The isometric contraction is maintained for several counts.

The therapist must give a transitional command ("Now don't let me pull you the other way") before sliding the hands to resist the opposite muscles; this allows the patient an opportunity to make appropriate preparatory postural adjustments.

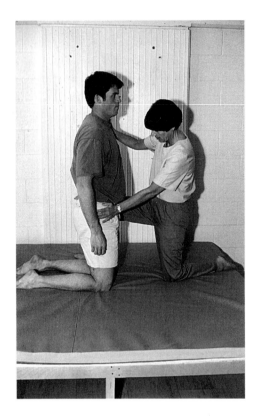

Figure 11–1. Kneeling: holding—alternating isometrics.

Theraband tubing can be placed around the distal thighs to increase the proprioceptive loading and contraction of the lateral hip muscles (gluteus medius).

Resistance can also be applied in anterior/posterior directions (Fig. 11–1). Because of the limited BOS in front, the patient will be able to take very little resistance anteriorly, and more resistance posteriorly. The patient can be positioned in the step position (with one knee slightly front of the other) and resistance can be applied on the diagonal. The position of the therapist will vary according to the direction of the line of force applied. The activity can be altered by offering resistance with one hand at the pelvis and the other hand at the upper trunk/shoulder to applying resistance with both hands at the upper trunk/shoulders.

Rhythmic Stabilization

In rhythmic stabilization (RS) the patient is asked to hold the kneeling position while the therapist applies rotational resistance to the trunk. The therapist places one hand on the posterior pelvis on one side and pushes forward while the other hand is on the anterior upper trunk, pulling backward on the opposite side. **Verbal commands** for RS are "Don't let me twist you; hold, now don't let me twist you the other way."

Motor control goal. Stability, static postural control.

Indications. Weakness of postural extensors (trunk and hip muscles). Kneeling is an important lead-up activity to upright stance in plantigrade and standing.

Functional outcomes. The patient is able to independently stabilize during upright kneeling.

Position/Activity: Kneeling, Weight Shifting

The patient actively shifts the pelvis from side to side with the knees in a symmetrical-stance position or diagonally forward and backward with the knees in a step position. Small-range shifts are stressed and are important lead-up skills for normal gait.

Active reaching activities can be used to promote weight shifting in all directions or in the direction of an instability (for example, in the patient with hemiplegia). The therapist provides a target ("Reach out and touch my hand,") or uses a functional task such as cone stacking to promote reaching. With the hands placed on a large ball, the patient can also practice moving the ball from side to side or forward and backward.

TECHNIQUES

Slow Reversals, Medial/Lateral Shifts

The therapist is positioned in kneeling or half-kneeling at the side of the patient. The movement of the hips is assisted for a few repetitions to ensure the patient knows the movements expected. Side-to-side movements (medial/lateral shifts) are then lightly resisted. The therapist alternates hand placement, first on one side of the pelvis resisting the pelvis as it pulls away, then on the opposite side as the pelvis pushes back. Smooth reversals (SRs) of antagonists are facilitated by well-timed **verbal commands** ("Pull away" or "Push back.")

Slow Reversals, Diagonal Shifts

The patient is kneeling with the knees in step position (one knee is advanced in front of the other, simulating normal step length). The therapist half-kneels diagonally in front of the patient. Resistance is applied to the pelvis as the patient weight-shifts diagonally forward over the knee in front, then diagonally backward over the other knee (Fig. 11–2). **Verbal commands** are "Shift forward and toward me; now shift back and away from me."

Slow Reversals, Diagonal Shifts with Rotation

Once control is achieved in diagonal shifts, the patient then is instructed to shift weight diagonally forward onto the knee in front while rotating the pelvis forward on opposite side; then diagonally backward while rotating the pelvis backward. **Verbal commands** are "Shift forward and twist, now shift back and twist."

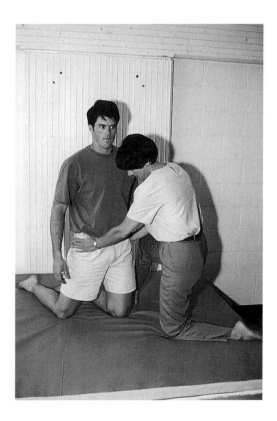

Figure 11–2. Kneeling: diagonal weight shifts— slow reversals.

If the upper trunk moves forward as the pelvis rotates forward, producing an ipsilateral trunk pattern, the therapist can isolate the pelvic motion by having the patient put both hands forward on the therapist's shoulders (Fig. 11–3) or on a wall in front. The patient is instructed to keep both elbows straight and move only the pelvis forward and backward during the weight shifts. The support for the UEs effectively locks up the upper trunk and allows the patient to move the pelvis in isolation.

Motor control goal. Controlled mobility.

Indications. Weakness and incoordination of postural muscles (trunk and hip muscles). Weight shifting in kneeling position is an important lead-up skill for the weight transfers and pelvic rotation needed for normal gait.

Functional outcomes. The patient is able to weight-shift independently in kneeling position.

Movement Transitions

Kneeling to Heel-Sitting
The patient is in kneeling, with the knees in normal stance position. The patient lowers the hips down to a sitting position on both heels. The patient then flexes the trunk forward and moves up into the kneeling position by extending both hips. As in sit-to-stand transitions, the forward trunk lean is important to ensure success in assuming the upright position and should be verbally cued. The therapist should encourage the patient to lower the body slowly rather than "plopping" or collapsing down. **Verbal commands** are "Go down slowly into sitting. Now come up into kneeling."

Achieving full hip extension in kneeling is a common problem. The therapist can verbally cue the patient or tap over the gluteal muscles to facilitate muscle contraction.

A prayer seat can be used to decrease the range for patients with weak hip extensors who may not be able to go down slowly or get up from the full heel-sitting position. A

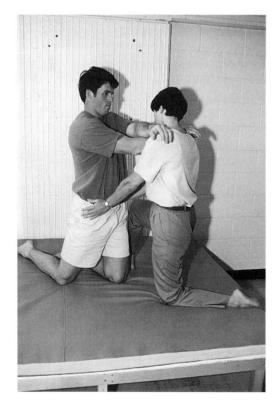

Figure 11–3. Kneeling: diagonal weight shifts with pelvic rotation—slow reversals.

prayer seat is a small wooden seat developed for individuals who practice yoga or meditate on their knees for long periods. The individual's legs fit underneath the seat while the person sits. Since the seat is only part way down, the range of excursion is decreased.

Kneeling to Side-Sitting

From kneeling the patient lowers both hips down to a side-sitting position. The trunk elongates on one side and the patient rotates the head and upper trunk slightly to keep the upper extremities (UEs) in the forward, weight-bearing position (Fig. 11–4). The patient then flexes the trunk forward, extends both hips, and moves back up into the kneeling position. The UEs are held in front of the patient or in a hands clasped, prayer position. The therapist can assist the movement by guiding the upper trunk rotation and providing verbal and tactile cues.

Patients with weak hip extensors or decreased lower trunk/hip flexibility may not be able go down into or up from the full side-sitting position. A side seat (sandbag or firm cushion) placed at the patient's side can be used to decrease the range of excursion and provide a platform for sitting.

Moving from kneeling to side-sitting is a useful treatment activity for the patient with decreased lower trunk/pelvic mobility (for example, the postacute patient with low back dysfunction) or the patient recovering from stroke with shortened or spastic side flexors). Side-sitting on the affected side with the hemiplegic UE weight bearing (shoulders flexed slightly, elbows and wrists extended, and hands open) inhibits the spastic muscles of the trunk and arm and provides joint compression to shoulder stabilizers.

Kneeling to Heel-Sitting Using the PNF Bilateral Symmetrical D2F Pattern

Transitions from kneeling to heel-sitting can be performed with bilateral symmetrical UE PNF patterns. The patient starts with both UEs overhead with the shoulders flexed, abducted, and externally rotated and the elbows extended and hands open (D2F). The hands close and the arms move down and across the body toward the opposite hips in D2E as the patient moves down into heel-sitting position. The patient then returns to kneeling with

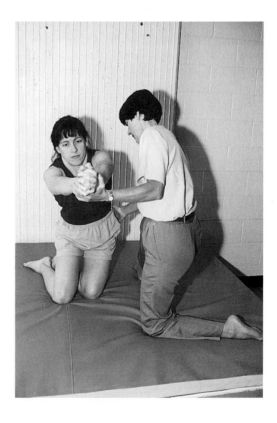

Figure 11–4. Kneeling to side-sitting—
active-assistive movements.

the arms moving back into D2F. This activity recruits upper trunk flexors as the patient moves down into heel-sitting and the upper trunk extensors as the patient moves up into kneeling. The UE patterns can be performed as active movements (the resistance of gravity is usually sufficient). The therapist can also apply light resistance by standing directly behind the patient (Fig. 11–5).

Kneeling to Heel-Sitting Using the PNF Reverse Lift Pattern

Kneeling to heel-sitting transitions can be performed with lift and reverse lift PNF patterns. In kneeling position, the patient starts with the lead limb in D2F (flexion, abduction, and external rotation) and the hand of the assist limb holding on to the wrist (Fig. 11–6A). The lead limb moves down and across into D2E (extension, adduction, internal rotation) as the patient moves down into heel-sitting or side-sitting position (Fig. 11–6B). The lead limb then moves back up into D2F as the patient returns to kneeling. This pattern recruits upper trunk rotators and flexors as the patient moves into heel-sitting and upper trunk rotators and extensors as the patient moves into kneeling. It also involves crossing the midline, making it a useful activity for patients with unilateral neglect (for example, the patient with stroke). The UE patterns can be performed as active movements or lightly resisted with the therapist standing behind and to the side of the patient. Chop and reverse chop PNF patterns can also be used.

TECHNIQUES

Agonist Reversals

This is an important lead-up activity for the patient with poor eccentric control who has difficulty sitting down slowly or going down stairs slowly. The therapist is in kneeling in front of the patient with both hands positioned on the anterior pelvis. The patient lowers both hips down into the heel-sitting position, then moves up into kneeling. The therapist applies resistance to the anterior pelvis during both the lowering and elevation phases of agonist reversals (ARs), thus both eccentric (lengthening) contraction and the concentric (shortening) contractions are resisted. Resistance is variable in different parts of the range: It is greatest initially, as the patient starts to sit down, and minimal during middle and end ranges, where the maximum effects of gravity take hold. In the reverse heel-sitting to kneeling transition, resistance is minimal through the early and middle range and builds up by the end of the transition as the patient moves into the shortened range to emphasize hip extensors. **Verbal commands** for ARs are "Go down slowly into sitting on your heels. Now push up into kneeling."

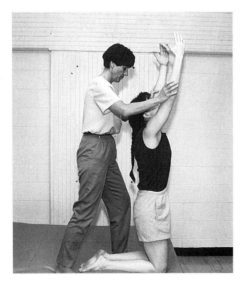

Figure 11–5. Heel-sitting to kneeling using PNF UE bilateral symmetrical D2 flexion patterns—slow reversals.

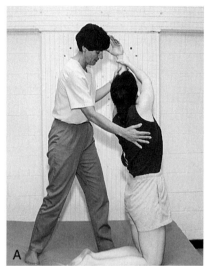

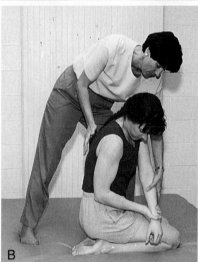

Figure 11–6*A* and *B*. Kneeling to heel-sitting using PNF lift/reverse lift patterns—slow reversals.

Motor control goal. Controlled mobility, static-dynamic control.

Indications. Weakness and incoordination of postural muscles (trunk and hip muscles). These activities are important lead-up skills for assumption of upright stance (floor-to-standing transfers).

Functional outcomes. The patient is able to assume kneeling position independently.

Position/Activity: Kneeling, Forward or Backward Progression (Kneel-Walking)

In the kneeling position, the patient moves forward or backward in small steps while weight bearing on the knees. The therapist can assist the timing and the sequence of the motion by providing verbal or tactile cues. Weight shifting with pelvic rotation is stressed. Overall timing can be facilitated with appropriate verbal commands ("On three I want you to step forward. One, two, and step, step, step.") If the patient is initially unstable, the therapist can be positioned in kneeling directly in front of the patient. The patient's hands should be placed on the therapist's shoulders for light support. The therapist then takes reverse steps in time with the patient's movements.

This is an activity that is generally limited to a small number of patients. Patients with bilateral LE extensor spasticity may benefit from training in kneel-walking. Inhibition is provided to the knee extensors while the patient is free to practice the elements needed for trunk and hip control. Patients with paraplegia and intact hip control (cauda equina injury) may also benefit from initial gait training in kneel-walking. Assistive devices (for example, bilateral mat crutches or canes) can be appropriately sized for this activity.

TECHNIQUES

Resisted Progression

The therapist provides steady resistance to the forward or backward progression (RP) by placing both hands on the pelvis. Resistance should be light (facilitatory) to encourage proper timing of the pelvic movements. Approximation can be applied down through the top of the pelvis to assist in stabilizing responses as weight is taken on the stance limb. Alternate hand placements for RP can include the pelvis and opposite shoulder, both shoulders, or the shoulder/head.

Motor control goal. Skill.

Indications. Kneel-walking is a lead-up activity for bipedal (upright) walking.

Functional outcomes. The patient is able to move independently in kneeling by using a reciprocal trunk and limb pattern.

Position/Activity: Kneeling, Balance Training Activities

Balance training begins with static holding (static postural control) and progresses to weight shifting or reaching activities in all directions (dynamic postural control). Additional activities that challenge anticipatory balance in the kneeling position include look-arounds (head and trunk rotation) and UE reaching and elevation activities.

Activities that can be used to challenge reactive balance include manual perturbations (disturbances of the patient's center of mass) in kneeling position and balance training in kneeling on an equilibrium board (disturbances of the patient's base of support).

Kneeling, Manual Perturbations

The patient is kneeling on a stationary surface (mat). The therapist provides a displacing force (manual perturbation) to the trunk. It is important to ensure appropriate compensatory responses with perturbations (disturbing the patient's center of mass) in varying directions. With backward displacements, hip and trunk flexor activity is required. With forward displacements, hip and trunk extensor activity is required. Lateral displacements require head and trunk inclination. Rotational displacements (twisting and displacing the trunk) require movement combinations of the trunk. Protective extension of the UEs can be initiated if the displacements move the center of mass near the limits of stability or outside of the base of support. If patient responses are lacking, the therapist may need to guide the initial attempts either verbally or manually. The patient can then progress to active movements.

Perturbations should be appropriate for patient's range and speed of control. It is important to use gentle disturbances with varied, asymmetrical manual contacts (tapping the patient out of position). Violent perturbations (pushes or shoves) are not necessary to stimulate balance responses. The therapist can vary the patient's base of support to increase or decrease difficulty (for example, by moving the knees apart or together).

Kneeling on an Equilibrium Board—Balance Training

The patient is positioned in kneeling on the equilibrium (balance) board with knees apart; the position is changed to provide for both anterior/posterior and medial/lateral (side-to-side) tilts. A folded towel can be placed under the knees to decrease discomfort. Initial activities include having the patient maintain a balanced or centered kneeling position (holding the board steady). The patient can then progress to active weight shifts, tilting the board in varying directions to stimulate balance responses. These patient-initiated challenges to balance stimulate both feed-forward (anticipatory) and feedback-driven (reactive) adjustments to balance.

The therapist can manually tilt the board to stimulate balance responses (evoking feedback-driven responses). The therapist varies the speed and range of displacements depending on the control exhibited by the patient. The direction of the displacements should be varied and unpredictable. It is important to observe the patient's responses carefully and use appropriate safety precautions.

Kneeling—Swiss Ball Activities

Prone to Kneeling on a Swiss Ball

This is a useful activity to strengthen lower abdominals and UEs and improve stabilizing and balance responses of the trunk muscles. The patient begins in quadruped position over a ball that is large enough to support the patient's chest. The patient walks out with both hands until the ball is positioned under the thighs (Fig. 11–7A). The patient then flexes both hips and knees, bringing the knees up toward the chest and the ball underneath. The patient is now kneeling on the ball in a tucked position with the UEs extended and weight bearing on the mat (Fig. 11–7B). The movements are reversed to return to the

Figure 11–7A and B. Prone to kneeling on a Swiss ball— active-assistive movements.

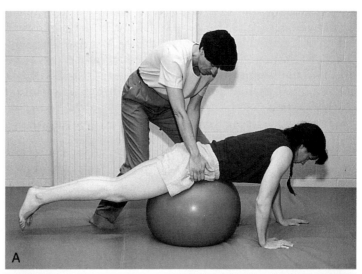

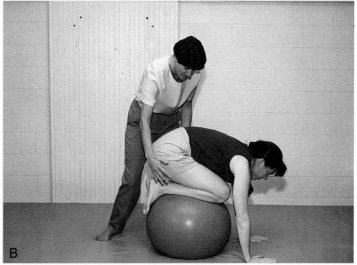

start position. The therapist can initially assist the movement into the tucked position by lifting the patient's hips up. Active movement control is stressed.

Variations can include having the patient bring both knees up into a tucked position to one side (moving into a side-sitting position on the ball). The patient can also move up into side-sitting on one side, then into kneeling in a tucked position, and finally into side-sitting on the other side (in clockwise or counterclockwise motions). This is a very difficult activity that requires a great deal of lower trunk flexibility and postural control. It is important to observe the patient's responses carefully and use appropriate safety precautions, guarding the patient while on the ball.

Motor control goals. Static and dynamic balance control.

Indications. Impaired balance control.

Functional outcomes. The patient demonstrates appropriate functional balance in kneeling position.

MOVEMENT TRANSITIONS INTO HALF-KNEELING

Kneeling to Half-Kneeling

From kneeling, the patient brings one limb up into the foot-flat position with both the hip and knee flexed while keeping the other knee weight bearing. The therapist is half-kneeling to the side and slightly behind the patient. Manual contacts are on the pelvis. The therapist assists the patient's weight shift onto the static limb by rotating the pelvis laterally and backward onto the weight-bearing limb. This unweights and facilitates movement of the dynamic limb into the hip flexion, foot-flat position. An alternate position for the therapist is standing with manual contacts on the upper trunk (under both axillae). This may be necessary for the patient who demonstrates upper trunk instability.

Motor control goals. Controlled mobility (active-assistive movements to active movements).

Indications. Weakness of trunk and hip muscles; postural instability, impaired balance, frequent falls. This is an important lead-up skill to independent floor-to-standing transfers.

Functional outcomes. The patient is able to assume the half-kneeling position independently.

HALF-KNEELING

General Characteristics

- The base of support (BOS) is greater than in kneeling and occurs on a diagonal.
- The center of mass (COM) is intermediate, similar to the COM in kneeling.
- This posture is more stable than kneeling as long as resistance or movements occur within the BOS (on a diagonal); the posture is unstable to resistance or movements outside the BOS.
- Half-kneeling involves head, trunk, and hip muscles for upright postural control.
- The head and trunk are maintained on the vertical in midline orientation, with normal spinal lumbar and thoracic curves.
- The pelvis is maintained in midline orientation with the hip fully extended on the posterior, knee-down support limb.
- The hip and knee are flexed to 90 degrees, with slight abduction on the anterior, foot-flat support limb.

- Normal righting reactions contribute to upright head position (face vertical, mouth horizontal).
- Static postural control is necessary for maintenance of upright posture. Dynamic postural control is necessary for control movements in the half-kneeling posture (for example, weight shifting or reaching).
- Reactive balance control is needed for adjustments in response to changes in the COM (perturbation) or changes in the support surface (tilting).
- Anticipatory balance control is needed for preparatory postural adjustments that accompany voluntary movements.
- Effects of tonic reflex activity are minimal if the head is maintained in a neutral position.

Treatment Strategies and Considerations

- Holding in the posture and weight-shifting activities in half-kneeling position provide early partial weight bearing for the foot and can be used to effectively mobilize foot and ankle muscles (for example, in the patient with ankle injury).
- The asymmetrical limb positioning (one knee down, one knee up with foot flat) can be used to disassociate (break up) symmetrical limb patterns. Half-kneeling is a useful activity for the patient with spastic diplegia.
- Inhibitory influences are in effect for the knee-down support limb (as in kneeling).
- Patients may demonstrate difficulties maintaining hip extension on the knee-down support limb (as in kneeling).
- Patients may demonstrate difficulties maintaining the flexed hip position of the foot-flat support limb.
  - Patients with strong extensor spasticity will have a tendency to adduct this limb and pull it down into extension (scissoring). The therapist can increase the amount of abduction to counteract this problem.
- Half-kneeling may be contraindicated in some patients (for example, individuals with osteoarthritis of the knee or those recovering from recent knee surgery).

Therapeutic Activities and Techniques

Position/Activity: Half-Kneeling, Holding

The patient is half-kneeling and bearing weight equally on the posterior, knee-down and anterior, foot-flat support limbs. The head and trunk are upright. The therapist is also half-kneeling in front of the patient in a reversed (mirror-image) position. During initial training the patient with instability may benefit from support provided by placing the hands on the therapist's shoulders. Alternately, both hands can be positioned on the patient's elevated anterior knee for support.

TECHNIQUES

Alternating Isometrics
In alternating isometrics (AI) the patient is asked to hold the half-kneeling position while the therapist applies resistance to the pelvis, first pushing the pelvis diagonally back toward the posterior, knee-down limb, then pulling the pelvis forward toward the anterior, foot-flat limb. The resistance is built up gradually from very light resistance to the patient's maximum. The isometric contraction is maintained for several counts. Resistance is applied only diagonally, in the direction of the BOS.

The therapist must give a transitional command ("Now don't let me move you the other way") before sliding the hands to resist the opposite muscles. This allows the patient an opportunity to make appropriate preparatory postural adjustments.

Motor control goal. Stability, static postural control.

Indications. The more unstable patient may benefit from training in half-kneeling before progressing to kneeling because of the wider BOS.

Functional outcome. The patient is able to stabilize independently in the half-kneeling position.

Position/Activity: Half-Kneeling, Weight Shifting

The patient actively weight shifts diagonally forward over the foot-flat support limb; then diagonally backward over the knee-down support limb.

TECHNIQUES

Slow Reversals, Diagonal Shifts
The patient is positioned in half-kneeling. The therapist is diagonally in front of the patient. Light resistance is applied to the pelvis as the patient weight-shifts diagonally forward over the support foot, then diagonally backward over the support knee (Fig. 11–8). Verbal commands are "Shift forward and toward me; now shift back and away from me."

Position/Activity: Half-Kneeling, Advanced Stabilization Activities

Half-Kneeling on the Swiss Ball
The patient is sitting on a ball with the hips and knees flexed to 90 degrees and the feet flat on the floor. The patient shifts weight over onto one side, freeing up the opposite limb for dynamic movement. The patient moves the limb down into the kneeling position and shifts weight over onto this knee. The ball is still underneath (partially supporting) the patient as the patient half-sits and the half-kneeling position is assumed (Fig. 11–9). The movements can then be reversed to return to sitting position. This is a useful activity to assist the patient with instability into the half-kneeling position.

The level of difficulty can be increased by having the patient practice alternate movements, moving down into half-kneeling on one side, then to sitting, then to half-kneeling on the other side.

Motor control goals. Controlled mobility, static-dynamic control.

Indications. Half-kneeling promotes control in a stable posture with a wide BOS.

Functional outcomes. The patient is able to weight-shift independently in half-kneeling position.

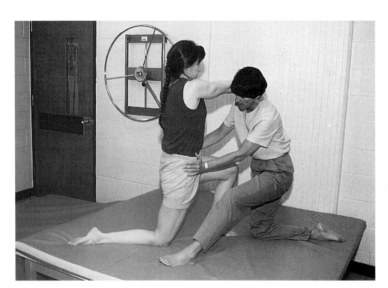

Figure 11–8. Half-kneeling: diagonal weight shifts— slow reversals.

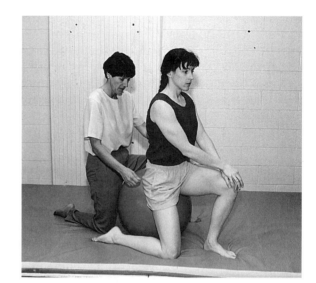

Figure 11–9. Half-kneeling on a Swiss ball: active-assistive movements.

Movement Transitions

Half-Kneeling to Standing

In the half-kneeling position, the patient flexes and rotates the trunk, transferring weight diagonally forward over the foot. The patient then comes up into the standing position by extending the hip and knee and placing the other foot parallel to the weight-bearing foot. This activity can be practiced with UE support: The patient places both hands on the elevated knee to assist in the rise to standing by pushing off (Fig. 11–10). The UEs can also be held in a forward prayer position. This helps get the weight forward over the anterior limb.

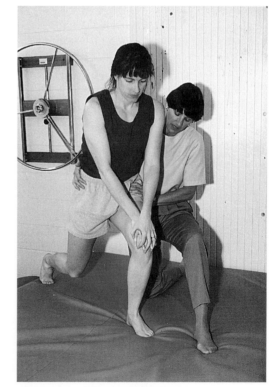

Figure 11–10. Half-kneeling to standing transfers—active-assistive movements.

The therapist stands behind the patient and assists the forward weight transfer by placing both hands on the upper trunk under the axillar. Alternately, in the half-kneeling position next to the patient, the therapist can place both hands on the patient's pelvis and assist the forward weight shift. Since the upward movement is largely unassisted, this requires more independent control by the patient.

If the patient is unsteady and demonstrates anxiety about this activity, it can be initially practiced with a chair or low table in front of the patient. The patient then comes up into standing position using both UEs for weightbearing and push-off. Practice can then progress to unassisted transfers (no UE support).

Motor control goals. Controlled mobility (active-assistive movements progressing to active movements).

Indications. Practicing half-kneeling-to-standing transfers is generally a late-stage training activity undertaken after the patient is walking. Functionally, this activity is important to ensure that the patient who falls can get up independently.

Functional outcome. The patient is able to independently transfer from floor to standing.

Modified Plantigrade Activities

MODIFIED PLANTIGRADE

General Characteristics

- The patient is standing with both elbows extended, hands open and weight bearing on a treatment table or plinth.
- The base of support (BOS) is wide: the hands are on the treatment table and the feet are in symmetrical stance.
- The center of mass (COM) is high.
- This posture is more stable than standing because of the four-limb support.
- Standing in modified plantigrade involves using the head, trunk, UE and LE muscles for upright postural control.
- The head and trunk are angled forward with weight borne over the UEs; the elbows are extended, shoulders flexed (typical ranges are 45 to 70 degrees).
- The hips are flexed with the knees extended; the ankles are dorsiflexed.
- Normal righting reactions contribute to an upright head position (face vertical, mouth horizontal).
- Static postural control is necessary for maintenance of upright posture.
- Dynamic postural control is necessary for control of movements in the posture (for example, weight shifting or reaching).

Treatment Strategies and Considerations

- The BOS can be increased or decreased by varying the distance the patient is standing from the table and the degree of shoulder flexion.
- The wider BOS in supported standing makes this an ideal safe posture for initial training in the fully upright position.
- Plantigrade is a better choice than standing in the parallel bars for patients who demonstrate UE flexor hypertonicity (for example, the patient with traumatic brain injury); holding onto the bars (pulling) encourages increased flexor tone while plantigrade promotes UE extension.
- The patient need not demonstrate the complete LE knee extensor control required for upright standing.
  - Weight bearing is shared through both UEs and LEs.
  - The slightly forward body position creates an extension moment at the knee, assisting in knee extension.
- The amount of weight bearing through forward placement of the UEs is intermediate between (1) sitting with the elbows extended and UEs weight bearing at the sides and (2) quadruped.
- Modified plantigrade posture may be used as a lead-up to more challenging weight bearing in quadruped for the patient with shoulder or elbow instability (for example, the patient with recent surgical repair of the shoulder).

- Weight-shifting activities forward and backward in plantigrade can be used to increase range of motion (ROM); this activity may be ideal for patients who are anxious about ROM exercises.
  - Improved ROM in shoulder flexion can be achieved by shifting the weight backward; positioning the feet farther from the treatment table increases the flexion range obtained.
  - Improved ROM in ankle dorsiflexion can be achieved by weight shifts forward.
  - Weight shifts with the patient facing a corner, both hands on the wall can be used to improve upper trunk extensor range, (for example, in the patient with dorsal kyphosis).
- Weight shifts can be combined with UE wall push-ups to increase the strength of the elbow extensors.
- In plantigrade position the hip is flexed with the knee extended; thus it is a useful treatment activity for the patient with stroke who demonstrates strong abnormal LE synergies because plantigrade combines muscles in an out-of-synergy pattern.

Therapeutic Activities and Techniques

Position/Activity: Modified Plantigrade, Holding

The patient is in modified plantigrade position, with weight borne equally on both UEs and LEs. The LEs can be positioned in a symmetrical stance or in a step position. During initial training, the patient with instability benefits from the bilateral upper limb support in this posture. As control develops, the patient can progress from bilateral to single-limb support to free standing.

Alternate arm positions include flexing both shoulders to 90 degrees with the elbows extended and the hands placed on a wall. This position allows for increased shoulder flexion range and increases the weight borne on the LEs. The patient can also be positioned sideways next to a treatment table or a wall with the arm in abduction. Both of these positions are useful in maintaining the UE out of the typical position of UE spasticity (flexion, adduction).

TECHNIQUES

Alternating Isometrics
The patient is asked to hold the plantigrade position while therapist stands behind the patient and applies resistance to the trunk (Fig. 12–1). The therapist's hands can be placed on the patient's pelvis, pelvis and contralateral upper trunk, or on the upper trunk. In alternating isometrics (AI), the resistance is applied first in one direction, then the other (anterior/posterior, medial/lateral, or on a diagonal with the LEs in the step position). The position of the therapist will vary according to the direction of the line of force. Resistance is built up gradually from very light resistance to the patient's maximum. The isometric contraction is maintained for several counts.

The therapist must give a transitional **verbal command** ("Now don't let me move you the other way") before sliding the hands to resist the opposite muscles; this allows the patient an opportunity to make appropriate preparatory postural adjustments.

Theraband tubing can be placed around the thighs (with the LEs in a symmetrical stance) to increase the proprioceptive loading and contraction of the lateral hip muscles (gluteus medius).

Rhythmic Stabilization
The patient is asked to hold the plantigrade position while the therapist stands behind the patient and applies rotational resistance to the trunk. In rhythmic stabilization (RS), one hand is placed on the posterior pelvis on one side, pushing forward, while the

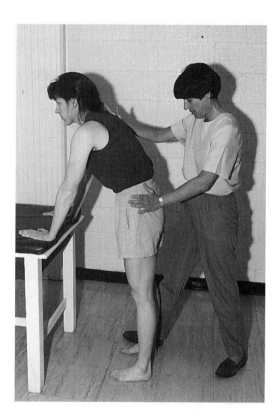

Figure 12–1. Modified plantigrade position: holding—alternating isometrics.

other hand is on the anterior upper trunk, contralateral side, pulling backward. **Verbal commands** are "Don't let me twist you—hold, hold; now don't let me twist you the other way."

Motor control goal. Stability, static postural control.

Indications. Modified plantigrade (supported standing) is a good initial standing posture for the patient who lacks the stability control needed for free standing in an upright posture.

Functional outcomes. The patient is able to independently stabilize in the modified plantigrade position.

Position/Activity: Modified Plantigrade, Weight Shifting

The patient actively shifts weight first forward (increasing loading on the UEs), then backward (increasing loading on the LEs). Weight shifts can also be performed from side to side (medial/lateral shifts), with the LEs in a symmetrical stance, or diagonally forward and backward, with the LEs in a step position.

   Active reaching activities can be used to promote weight shifting in all directions, or in the direction of an instability (for example, in the patient with hemiplegia). The therapist provides a target ("Reach out and touch my hand") or uses a functional task like cone stacking to promote reaching.

Plantigrade, Hands on a Swiss Ball
The patient is in plantigrade position with both hands open and resting on a large ball. Alternately, a medium-size ball can be placed on top of a flat treatment table (Fig. 12–2). The patient places both hands on the ball and actively moves it in all directions: side to side, forward and backward, or diagonally forward and backward. This activity requires advanced stabilization of the trunk and extremities and promotes weight shifting in plantigrade position.

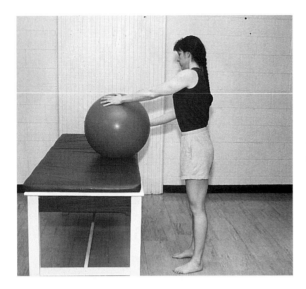

Figure 12–2. Modified plantigrade position: weight shifts, hands moving a Swiss ball—active movements.

TECHNIQUES

Slow Reversals
The therapist is standing at the patient's side (for medial/lateral shifts), or behind the patient (for anterior/posterior shifts). Manual contacts can be placed on the pelvis, the pelvis/contralateral upper trunk, or on the upper trunk. The slow reversals (SRs) are assisted for a few repetitions to ensure the patient knows the movements expected. Movements are then lightly resisted. The therapist alternates hand placement, resisting the movements first in one direction, then the other. Smooth reversals of antagonists are facilitated by well-timed **verbal commands** ("Pull away—now push back.")

Slow Reversals—Diagonal Shifts
The patient is positioned in plantigrade with the LEs in step position. The therapist stands diagonally behind the patient. Resistance is applied to the pelvis as the patient weight-shifts diagonally onto the forward LE, then diagonally backward onto the other LE. **Verbal commands** are "Shift forward and away from me; now shift back and toward me."

Slow Reversals—Diagonal Shifts with Rotation
Once control is achieved in diagonal shifts, the patient then is instructed to shift weight diagonally onto the forward LE while rotating the pelvis forward on the opposite side; then the weight is shifted diagonally backward while rotating the pelvis backward. The therapist resists the motion at the pelvis. **Verbal commands** are "Shift forward and twist, now shift back and twist."

   If the elbows flex, the upper trunk may move forward as the pelvis rotates forward, producing an ipsilateral trunk rotation pattern. The therapist can isolate the pelvic motion by instructing the patient to keep both elbows fully extended.

Slow Reversals—Diagonal Shifts with Stepping Movements
The patient progresses to taking a step with the dynamic limb while weight shifting diagonally forward or backward onto the static limb. The therapist maintains manual contacts on the pelvis to facilitate the accompanying pelvic rotation. **Verbal commands** are "Shift forward and step; now shift back and step."

Motor control goals.   Controlled mobility (weight shifts), static-dynamic control (stepping).

Indications.   Absent or diminished isolated pelvic control needed for weight shifting and stepping. These activities are important lead-up skills for bipedal gait.

Functional outcomes. The patient is able to weight-shift and step forward and backward in plantigrade position.

Position/Activity: Modified Plantigrade, Upper Extremity Patterns

The patient is in plantigrade position with only one arm used for support. The static (support) limb is positioned in weight bearing near the end of the treatment table to free up the dynamic limb for movement.

Upper extremity PNF patterns are used to provide a dynamic challenge to the stabilizing extremities and trunk. The patient can be instructed to actively move the dynamic limb in the pattern(s) or light resistance can be imposed. Resistance can be manual (from the therapist's hands) or the patient can use free weights (for example, a wrist cuff).

Benefits to the dynamic limb include diagonal and rotational movements occur in natural synergistic combinations. PNF patterns also allow crossing the midline, an important activity for patients with unilateral neglect. The patient focuses full attention on the correct UE movements and not on the stabilization of the trunk and limbs. Therefore, the PNF patterns assist in promoting automatic postural control.

PNF UNILATERAL UE D1 PATTERNS

D1F, Flexion-Adduction-External Rotation
The hand of the dynamic limb is positioned near the side of the ipsilateral hip with the hand open and the thumb facing down. The patient is instructed to close the hand, turn, and pull the arm up and across the face.

D1E, Extension-Abduction-Internal Rotation
The patient opens the hand, turns, and pushes the arm down and out to the side.

PNF UNILATERAL UE D2 PATTERNS

D2F, Flexion-Abduction-External Rotation
The hand of the dynamic limb is positioned across the body on the opposite hip with the hand closed and the thumb facing down. The patient is instructed to open the hand, turn, and lift the arm up and out (Fig. 12–3).

D2E, Extension-Adduction-Internal Rotation
The patient closes the hand, turns, and pulls the arm down and across the body. The patient is instructed to follow the movements of the arm by looking at the hand. This encourages head and neck rotation.

When using resisted patterns, the level of resistance is determined by the ability of the static limbs and trunk to stabilize and maintain the plantigrade posture, not the strength of the dynamic limb. If stabilization is lacking, resistance may be contraindicated. Active movements should be promoted.

Position/Activity: Modified Plantigrade, Lower Extremity Patterns

Plantigrade, Leg Lifts
The patient is in plantigrade position with bilateral UE support. Lower extremity movements are used to provide a dynamic challenge to the stabilizing extremities and trunk. Leg lifts (hip and knee extension) or bent-knee lifts (knee flexion with hip extension) can be used. The patient is instructed to weight-shift onto the static limbs and lift the dynamic limb posteriorly. The movements can be lightly resisted, either manually or with an ankle cuff.

Posterior bent-knee lifts are an important activity for the patient with stroke who demonstrates obligatory synergies. Hip extension with knee flexion is a difficult out-of-synergy combination needed for bipedal gait (specifically, end-stance control and toe-off).

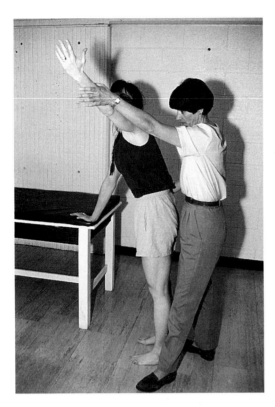

Figure 12–3. Modified plantigrade position: PNF UE D2 flexion patterns— slow reversals.

Motor control stages. Controlled mobility, static-dynamic control.

Indications. Dynamic limb movements increase the static challenge on the weight-bearing limbs and trunk.

Functional outcomes. The patient is able to independently shift weight and move the limbs in a supported standing (plantigrade) position; the patient is able to perform functional activities in supported standing position (reaching, grooming, and bathing).

Standing Activities

STANDING

General Characteristics

- The base of support (BOS) in standing is small.
- The center of mass (COM) is high.
- Limits of stability are determined by the distance between the feet and the length of the feet as well as the height and weight of the individual.
  - The normal anterior/posterior limit of stability (LOS) is approximately 12 degrees.
  - The normal medial/lateral LOS is approximately 16 degrees.
- There is normally a small amount of spontaneous postural sway back and forth and side to side within a sway envelope.
  - Sway cycles intermittently.
  - The midpoint of sway is the center of LOS.
- Postural stability is maintained by normal postural alignment.
  - Vertical alignment is present in all body segments.
  - The line of gravity (LOG) falls close to most joint axes: slightly anterior to the ankle and knee joints; slightly posterior to the hip joint; posterior to the cervical and lumbar vertebrae and anterior to the thoracic vertebrae and atlanto-occipital joint.
  - Natural spinal curves are present but flattened in upright stance depending upon the level of postural tone, lumbar and cervical lordosis, and thoracic or dorsal kyphosis.
  - The pelvis is in neutral position, with no anterior or posterior tilt.
  - Normal alignment minimizes the need for muscle activity during erect stance.
- Postural stability is maintained by muscle activity that includes:
  - Postural (muscle) tone in the antigravity muscles throughout the trunk and lower extremities (LEs).
  - Contraction of antigravity muscles—the gluteus maximus and hamstrings contract to maintain pelvic alignment; the abdominals contract to flatten the lumbar curve; and the paravertebral muscles contract to extend the spine.
- Vertical postural orientation is maintained by multiple and overlapping sensory inputs; the central nervous system (CNS) organizes and integrates sensory information and generates responses for controlling body position.
- The vestibular system responds to gravity acting on the head:
  - It stabilizes gaze during movements of the head using the vestibulo-ocular reflex (VOR).
  - It provides input to labyrinthine righting reactions (LRR) of the head, trunk, and limbs, and contributes to upright head position and normal alignment of the head and body.
  - It regulates postural tone.
- The somatosensory (tactile and proprioceptive) systems respond to support-surface inputs about the relative orientation of body position and movement. The somatosensory systems influence postural responses through the stretch reflexes and automatic postural reactions.
- The visual system responds to visual cues about the environment and the relationship of the body to objects in the environment:

- ◦ It provides input to optical righting reactions of the head, trunk, and limbs; contributes to upright head position and normal alignment of the head and body.
  - ◦ It regulates postural tone.
  - ◦ It guides safe movement trajectories.
- Normal postural strategies for maintaining upright stability and balance include:
  - ◦ The ankle strategy, which involves small shifts of the COM by rotating the body about the ankle joints; there is minimal movement of the hip and knee joints.
  - ◦ The hip strategy, which involves larger shifts of the COM by flexing or extending at the hips.
  - ◦ The support or stepping strategy, which involves large shifts of the COM outside the BOS; realignment of the BOS under the COM is achieved by rapid steps, hops, or stumbles in the direction of the instability.
- Hip abductors are important in maintaining upright stability for lateral displacements.
- Static postural control is necessary for maintenance of upright posture.
- Dynamic postural control is necessary for control movements in the posture (for example, weight shifting or reaching).
- Reactive balance control is needed for adjustments in response to changes in the COM (perturbations) or changes in the support surface (tilting):
  - ◦ Postural fixation reactions stabilize the body against a force thrust (for example, a perturbation or push).
  - ◦ Tilting reactions reposition the COM within the BOS in response to changes in the support surface (for example, standing on an equilibrium board).
- Anticipatory postural control occurs in advance of the execution of skill movements. The postural system is pretuned to stabilize the body; for example, an individual readies his or her posture before lifting a heavy weight.
  - ◦ Postural responses are highly adaptable to the specific task and environmental conditions at the time of the task.
  - ◦ Prior experience influences the adaptability of an individual.

Treatment Strategies and Considerations

- Changes in normal alignment result in changes in other body segments; malalignment or poor posture results in increased muscle activity, energy expenditure, and postural stress.
  - ◦ A flexed-knee posture increases the need for quadricep activity; it also requires increased hip extensor and soleus activity for accompanying increases in hip flexion and dorsiflexion.
  - ◦ Excessive anterior tilt of the pelvis increases lumbar lordosis and produces a compensatory increase in thoracic kyphosis; lumbar interdiscal pressures are increased. The abdominals are stretched and the iliopsoas becomes shortened.
  - ◦ Excessive lumbar lordosis produces shortening of the lumbar extensors.
  - ◦ Excessive dorsal kyphosis produces stretching of the thoracic back extensors and shortening of the anterior shoulder muscles.
  - ◦ Excessive cervical lordosis produces shortening of the neck extensors.
  - ◦ Genu valgum produces medial knee joint stresses and pronation of the foot with increased stress on the medial longitudinal arch of the foot.
  - ◦ Pes planus (flat foot) results in depression of the navicular bone and compressive forces laterally; increased weight is borne on the metatarsal heads.
  - ◦ Pes cavus (high-arched foot) results in increased height of the longitudinal arch with a depressed anterior arch and plantarflexion of the forefoot; toe deformity (claw toes) is also present.
- Asymmetric standing with weight borne primarily on one LE with little weight on the other results in increased ligament and bony stress on the weight-bearing side; the knee is usually fully extended on the stance limb.

- Changes in muscle activity result in changes in standing posture:
  - Gastrocnemius-soleus paralysis results in limited sway and wide BOS.
  - Quadriceps paralysis results in unstable sway; the knees are hyperextended (genu recurvatum) and the trunk may be inclined forward to increase stability.
  - The patient without active knee control (for example, the patient with bilateral above-knee amputations) compensates by keeping the hips slightly flexed, with increased lordosis.
  - The patient with bilateral LE paralysis (for example, the patient with paraplegia) can obtain foot/ankle and knee stability through orthotics; the hip can be stabilized by leaning forward on the iliofemoral (Y) ligament.
  - The patient with hypertonicity of the lower extremities demonstrates decreased mobility; the action of the foot/ankle muscles and balance reactions are compromised.
- BOS can be varied to decrease or increase difficulty in maintaining standing:
  - A wide-based stance is a common compensatory change in patients with decreased postural control.
  - A decreased stance (feet together) can be used to increase the challenge to postural control.
  - Tandem stance (heel-toe position) increases the difficulty of standing even further.
- Visual inputs can be varied to increase difficulty in maintaining standing: eyes open (EO) to eyes closed (EC).
- Somatosensory inputs can be varied to increase difficulty in maintaining standing: feet in contact with flat surface to feet on dense foam.

Therapeutic Activities and Techniques

Position/Activity: Standing, Holding

The patient is standing, with equal weight on both LEs. The feet are positioned parallel and slightly apart (a symmetrical stance position); knees are slightly flexed, not hyperextended. The pelvis is in neutral position. An alternate standing position is with one foot slightly advanced of the other in a step position. Theraband tubing can be placed around the thighs (LEs in a symmetrical stance position) to increase the proprioceptive loading and pelvic stabilization by lateral hip muscles (gluteus medius).

Knee instability in which the knee buckles due to quadriceps weakness can be managed by having the patient stand on an inclined surface facing forward. The forward tilt of the body and anterior displacement of the COM provide a posteriorly directed moment (force) at the knee, stabilizing it in extension.

TECHNIQUES

Alternating Isometrics
The patient is asked to hold the standing position while the therapist applies resistance to the trunk. As in plantigrade, the hands can be placed on the pelvis, pelvis/contralateral upper trunk, or on the upper trunk. In alternating isometrics (AI), resistance is applied first in one direction, then the other (anterior/posterior, medial/lateral, or on the diagonal with the LEs in the step position). The position of the therapist will vary according to direction of the line of force applied. Resistance is built up gradually from very light resistance to the patient's maximum. The isometric contraction is maintained for several counts. Light approximation can be given to the tops of the shoulders, pelvis, or head to increase stabilizing responses.

The therapist must give a transitional command ("Now don't let me move you the other way") before sliding the hands to resist the opposite muscles; this allows the patient the opportunity to make appropriate preparatory postural adjustments.

Rhythmic Stabilization

In rhythmic stabilization (RS), the patient holds the symmetrical standing position while the therapist applies rotational resistance to the trunk. One hand is placed on the anterior pelvis on one side pushing backward while the other hand is on the posterior upper trunk on the contralateral side, pulling forward (Fig. 13–1). **Verbal commands** for RS are "Don't let me twist you—hold, hold; now don't let me twist you the other way."

Motor control goal. Stability, static postural control.

Indications. Weakness of postural (antigravity) muscles.

Functional outcomes. The patient is able to independently perform static standing. Stabilization control in standing is an important lead-up activity to unilateral stance and bipedal gait.

Position/Activity: Standing, Weight Shifts

The patient actively shifts weight first forward, then backward. Weight shifts can also be performed side to side (medial/lateral shifts) with the LEs in a symmetrical stance position or diagonally forward and backward with the LEs in a step position.

Active reaching activities can be used to promote weight shifting in all directions, or in the direction of an instability (for example, in the patient with hemiplegia). The therapist provides a target ("Reach out and touch my hand") or uses a functional task like cone stacking to promote reaching.

TECHNIQUES

Slow Reversals

The therapist is standing at the patient's side (for medial/lateral shifts), or behind (for anterior/posterior shifts). As when slow reversals (SRs) were performed in plantigrade, manual contacts can be placed on the pelvis, the pelvis/contralateral upper trunk, or on the upper

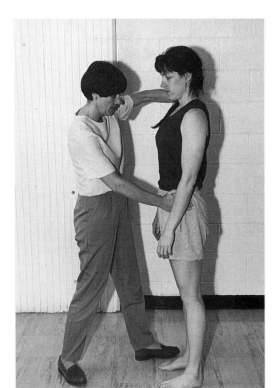

Figure 13–1. Standing: holding—rhythmic stabilization.

trunk. The movement is assisted for a few repetitions to ensure that the patient knows the movements expected. Movements are then lightly resisted. The therapist alternates hand placement, resisting the movements first in one direction, then the other. Smooth reversals of antagonists are facilitated by well-timed **verbal commands,** "Pull away. Now push back."

Slow Reversals, Diagonal Shifts

The patient is in standing with the LEs in step position. The therapist is diagonally in front of the patient, either sitting on a stool or standing. Resistance is applied to the pelvis as the patient shifts weight diagonally forward over the limb in front, then diagonally backward over the opposite limb. **Verbal commands** for the shifts are "Shift forward and away from me; now shift back and toward me."

Slow Reversals, Diagonal Shifts with Rotation

Once control is achieved in diagonal shifts, the patient then is instructed to shift weight diagonally forward onto the limb in front while rotating the pelvis forward on opposite side (Fig. 13–2). Weight is then shifted diagonally backward while rotating the pelvis backward. The therapist resists the motion at the pelvis. **Verbal commands** are "Shift forward and twist; now shift back and twist."

The upper trunk may move forward as the pelvis rotates forward, producing an ipsilateral trunk rotation pattern. The therapist can isolate the pelvic motion by providing verbal or manual cues. The patient can also hold the UEs directly in front with the hands clasped in a prayer position to stabilize upper trunk motion.

The activity can be progressed to a contralateral trunk pattern. The upper extremities are resting in midline with the trunk. As the pelvis moves forward on one side, the patient is instructed to swing the opposite arm forward. This promotes contralateral trunk rotation and normal arm swing needed for gait.

Motor control goal. Controlled mobility, dynamic postural control.

Indications. Weight shifts promote dynamic standing with normal timing and sequencing of movements of the pelvis.

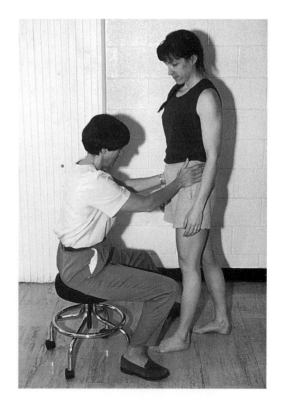

Figure 13–2. Standing: diagonal weight shifts with pelvic rotation—slow reversals.

Functional outcomes. The patient is able to independently transfer weight from one limb to the other while standing.

Position/Activity: Standing, Stepping

This activity is initiated with the LEs in step position. The patient shifts weight diagonally forward over the anterior support limb (stance limb) and takes a step forward with the dynamic (swing) limb. The movements are then reversed: the patient shifts diagonally back and takes a step backward using the same dynamic limb.

Slow Reversals, Stepping

The therapist is in front of the patient, either sitting on a rolling stool or standing. Manual contacts are on the pelvis. The therapist applies a light stretch and resistance to facilitate the forward pelvic rotation as the swing limb moves forward (Fig. 13–3A and B). Approximation can be given as needed over the top of the pelvis as the dynamic limb comes into extension and weight bearing. **Verbal commands** for the slow reversals (SRs) are "Shift forward and step; now shift back and step."

Standing, Stepping-up

From a symmetrical stance position, the patient weight shifts laterally toward the support limb and places the dynamic limb up on a step positioned directly in front of the patient (Fig. 13–4). The limb is then returned to the original stance position; the patient does not move up onto the step. Normal postural alignment is maintained during the activity. Excessive trunk flexion is not permitted.

The height of the step can be varied to increase or decrease the difficulty of this activity. For example, a 4-inch (10-cm) aerobic step can be used initially. The height can then be progressed to a standard 7-inch (17.5-cm) step. As control develops, the patient can progress to stepping up onto the step, then stepping up and over the step.

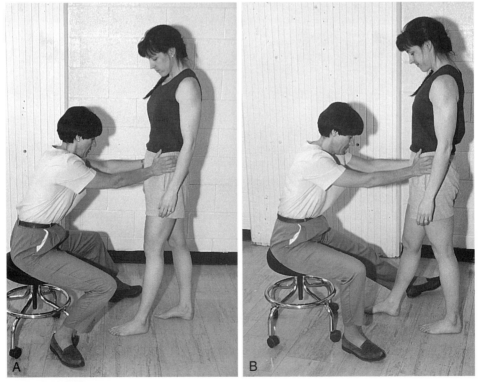

Figure 13–3A and B. Standing: stepping—slow reversals.

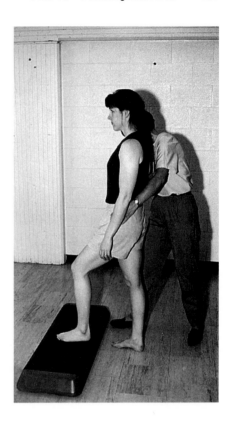

Figure 13–4. Standing: stepping up—active-assistive movements.

Standing, Side-stepping
The patient shifts weight laterally over the support limb and takes a side-step with the dynamic limb. This activity recruits hip abductors (gluteus medius) and is therefore useful for the patient with abductor weakness.

Lateral Step-ups
The patient can also place the dynamic limb up on a low step positioned to the side (Fig. 13–5).

Motor control goal. Static-dynamic control.

Indications. Stepping is an important lead-up activity for bipedal gait and independence in community ambulation.

Functional outcomes. The patient independently ambulates up and down stairs.

Position/Activity: Standing, Advanced Stabilization Activities

Standing, Single-Limb Support
The patient lifts one limb off the ground and maintains the standing position using single limb support. The patient is instructed to maintain the pelvis level. A pelvis that drops on the side of the dynamic limb is indicative of hip abductor weakness on the opposite (static-limb) side.

Standing, Single-Limb Support with Abduction
The patient stands sideways next to a wall but does not lean on the wall. The lower limb closest to the wall becomes the dynamic limb while the other lower limb becomes the support limb. The patient flexes the knee and abducts the dynamic limb, pushing the knee against the wall. The static limb maintains the upright posture during unilateral stance with the knee flexed slightly (Fig. 13–6).

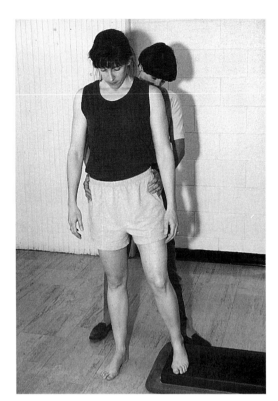

Figure 13–5. Standing: lateral step-ups—active-assistive movements.

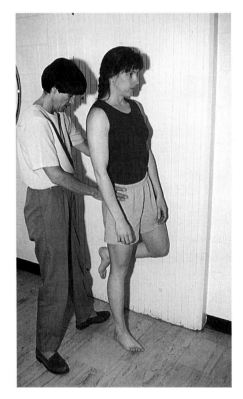

Figure 13–6. Standing: single-limb support with abduction—active-assistive movements.

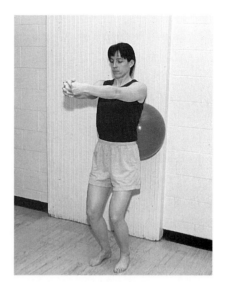

Figure 13–7. Standing: partial wall squats with a Swiss ball—active movements.

Initially the weaker limb is the dynamic limb. As control develops, the patient turns so that the weaker limb is used as the static or support limb. The abductors on both sides are working strongly to push into the wall and to maintain the unilateral stance position. Overflow from one side to the other is strong, because of reciprocal innervation effects.

Motor control stage. Static-dynamic control.

Indications. Hip abductor weakness. Trendelenburg gait pattern.

Functional outcomes. The patient ambulates independently without pelvic instability.

Standing, Partial Squats

The patient stands with the back next to a wall, feet about 4 inches (10 cm) from the wall. The patient is instructed to bend both knees while sliding the back down the wall. Movement is restricted to partial range; the patient is instructed to stop when no longer able to see the tips of the toes. The hip is maintained in neutral rotation to ensure proper patellar tracking. The pelvis is also maintained in neutral, or squats can be performed with a slight posterior pelvic tilt (for example, if the patient suffers from low back pain).

The patient can also stand with the back supported by a medium-size Swiss ball placed in the lumbar region; the feet are positioned directly underneath the body, trunk upright. The ball is resting on the wall. As the patient moves down into the partial squat position, the movement is facilitated by the ball rolling upward (Fig. 13–7).

A small towel roll can be placed between the knees. The patient is instructed to hold the towel roll in position by squeezing both knees together during the squat. This can be used to enhance contraction of the vastus medialis and improve patellar tracking.

Theraband tubing placed around the thighs can be used to increase the stabilizing activity of the hip abductors during partial wall squats. The activity can progress to unilateral (single-limb) squats.

Motor control stage. Controlled mobility.

Indications. Quadriceps weakness. Partial wall squats are an important lead-up activity for independent sit-to-stand transitions or stair climbing.

Functional outcomes. The patient is able to perform dynamic standing activities independently.

Gait Activities

THE GAIT CYCLE

Phases of the Gait Cycle

The **stance phase** is the portion of the cycle when the foot is in contact with the ground (60 percent of the cycle); the **swing phase** is the portion of the cycle when the limb is off the ground and moving forward (or backward) to take a step (40 percent of the cycle). Traditional terminology is presented here. For descriptions of the gait cycle using the Rancho Los Amigos (RLA) terminology, please refer to the chapter on gait analysis by Norkin in O'Sullivan and Schmitz.[1]

Traditional Gait Terminology

- **Heel strike** is the point when the heel of the reference or support limb contacts the ground at the beginning of stance phase.
- **Foot flat** is the point when the sole of the foot of the reference or support limb makes contact with the ground; foot flat occurs immediately after heel strike.
- **Midstance** is the point at which full body weight is taken by the reference or support limb.
- **Heel off** occurs after midstance as the heel of the reference or support limb leaves the ground.
- **Toe off** is the last portion of stance following heel off, when only the toe of the reference or support limb is in contact with the ground.
- **Swing-phase acceleration** is the first portion of the swing phase, from toe off of the reference limb until midswing.
- **Midswing** is the midportion of the swing phase, when the reference extremity moves directly below the body.
- **Swing-phase deceleration** is the end portion of the swing phase, when the reference extremity is slowing down in preparation for heel strike.

Muscle Activation Patterns

- Heel strike: The knee extensors (quadriceps) are active at heel strike through early stance to control small amount of knee flexion for shock absorption; ankle dorsiflexors (anterior tibialis, extensor hallucis longus, extensor digitorum longus) decelerate the foot, slowing the plantarflexion from heel strike to foot flat.
- Foot flat: The gastrocnemius-soleus muscles are active from foot flat through midstance to eccentrically control forward tibial advancement.
- Midstance: The hip, knee, and ankle extensors are active throughout stance to oppose antigravity forces and stabilize the limb; hip extensors control forward motion of the trunk; hip abductors stabilize the pelvis during unilateral stance; plantarflexors propel the body forward.
- Heel off: Peak activity of the plantarflexors occurs just after heel off, to push off and generate forward propulsion of the body.

- Toe off: Hip and knee extensors (hamstrings and quadriceps) contribute to forward propulsion with a brief burst of activity.
- Swing-phase acceleration: Forward acceleration of the limb during early swing is achieved through the action of the quadriceps; by midswing the quadriceps is silent and pendular motion is in effect; hip flexors (the iliopsoas) aid in forward limb propulsion.
- Midswing: Foot clearance is achieved by contraction of the hip and knee flexors, and ankle dorsiflexors.
- Swing-phase deceleration: The hamstrings act during late swing to decelerate the limb in preparation for heel strike; quadriceps and ankle dorsiflexors become active in late swing to prepare for heel strike.

Pelvic and Thoracic Motions during Gait

- The pelvis moves forward and backward approximately 8 degrees (transverse pelvic rotation). Forward rotation (4 degrees) occurs on the side of the unsupported or swing LE; backward rotation (4 degrees) occurs on the side of the stance LE.
- As the ipsilateral thorax rotates forward or backward, the contralateral thorax rotates simultaneously in the opposite direction; the arm swings forward with the forward motion of the thorax.
- The pelvis moves up and down on the unsupported or swing side approximately 5 degrees (lateral pelvic tilt); the movement is controlled by the hip abductor muscles. The high point is at midstance; the low point is during the period of double support.
- The pelvis moves side to side about 1½ inch (4 cm); follows the stance or support limb.

Step

Step is defined by the following parameters:

- **Step length** is the linear distance between point of foot contact (preferably heel strike) of one extremity to the point of heel strike of the opposite extremity (in centimeters or meters).
- **Step time** is the number of seconds that elapses during one step.
- **Step width** is the distance between feet (base of support), measured from one heel to the same point on the opposite heel; normal step width ranges between 1 inch (2.5 cm) and 5 inches (12.5 cm). Step width increases as stability demands rise (for example, in older adults or very young children).

Stride

Stride is defined by the following parameters:

- **Stride length** is the linear distance between two consecutive points of foot contact (preferably heel strike) of the same extremity (in centimeters or meters).
- **Stride time** is the number of seconds that elapse during one stride (one complete gait cycle).
- **Step width** is the side-to-side distance between the two feet. Step width is increased in instability.
- Increased foot angle (turning the foot outward) can also result from decreased stability (for example, in an older adult's foot).

Cadence/Velocity

- Normal **cadence** is the number of steps taken per unit of time; the normal range for cadence is 91 to 138 steps per minute. Increased cadence is accompanied by a shorter step length and decreased duration of the period of double support. Running occurs when the period of double support disappears, typically at a cadence of 180 steps per minute.
- **Velocity** (walking speed) is the distance covered per unit of time (meters/minute). Average walking speed is 82 meters per minute, or approximately 3 miles per hour. Speed is increased by lengthening stride. Speed or velocity is affected by physical characteristics such as height, weight, and gender; it decreases with age, physical disability, and so forth.
- **Acceleration** is the rate of change of velocity with respect to time.
- **Energy requirements** may vary widely depending on speed of walking, stride length, body weight, type of surface, gradient, and activity (for example, stair climbing).
  - The energy cost of normal walking (at average walking speed) is 12 milliliters per kilogram of body weight per minute (mL/kg/min).
  - Increased energy costs occur with age, abnormal gait (owing to disease, muscle weakness or paralysis, or physical disability), or with the use of functional devices such as crutches, orthoses, or prostheses.
- Gait is an automatic postural activity. Neural control of gait arises from subcortical and spinal centers (spinal pattern generators). The cortex intervenes to adapt gait to environmental changes and correct motor patterns following inputs from the cerebellum.

TREATMENT STRATEGIES AND CONSIDERATIONS

- Common gait deviations involving the trunk and hip that occur during the **stance phase** include:
  - Lateral trunk bending caused by a weak gluteus medius; bending occurs to the same side as the weakness.
  - Trendelenburg gait—the pelvis drops on the contralateral side of a weak gluteus medius; a compensatory strategy is lateral trunk bending.
  - Backward trunk lean—the result of a weak gluteus maximus; the patient also has difficulty going up stairs or ramps.
  - Forward trunk lean—the result of weak quadriceps (the forward trunk lean decreases flexor moment at the knee) and hip and knee flexion contractures.
  - Excessive hip flexion—the result of weak hip extensors or tight hip and/or knee flexors.
  - Limited hip extension—the result of tight or spastic hip flexors.
  - Limited hip flexion—the result of weak hip flexors or tight extensors.
  - Abnormal synergistic activity (as in patients with stroke)—excessive hip adduction combined with hip and knee extension and plantarflexion produces a scissoring or adducted gait pattern.
  - Antalgic gait (painful gait)—stance time is abbreviated on the painful limb, resulting in an uneven gait pattern (limping); the uninvolved limb has a shortened step length, since it must bear weight sooner than normal.
- Common gait deviations involving the knee during the stance phase include:
  - Excessive knee flexion—the result of weak quadriceps (the knee wobbles or buckles) or knee flexor contractures; the patient also has difficulty going down stairs or ramps; forward trunk bending can compensate for weak quadriceps.
  - Hyperextension—the result of a weak quadriceps, plantarflexion contracture, or extensor spasticity (quadriceps and/or plantarflexion).
- Common gait deviations involving the ankle/foot during the stance phase include:
  - Toes first: the toes make contact at heel strike—the result of weak dorsiflexors, spastic or tight plantarflexors; toes first may also be due to a shortened leg (leg-length discrepancy), painful heel, or a positive support reflex.

- ◦ Foot slap: the foot makes floor contact with an audible slap—the result of weak dorsiflexors or hypotonia; the slap is compensated for with steppage gait.
  - ◦ Foot flat: the entire foot contacts ground—the result of weak dorsiflexors, limited range of motion, or an immature gait pattern.
  - ◦ Excessive dorsiflexion with uncontrolled forward motion of the tibia—the result of weak plantarflexors.
  - ◦ Excessive plantarflexion (equinus gait): the heel does not touch the ground—the result of spasticity or contracture of the plantarflexors; eccentric contraction is poor, as in tibia advancement.
  - ◦ Varus foot: at foot contact, the lateral side of the foot touches first; the foot may remain in varus throughout the stance phase—the result of spastic anterior tibialis or weak peroneals.
  - ◦ Claw toes—the result of spastic toe flexors, possibly a plantar grasp reflex.
  - ◦ Inadequate push-off—the result of weak plantarflexors, decreased range of motion, or pain in the forefoot.
- Common gait deviations involving the trunk and hip that occur during the **swing phase** include:
  - ◦ Insufficient forward pelvic rotation (pelvic retraction)—the result of weak abdominal muscles and/or weak hip flexor muscles (for example, in the patient with stroke).
  - ◦ Insufficient hip and knee flexion—the result of weak hip and knee flexors or strong extensor spasticity, resulting in an inability to lift the leg and move it forward.
  - ◦ Circumduction: the leg swings out to the side (abduction/external rotation followed by adduction/internal rotation)—the result of weak hip and knee flexors.
  - ◦ Hip hiking (quadratus lumborum action)—a compensatory response for weak hip and knee flexors, or extensor spasticity.
  - ◦ Excessive hip and knee flexion (steppage gait)—a compensatory response to shorten the limb—the result of weak dorsiflexors (for example, resulting from neuritis of the peroneal nerve in the patient with diabetes).
  - ◦ Abnormal synergistic activity (for example, in the patient with stroke): use of a strong flexor synergy pattern, resulting in excessive hip and knee flexion with abduction.
- Common gait deviations involving the knee that occur during the swing phase include:
  - ◦ Insufficient knee flexion—the result of extensor spasticity, pain, decreased range of motion, or weak hamstrings.
  - ◦ Excessive knee flexion—the result of flexor spasticity; flexor withdrawal reflex.
- Common gait deviations involving the ankle and foot that occur during the swing phase include:
  - ◦ Foot-drop (equinus)—the result of weak or delayed contraction of the dorsiflexors or spastic plantarflexors
  - ◦ Varus or inverted foot—the result of spastic invertors (anterior tibialis), weak peroneals, or an abnormal synergistic pattern (for example, in the patient with stroke)
  - ◦ Equinovarus—the result of spasticity of the posterior tibialis and/or gastrocnemius/soleus; or structural deformity (club foot).
- A common gait deviation involving the trunk and pelvis that occurs during the swing phase is decreased amplitude in trunk and pelvic rotation, which is seen in the elderly and in patients with disabilities (for example, the patient with Parkinson's disease).
- Gait that requires constant cognitive monitoring (conscious thought) is mentally fatiguing and prone to errors when the patient becomes distracted or is required to do simultaneous (dual) motor tasks such as walking while carrying an object or bouncing a ball.

THERAPEUTIC ACTIVITIES AND TECHNIQUES

Activity: Walking Forward and Backward

During initial walking, the therapist analyzes the patient's gait for deviations that interfere with walking. The patient practices walking forward and backward as a progression from stepping in place (standing, stepping). The therapist focuses on the proper timing and sequencing, beginning with the weight shift diagonally forward or backward onto the stance limb and pelvic rotation with advancement of the swing limb. It is important to ensure that knee extension (not hyperextension) occurs with hip flexion during forward progression and that knee flexion occurs with hip extension during backward progression. The movements are repeated to allow for a continuous movement sequence. **Verbal commands** are "Shift forward, and step, step, step."

Manual contacts can be used to guide movements and facilitate missing elements. For example, the therapist can assist forward pelvic rotation during swing by placing the hands on the anterior pelvis. This is an effective strategy in managing a retracted and elevated pelvis, a problem that exists for many patients with lower extremity (LE) spasticity. For backward progression, the therapist's hand can be placed posteriorly over the gluteal muscles to facilitate hip extension and weight acceptance on the stance leg. This also helps prevent the knee on the stance limb from hyperextending.

Upper extremity (UE) flexor spasticity can be reduced by using an inhibition pattern; the therapist holds the spastic limb out into extension, abduction, and external rotation.

As training progresses, the therapist can alter:
- The level of assistance or supervision: progressing from walking in the parallel bars or with assistive device(s) to unassisted walking
- The step length: from reduced to normal
- The speed of walking: from reduced to normal to increased, progressing to treadmill walking
- The base of support: from feet apart (wide based) to normal to feet together to tandem (heel-toe)
- Acceleration or deceleration: the patient practices stopping and starting or turning on command

The environment can be changed to (1) vary the support surfaces from flat to carpeted to irregular (outdoors); (2) include anticipatory timing demands such as crossing the street at a light, crossing in traffic, and catching a bus or train; and (3) include occupational requirements (return-to-work skills).

The tasks can be varied to include dual-task walking such as walking and talking, walking and turning the head (right or left and up or down), and walking and bouncing a ball.

TECHNIQUES

Resisted Progression
The therapist is in front of the patient, either standing (Fig. 14–1) or sitting on a rolling stool (Fig. 14–2). As the patient moves forward, the therapist also moves in a reverse or mirror image of the patient's movements. The therapist provides maintained resistance to the forward progression (RP) by placing both hands on the pelvis. Resistance should be light (facilitatory) to encourage proper timing of the pelvic movements. Approximation can be applied down through the top of the pelvis to assist in stabilizing responses as weight is taken on the stance limb. A stretch to the pelvic rotators can be added as needed to facilitate the initiation of the pelvic motion. Resistance can also be applied with manual contacts on the pelvis and contralateral shoulder. The position and movements are reversed for backwards walking.

Problems can arise if the therapist's movements are not synchronized with the patient's. The pacing of the activity is dependent upon the timing of the therapist's verbal commands. Movements can become uncoordinated or out of synchronization if the manual resistance on the pelvis is too great. The patient will feel as if he or she is "walking uphill" and may respond with exaggerated movements of the trunk (for example, forward head and trunk flexion). This defeats the overall purposes of facilitated walking; that is, to improve timing and sequencing of gait and to decrease effort.

Figure 14–1. Walking forward—resisted progression.

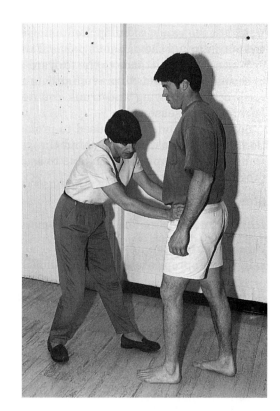

Figure 14–2. Walking forward—resisted progression (therapist seated on a rolling stool).

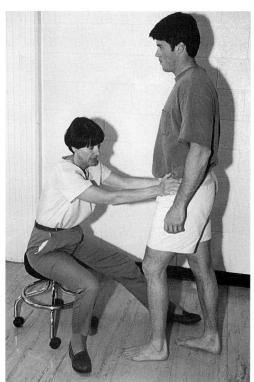

TECHNIQUES

Resisted Progression

The therapist is behind the patient, standing slightly to side in the direction of the movement. As the patient moves sidewards in braiding, the therapist moves in the same sequence and timing with the patient. The therapist provides maintained resistance to the sidewards progression (RP) by placing one hand on the side of the pelvis. The other hand alternates, first on the anterior pelvis resisting the forward pelvic motion and crossed step in front. It then slides to the posterior pelvis to resist the backward pelvic motion and crossed step behind (Fig. 14–5A and B). Resistance should be light (facilitatory) to encourage proper timing of the pelvic movements. A stretch to the pelvic rotators can be added as needed to facilitate the initiation of the pelvic motion.

Motor control stage. Skill.

Indications. RP can be used to facilitate lower trunk rotation and LE patterns with upright postural control; it helps the patient develop protective stepping strategies for balance.

Functional outcomes. The patient ambulates independently using complex stepping patterns.

Activity: Stair Climbing

Normal stair climbing involves a step-over-step pattern. The patient transfers weight onto the stance limb and lifts the dynamic limb up and onto the step. Weight is then transferred onto this limb as it extends and moves the body up and onto the step. Quadriceps and gastrocnemius activity powers the elevation of the body. Going down stairs involves a similar weight transfer onto the stance limb with an accompanying eccentric contraction of hip and knee extensors to lower the body to the next step. Weight is then transferred

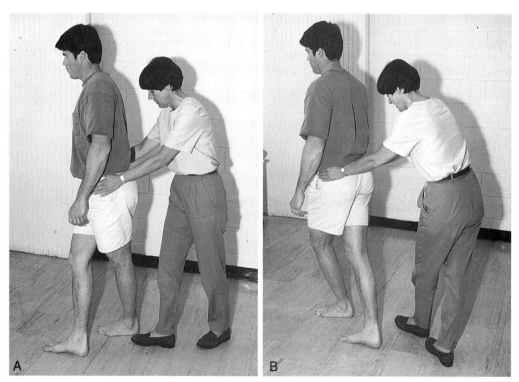

Figure 14–5A and B. Braiding—resisted progression.

onto this limb as it extends and accepts weight. The patient needs to shift weight diagonally forward over the stepping limb. The therapist should watch for, and prevent, excessive trunk bending. The sequence is repeated to allow for completion of a set of steps.

Arm support using a handrail is typically needed during early stair-climbing training to steady the body. The patient should not be allowed to pull the body up the stairs. Progression should be from light, touch-down support to no UE support.

Initial training can be facilitated by using low-rise steps and progressing to higher and finally normal-rise (7-inch—17.5 cm) steps.

The therapist provides assistance as needed. Typically, assistance to the diagonal weight shifts is required and can be accomplished by a manual contact placed on the patient's pelvis. A UE prayer position (hands clasped together with shoulder flexion and elbow extension) may be helpful in initially facilitating forward weight transfer. This position is also helpful in controlling UE spasticity. Additionally the knee extensors may require assistance. The therapist can place the other hand over the lower thigh and press downward over the quadriceps.

Motor control stage. Skill.

Indications. LE weakness of hip and knee extensors and ankle plantarflexors. Bridging, sit-to-stand transfers, kneeling to heel-sitting transfers, partial squats, and stepping activities are all important lead-up activities for stair climbing.

Functional outcomes. The patient ambulates independently up and down stairs and ambulates independently in the community, including up and down curbs.

Balance Training Activities

BENEFITS OF BALANCE TRAINING

Balance training activities can be used to:

- Improve trunk stability, biomechanical alignment, and symmetrical weight distribution
- Improve awareness and control of center of mass (COM) and limits of stability (LOS)
- Improve musculoskeletal responses necessary for balance including functional range of motion (ROM) and strength
- Promote use of normal balance strategies and synergies during static and dynamic activities
- Improve utilization of sensory (somatosensory, visual, vestibular) systems for balance and challenge CNS sensory integration mechanisms
- Teach safety awareness and compensation

Motor control goals. Skill level, static and dynamic balance control.

Functional outcomes

- The patient demonstrates appropriate functional balance during standing and walking.
- The patient performs activity-of-daily-living skills (ADLs) safely during standing and walking without loss of balance or falls.

TREATMENT STRATEGIES AND CONSIDERATIONS

- Repetition and practice are important to assist the CNS in modification and compensation of balance dysfunction.
  - Effective practice schedules can improve responsiveness of postural muscles and overall balance performance.
  - Repetition and practice provide appropriate feedback about sensory information, muscle recruitment, coordination, and postural patterns.
- Some activities may cause the patient distress initially. The patient will feel threatened when placed in situations where he or she is in jeopardy of losing balance.
  - The therapist should give a clear explanation of what is going to be done, and explain what is expected of the patient in terms that are easy to understand.
  - The therapist should ensure patient confidence and patient safety.
  - The patient should practice under close supervision at first, then progress to independent practice (a home exercise program).
- The patient needs to develop and maintain adequate lower extremity ROM and strength to withstand challenges to balance. Activities should include:
  - Standing, heel-cord stretches (wall push-ups)—for the Achilles tendon ROM
  - Standing, heel-rises—for the gastrocnemius-soleus muscles
  - Standing, toe offs—for the anterior tibial muscles
  - Standing, partial wall squats and chair rises—for the quadriceps and hip extensors
  - Side kicks, single-leg stance, or single-leg stance with the dynamic leg pushing into the wall—for the hip abductors

- ◦ Back kicks—for the hip extensors
- ◦ Marching in place—for the hip and knee flexors
- The therapist should focus on obtaining the responses necessary to maintain static balance in a symmetrical stance:
  - ◦ The therapist should help the patient improve sway in the direction of an instability (for example, the patient recovering from stroke typically needs to shift weight from the sound side toward the affected side).
- The therapist should focus on obtaining the correct postural synergies in response to disturbances of the COM:
  - ◦ Small shifts in COM alignment or slow sway movements should result in activation of an ankle strategy.
  - ◦ Larger shifts in COM alignment or faster sway movements should result in activation of a hip strategy.
  - ◦ Even larger shifts in which the COM exceeds the LOS should result in activation of stepping strategies; the patient should practice stepping in all directions.
  - ◦ Extraneous movements should be eliminated.
- Balance skills are highly task and context specific.
  - ◦ Balance control should be practiced using a variety of different functional tasks and environments.
  - ◦ Training on balance machines (for example, center of pressure biofeedback devices) should not be expected to transfer to functional balance tasks such as sit-to-stand transfers, walking, or stair climbing.
- A variety of training activities should be provided:
  - ◦ Training should progress with the patient holding in a posture (static balance) to moving in a posture (dynamic balance).
  - ◦ Training should progress with the patient standing on a stationary surface to a compliant surface (foam) or moveable surface (equilibrium or wobble board).
  - ◦ Training should progress from self-initiated voluntary challenges to posture (feed-forward and feedback-driven) to therapist-initiated (feedback-driven) challenges.
- A variety of environments should be provided:
  - ◦ Training should progress from a closed (fixed) environment to an open (variable or changing) environment.
  - ◦ Training should progress from simulated home, community, and work environments to real-life environments.
- The therapist should help the patient improve response latencies:
  - ◦ Slowed response times may result in inadequate postural responses or falls.
  - ◦ Sensory stimulation techniques (for example, quick stretch or tapping) can be used to increase responsiveness of postural muscles.
  - ◦ Functional electrical stimulation may be an effective training modality to improve responsiveness of postural muscles.

BALANCE TRAINING ACTIVITIES

The therapist appropriately varies challenges to balance, combining some activities that are relatively easy for the patient with some that are more difficult. Progression is not dependent upon successful attainment of all the activities listed at any given level. An effective motor learning strategy ensures that the patient experiences success. Thus, the therapist alternates easier activities with more difficult ones and begins and ends each treatment session with activities the patient can complete successfully.

Beginning-Level Balance Activities

These activities are appropriate for initial balance training for the patient with instability and significant disturbances in balance control.

Standing Activities

The patient is positioned in a bilateral stance on a level surface with normal or widened stance, eyes open (EO). Light touch-down support of both hands or one hand is achieved by having the patient stand near a support surface (treatment table, parallel bars, or a wall). Activities that can be practiced include:

Weight shifts in all directions—to foster re-education of the limits of stability (LOS), centered LOS.
Look-arounds—head and trunk rotation.
Head tilts—up and down, side to side.
Heel-rises—active plantarflexion.
Toe offs—active dorsiflexion. Toe offs are generally more difficult than heel offs because the COM is shifted posteriorly, where there is no effective BOS.
Single-leg stands—(Fig. 15–1).
Hip circles—body clock.

Gait Activities

The patient begins with assisted walking, using parallel bars or walking near a wall for light touch-down support; the base of support (BOS) is normal and the eyes are open (EO). Assistive devices (for example, a straight or slant cane) can be used to assist balance. A swimming pool provides an ideal supportive environment for initial walking for the patient with balance dysfunction (for example, the patient with ataxia).

Intermediate-Level Balance Activities

These activities are appropriate for the patient who is able to withstand moderate challenges to balance.

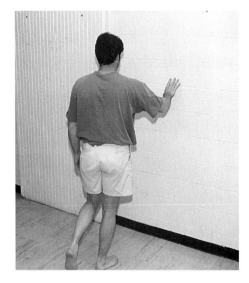

Figure 15–1. Standing: balancing, one-legged stands—light touch-down support.

Movement Transitions

Sit-to-stand transfers (chair rises) can be varied by changing the height of the seat from high to low, the speed of the transitions, or the UE support—from using a chair with armrests to no armrests.

Standing Activities

Activities that can be practiced at this level include:

Exaggerated arm swings
Functional reach activities
Reduced BOS—feet together
Eyes open (EO) to eyes closed (EC)—Romberg position
Heel offs, toe offs, or single-leg stands—holding on with light touch-down support
   of one hand, progressing to no hands
Marching in place (high stepping)—holding on with light touch-down support,
   progressing from both hands to one hand
Partial squats
Partial lunges—one foot advanced with the trunk upright and the hips in neutral
   position, with the knee flexed on the advanced limb (Fig. 15–2)

Gait Activities

Activities at the intermediate level include:

Gait with narrowed BOS
Gait with wide turns to right and left
Side-stepping—holding on with light touch-down support, progressing from both hands
   to one hand

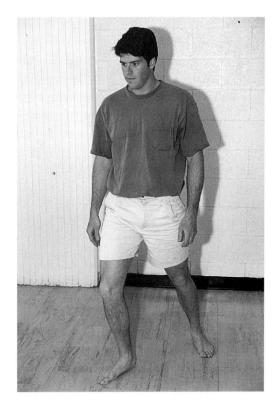

Figure 15–2. Standing: balancing, partial lunges—active movements.

Advanced-Level Balance Activities

These activities are appropriate for the patient who is able to withstand high-level challenges to balance.

Standing Activities

Activities that can be practiced at this level include:

Tandem stance (heel-toe position) progressing to sharpened or tandem Romberg (heel-toe position, eyes closed)
Single-leg stands:

   Heel offs, toe offs
   Partial squats
   Tracing the letters of the alphabet on the floor with a foot
   LE ball activities—kicking a ball

Dual-task activities—UE activities in standing:

   Bouncing a ball
   Catching or throwing a ball (vary the weight and size of the ball)
   Hitting a balloon, hitting a foam ball with a paddle

Games that involve stooping and/or aiming—bowling, shuffleboard
Squatting and lifting an object off the floor
Lunges to the half-kneeling position, progressing from UE support on a chair to no support
Floor-to-standing transfers

Gait Activities

Activities at the advanced level include:

Unassisted walking forward and backward, progressing from:

   Walking near a wall to walking in open space
   Eyes open (EO) to eyes closed (EC)
   Feet together to heel-toe/tandem walking
   Slow movements to fast while moving the head left and right

Side-stepping (without touch-down support)
Crossed-step walking, braiding
Line dancing
Gait with small turns to the right and left
Walking in 360-degree circles—first in one direction, then reversing direction
Walking in a figure-eight pattern
Stopping and starting, turning on command
Treadmill walking—progressing from slow to fast
Toe-walking, heel-walking
Walking over the rungs of a ladder—stepping through a grid
Dual-task walking—walking and bouncing or tossing a ball
Walking through an obstacle course
Walking while conversing (walkie-talkie test)—the patient's attention is diverted away from the activity of walking

Elevation Activities

Step-ups, lateral step-ups: ascend/descend platforms or steps
Vary step height from 1 inch (2.5 cm) to 8 inches (20 cm)

Stepping up and over a step or narrow platform
Stair climbing—ascent and descent
Ramps

Community Activities

Unassisted walking in a community (open) environment, including walking on uneven
  terrain
Finding solutions to real-life functional problems

  Pushing or pulling open doors
  Pushing a grocery cart
  Car transfers—getting into and out of a car
  Getting on and off a bus or other public transportation
  Carrying a bag of groceries

Anticipatory timing activities:

  Getting on an escalator or elevator
  Crossing at a busy intersection or at traffic lights

Center of Pressure Biofeedback

Force-platform retraining devices can be used to provide center of pressure (COP) feedback. The weight on each foot is computed and converted into visual feedback regarding
the locus and movement of the patient's COP. Some units also provide auditory feedback.
A computer provides data analysis and training protocols.

  Postural symmetry and limits of stability (LOS) measures can be provided to the patient. Postural sway movements can be shaped and modified to enhance symmetry, steadi-
ness, and dynamic stability. The patient can be instructed to increase or decrease his or
her sway movements or to move the COP cursor on the computer screen to achieve a designated range or to match a designated target.

  Force-platform biofeedback is an effective training device for patients who demonstrate
asymmetrical weight bearing (for example, the patient recovering from stroke who limits
weight bearing on the stroke side). Problems in force generation, producing either too
much force (hypermetria) or too little force (hypometria), can also be improved with force-
platform biofeedback. For example, the patient with Parkinson's disease who demonstrates hypometric responses can be encouraged to achieve larger and faster sway movements using force-platform training.

  A set of bathroom scales or bilateral limb-load monitors can also be used to provide
weight information and achieve symmetrical weight bearing.

Standing, Manual Perturbations

The therapist displaces the patient's center of mass (COM) in relation to the base of support (BOS). The patient is standing on a stationary surface and resists the disturbances of
the COM.

  The therapist should use manual contacts—for example, tapping the patient out of position or nudging the patient's sternum—to provide challenges that are appropriate for patient's range and speed of control. Violent perturbations—for example, pushes or shoves—
are neither necessary nor appropriate. The BOS can be varied to increase or decrease
difficulty. Perturbation training should be limited. Most demands for balance come with
normal everyday functional activities.

Standing on a Moveable Surface

The patient is standing on an equilibrium board or wobble board (see discussion of devices in section on sitting). The patient practices maintaining a centered balance position, without allowing the wobble board to touch down (Fig. 15–3) when the BOS is disturbed.

The therapist should then have the patient practice self-initiated tilts at first and then progress to therapist-initiated tilts. The therapist should observe the patient's responses carefully and use safety precautions, including appropriate spotting (guarding) to keep the patient from falling. The therapist can (1) vary the BOS to increase or decrease difficulty; or (2) vary the type of board to increase or decrease difficulty: A limited-motion board provides bidirectional challenges; a dome board provides multidirectional challenges. The profile of a domed-bottom board can be varied from low dome to high dome to increase the range of excursion. The patient can progress to unilateral (single-leg) standing—for example, on a biomechanical ankle platform system (BAPS) board. The patient can also practice standing on a foam roller.

Perturbation training can also be provided by some balance devices (for example, Equi-test by NeuroCom). Changes in the support surface provide the destabilizing challenges.

Single Limb Standing with One Foot on a Swiss Ball

The patient stands with one foot flat on the support surface and the other placed on a small Swiss ball (or roller). The patient actively rolls the ball (forward, backward, and diagonally) while maintaining upright balance (feedforward-driven balance responses). The therapist stands in front of the patient to assist as needed.

The therapist can also stand in a mirror-image position with one foot placed on the Swiss ball. Both the therapist and the patient hold onto a wand for stabilization (Fig. 15–4). The therapist's foot is used to move the ball and stimulate reactive balance challenges for the patient (feedback-driven balance responses).

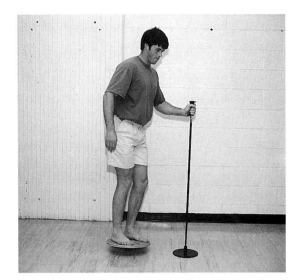

Figure 15–3. Standing: balancing on a balance board with UE support—active stabilization of a centered balance position.

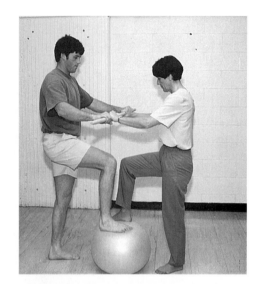

Figure 15–4. Standing: balancing with one foot on a Swiss ball—reactive balance challenges.

Sensory Training Activities

A complete sensory assessment is necessary prior to balance training in order to determine which sensory systems ar intact, disordered, or absent. CNS integration mechanisms should also be assessed (for example, using the Sensory Organization Test).

Vision Assessment

The patient should practice standing and walking with varying visual inputs:

Eyes open (EO) to eyes closed (EC)
Full lighting to reduced lighting
Goggles that reduce peripheral vision and prevent looking at feet
Petroleum-coated glasses that distort vision

Mirrors can be used to help the patient achieve upright alignment and postural control; they are contraindicated for patients with visual-perceptual deficits.

Somatosensory Assessment

The patient should practice standing and walking on varying surfaces, progressing from:

Flat surface to compliant surface—tile floor to carpet; low-pile carpet to high-pile
Foam cushion (firm density) of varying height—2 to 5 in. (Fig. 15–5)
Outside on relatively smooth terrain (sidewalks) to uneven terrain (such as grassy lawns)
Stationary to moving surfaces (escalator, elevator)

Vestibular Assessment

The patient should practice standing and walking with varying vestibular inputs:

Moving the head from side to side and up and down while standing and walking
Getting on and off a moving escalator or elevator
Standing on a moving bus, train, or subway

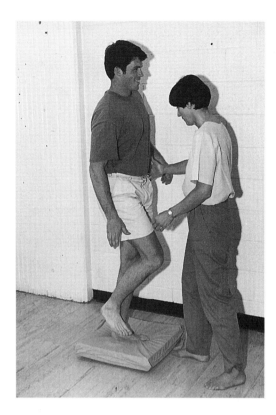

Figure 15–5. Standing: balancing on a foam cushion, single-limb support, eyes open.

Sensory Conflict Situations

The patient should practice standing and walking in sensory conflict situations:

Standing on a foam cushion with the eyes closed (EC) (Fig. 15–6)
Standing or walking on a balance instrument—for example, Equitest by NeuroCom

   As training progresses, more and more combinations of activities should be included:

Stepping in place on foam
Nodding the head up and down with the eyes closed (EC)
Walking in a busy environment

Compensatory Strategies

The patient should be instructed to:

Recognize ineffective postural strategies and superimpose voluntary (cognitive) control
   when appropriate
Maintain adequate BOS at all times:
• Widen BOS when turning or sitting down
• Widen BOS in direction of an expected force (for example, leaning into the wind)
Lower the COM when greater stability is needed—for example, crouching when a threat
   to balance is presented or a fall is imminent
Wear comfortable, well-fitting shoes with low heels and rubber soles for better friction
   and gripping
Use assistive devices—for example, (typically used by the individual who is blind) verti-
   cal or slant cane—for light touch-down support to increase somatosensory inputs

arm coupled with weakness and/or hypotonicity of rotator cuff muscles results in inferior subluxation (for example, in the patient with stroke).

- ◦ **Shoulder-hand syndrome** (reflex-sympathetic dystrophy—is associated with pain and swelling of the hands along with decreased ROM and pain at the shoulder. Dystrophic changes with severe pain may occur in the late stages; this is a debilitating condition that may be seen in the patient recovering from stroke.
- Weakness, spasticity, and abnormal synergistic patterns or reflexes may interfere with reaching.
  - ◦ Reaching may be affected by typical flexor (biceps) spasticity and corresponding triceps weakness.
  - ◦ Abnormal synergistic patterns in the UEs such as mass flexion or mass extension synergies link muscles in stereotyped, obligatory patterns:

    Mass flexion synergy links shoulder flexion, abduction, external rotation, elbow flexion, and forearm supination with wrist and finger flexion (mass grasp).
    Mass extension synergy links shoulder extension, abduction, internal rotation, elbow extension, and forearm pronation (the fingers typically remain flexed but may extend).

  - ◦ **Hyperactive traction response** is an abnormal reflex pattern in which a stretch applied to the flexor muscles of the UE at any joint results in contraction of the flexor muscles at all other joints of the same extremity (for example, in some patients recovering from stroke).
  - ◦ In the patient with stroke (hemispheric lesions), reaching is typically less affected and recovers earlier; grasping is typically more affected and recovery is less complete. The uninvolved limb may also demonstrate deficits in reaching tasks (for example, decreased accuracy and increased movement times).
- Weakness, spasticity, and abnormal synergistic patterns or reflexes may interfere with grasping movements:
  - ◦ Excess tone in the forearm leads to shortening of the finger flexors; the hand is fisted with the thumb typically adducted, making it difficult to open the hand and grasp and release.
  - ◦ When a hyperactive **grasp reflex** is present, pressure to the palm of the hand results in grasping of the object with a delayed or incomplete release.
  - ◦ Difficulty with grasping may arise from absent or weak wrist extensors; the wrist is unable to stabilize for grasping movements.
  - ◦ Difficulty with voluntary finger extension, flexion, or opposition may make the hand unable to position the fingers for grasp and release activities.
- Coordination deficits (for example, in patients with cerebellar ataxia) may produce **dysmetria**—problems with reaching movements:
  - ◦ In **hypermetria,** the patient overshoots the target during reaching movements.
  - ◦ In **hypometria,** the patient undershoots the target.
- Sensory deficits may impair both the reach and grasp components:
  - ◦ Visual deficits (for example, in the patient with optic ataxia) impair the accuracy of the reach endpoint and subsequently influence the effectiveness of grasp.
  - ◦ Somatosensory inputs are not essential for reaching movements as long as vision is intact.
  - ◦ The accuracy of complex, multijoint UE movements and grasp formation may be impaired (for example, in the patient with diabetic neuropathy).
- Motor planning disorders such as **dyspraxia** or **apraxia** may impair the execution and sequencing of reaching and grasp components. Deficits in functional performance of familiar tasks are common; for example, the patient is unable to initiate or properly sequence the steps in brushing teeth, eating, or dressing.
- Unilateral UE dysfunction may result in compensatory efforts of the sound or unaffected limb. The affected limb does not participate in functional tasks, resulting in learned nonuse of the limb; this condition is commonly seen during recovery from stroke.

○ The patient needs to be encouraged to use the affected limb even though efforts may be less successful than if the sound limb were used.
○ Continued practice increases the ease with which the affected limb moves and increases the likelihood of functional reintegration.

THERAPEUTIC ACTIVITIES AND TECHNIQUES

Eye, Head, and Hand Activities

Initial training may require beginning with eye and head movements for problems of target location (eye-hand control).

• The eyes are trained to locate a target within the central visual field, progressing to target location in the peripheral visual field.
• The eyes are trained to stabilize on a target while moving the head (vestibulo-ocular reflex control).
• The eyes and head are trained to follow a moving target.

Proximal Stabilization Activities

Initial training addresses the problems of postural stability and proximal UE control before focusing on difficulties with reach and grasp activities.

Non-Weight-Bearing Activities: Shoulder Stabilization

Active Holding
The patient is in supine position. The elbow is extended and the UE passively positioned at 90 degrees of shoulder flexion. The patient is asked to actively hold this position. This is a good initial position for stabilization training of the shoulder because of the minimized influence of gravity.

The patient can then be asked to maintain the position of the shoulder while flexing and extending the elbow. These simultaneous movements increase the difficulty of the task and promote independent or isolated joint activity. This is a useful training activity for the patient with abnormal synergistic activity (for example, the patient recovering from stroke).

The position can be modified to promote active holding in alternate positions such as sidelying, sitting, or standing. Upright positioning with the shoulder holding at 90 degrees of flexion with the elbow extended imposes a greater challenge because of the maximum effects of gravity acting on the shoulder and the increased demands for upright postural stability. The therapist can provide initial support (facilitation and assistance) and remove it as soon as the patient is able to assume voluntary control.

TECHNIQUES

Rhythmic Stabilization
The patient is positioned in supine and instructed to move in the PNF D1 flexion pattern—the UE moves up into flexion, adduction, and external rotation with the elbow held straight. As the UE moves up and across into D1F, the patient is asked to hold at approximately 90 degrees of flexion. The therapist applies isometric resistance to the shoulder flexors, adductors, and external rotators (D1 flexion pattern). The therapist then switches hands to the opposite side of the limb to resist the D1E pattern (resistance is now applied to shoulder extensors, abductors, and internal rotators) (Fig. 16–1). The therapist gives a **verbal command** ("Now hold here—don't let me move you up and across") before resistance is applied.

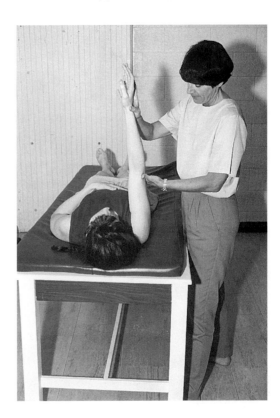

Figure 16–1. Supine: UE shoulder flexion to 90 degrees, holding—rhythmic stabilization.

Resistance is built up gradually; the patient is expected to hold the UE steady. The technique is continued for several repetitions. The patient is then asked to complete the D1E pattern and push the arm down and out to the side.

Isometric training is specific to the range of joint motion where it is applied. The therapist therefore must vary the shoulder-joint angle and apply resistance using rhythmic stabilization (RS) to the UE at various points in the range to ensure shoulder stability throughout the entire range of motion.

Rhythmic stabilization (RS) can also be applied in sitting and standing positions to increase the difficulty of the task. The upright postures require additional stabilization control of the trunk and LE muscles and recruit shoulder stabilizers in more functional postures.

Alternating isometrics (AI) is a technique that can also be used to promote shoulder stabilization. The difference between RS and AI is the absence of isometric resistance to rotators in AI.

Hold-Relax Active Motion

The patient is supine with the limb positioned in D1 extension; the shoulder is held at approximately 30 degrees of flexion. The position is similar to the UE position needed during ambulation with an assistive device or in the parallel bars. The patient is asked to hold while the therapist applies gradually increasing isometric resistance to the shoulder extensors, abductors, and internal rotators—the D1 extension pattern (Fig. 16–2). The patient is then asked to actively relax. The therapist moves the UE quickly in the opposite D1F pattern and provides a quick stretch and verbal command to push the arm down and out back to the original start position. The patient actively contracts and pushes the arm down and out. The sequence is then repeated. This is an effective procedure to improve shoulder stabilization within a functional position needed for weight bearing. Muscles needed for assisted ambulation or for push-up transfers (that is, the latissimus dorsi, teres minor, and triceps) are strengthened.

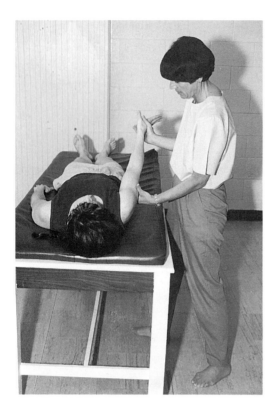

Figure 16–2. Supine: UE shoulder flexion to 30 degrees—hold-relax active motion.

Weight-Bearing Activities

Weight-bearing activities can be used to increase the challenge to shoulder stabilizers. An initial sitting position is used to reduce the degrees of freedom and overall challenges to upright posture. The elbow can be flexed (forearm weight bearing) or extended (UE weight bearing). The patient is asked to actively hold the position or may be passively assisted to hold the position. Joint compression (approximation) facilitates action of the shoulder stabilizers. The patient can actively shift weight onto the weight-bearing arm to increase proprioceptive loading or the therapist can apply approximation force down through the top of the shoulder. The therapist needs to assist the patient in correct alignment of the trunk and scapula during all weight-bearing activities.

Forearm Weight Bearing
Forearm weight bearing can be achieved with the elbow positioned on a table top in front of the patient (Fig. 16–3) or on a stool placed at the patient's side. Table-top forearm weight bearing has the added benefit of mobilizing the scapula out of a retracted position, a common problem for many patients with spasticity. This functional position can be used to gain stability for tasks such as eating, or to use the limb to stabilize paper during a writing task or a book while reading. The height and proximity of the table should be adjusted for comfortable weight bearing.

Progression is to UE weight-bearing activities with the elbows extended.

Sitting, UE Weight Bearing on Extended Elbow
With the hands still positioned anteriorly on a table top, the patient actively extends both elbows while keeping the hands stationary. This movement into a modified plantigrade (supported) position can be a useful lead-up activity to promote use of the UEs in sit-to-stand transitions.

Sitting with an extended UE bearing weight at the side is an important activity for many patients (Fig. 10–2). Either one or both UEs can be weight bearing, depending upon the stability needs of the patient. Demands for upright postural control are increased

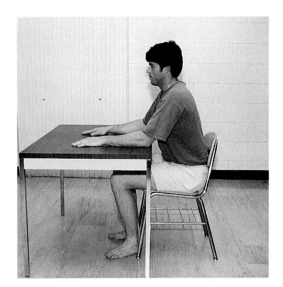

Figure 16–3. Sitting: holding, UE forearm weight bearing—active holding.

from the previous activity and extension of the trunk is promoted (especially with hands positioned to the side of the hips or behind the hips). This can be a useful lead-up activity during transfers, use of assistive devices during ambulation, or stair climbing with a rail.

Weight shifts (medial/lateral, anterior/posterior, rotational) increase the stability demands on the UE. Dynamic patterns with one limb (the dynamic limb moves in D1F and D1E) also increase the stability demands on the static limb, as does reaching forward toward the support surface.

Standing in Modified Plantigrade, UE Weight Bearing on Extended Elbows
The patient is standing with the hands open on an anteriorly placed treatment table with the shoulders flexed and the elbows extended (see Fig. 12–1). The amount of weight bearing through the UE and the range of shoulder flexion can be controlled by the position of the feet: close to the table decreases UE loading and shoulder flexion range; placement farther away from the table increases UE loading and shoulder flexion range.

The patient can also be positioned directly facing a wall, either in sitting or standing (Fig. 16–4) depending upon the degree of postural (trunk) control present. The shoulder is

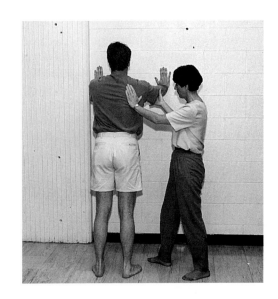

Figure 16–4. Modified plantigrade position: UEs extended and weight bearing against wall—active holding.

positioned in flexion and external rotation with the elbow extended and the hand rests anteriorly on a wall. The patient partially supports the body by leaning onto the UEs. The shoulders stabilize in a range that may be initially difficult to control (90 or 120 degrees of shoulder flexion). The therapist can assist upward rotation of the scapula and stabilization of the elbow in extension. The patient can also practice modified push-ups in this position to improve elbow extension control.

An alternate position is to have the patient face sidewards to the wall, stabilizing the UE in elbow extension with the shoulder in 90 degrees of abduction. This can be a useful training activity for the patient with stroke who is beginning to break out of flexion synergy dominance (flexion, abduction, external rotation with elbow flexion).

Prone-on-Elbows, Quadruped

The most difficult weight-bearing positions for shoulder stabilization are prone-on-elbows (see Fig. 8–5) and quadruped (see Fig. 8–10). Both positions require maximum loading on the shoulder at 90 degrees of shoulder flexion. Patients should be challenged in postures with decreased stabilization requirements prior to attempting these postures.

Comments

Scapular winging with movement of a portion of the scapula protruding off the thorax is an indication of serratus weakness and scapulothoracic instability. This situation must not be allowed to persist as it will likely further increase weakness and stability. The therapist must recognize the posture in which scapular winging is occurring is too stressful; the patient's position should be modified immediately. Weight-bearing demands should be reduced by selecting a less challenging posture.

Weight shifting during UE weight bearing can be used to increase glenohumeral range of motion and scapulothoracic mobility.

The presence of UE hypertonicity (typically elbow flexion with forearm pronation and wrist and finger flexion) can be effectively addressed by rocking while weight bearing (for example, sitting extended UE weight bearing). Slow vestibular stimulation coupled with inhibitory positioning (secondary stretch) provides relaxing input and promotes lengthening of spastic muscles. The patient's hand should be open and flat on the supporting surface. This position provides additional inhibitory pressure and relaxation to spastic wrist and finger flexors. Initially, a tightly fisted hand can be opened by grasping the thumb and moving it into extension and abduction using rhythmic rotation, then applying counter pressure to the tops of the fingers while gripping the fingertips. The patient's hand may need to be initially positioned on the therapist's knee to allow for slight wrist and finger flexion. As relaxation occurs with rocking, the patient's hand can be shifted to the flat surface of the mat.

Weakness of elbow extensors can be problematic in maintaining an extended elbow UE weight-bearing position. The triceps can be facilitated by tapping directly over the muscle belly. Rhythmic stabilization (RS) can also be applied directly to the UE with the elbow holding in slight flexion (hyperextension is avoided). This technique is used to facilitate stability control of the elbow. The therapist can also provide manual assistance to stabilize the position of the shoulder and elbow (generally by gripping the patient under the axillae). For patients in whom triceps control is absent, a forward shoulder with glenohumeral external rotation can be used to mechanically lock the elbow into extension (for example, for the patient with quadriplegia).

Motor control goal. Stability, static postural control.

Indications. Weakness, instability of the shoulder and UE stabilizing muscles.

Functional outcomes. The patient is able to independently stabilize the shoulder in all positions needed for UE function; the patient performs basic activities of daily living (BADLs—bathing, grooming, dressing, feeding).

Reach Training Activities

Training activities for reaching include initial practice of the reach component without the grasp component.

* Practice is focused on different directions and ranges of motion:
  ○ Forward reaching
  ○ Sideward reaching
  ○ Backward reaching
  ○ Reaching across the midline (Fig. 16–5)
  ○ Reaching away from the midline
* Practice is directed to different combinations of shoulder and elbow motions:
  ○ Reach with shoulder and elbow flexion (close to the body)
  ○ Reach with shoulder flexion and elbow extension (reaching away from the body)
  ○ Reach with shoulder extension and elbow flexion
  ○ Reach with shoulder external/internal rotation
  ○ Reach with forearm pronation/supination
* Practice is directed toward different functional tasks:
  ○ Reach and lift
  ○ Reach and move toward body
  ○ Reach to the top of the head (needed for BADLs such as combing the hair)
  ○ Reach to the opposite arm (needed for BADLs such as bathing)

The therapist must ensure normal trunk, scapula, and shoulder alignment during all reach training activities. Postural instability may need to be addressed initially by using supported positioning of the trunk. Progression is then made to sitting without support.

Difficulty in control of UE movement patterns can be reduced by controlling the degrees of freedom present with multijoint control. Manual assistance is given as needed to promote optimal limb function and reduce errors. Guided movements should be eliminated as soon as the patient is able to assume voluntary control of the movement.

Resistive Patterns

Resistance can be used to increase proprioceptive loading and kinesthetic awareness of limb movements. Resistance also improves strength and synergistic action (coordination)

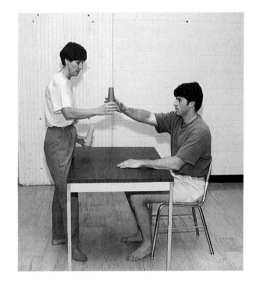

Figure 16–5. Sitting: UE reaching across midline—active movements.

of UE muscles. The patient can be positioned in sitting, modified plantigrade, or standing, depending upon the degree of postural control present. Theraband tubing, weight cuffs, or wall pulleys can be used to provide mechanical resistance.

The following synergistic PNF patterns can be lightly resisted to promote improved control in reaching:

PNF UE D2F (shoulder flexion, abduction, external rotation) with the elbow straight or extending promotes overhead reaching out to the side of the body, which is useful in instrumental activities of daily living (IADLs) such as reaching for cabinets overhead (see Fig. 12–2).

PNF UE D2F (shoulder flexion, abduction, external rotation) with elbow flexing promotes overhead reaching to the top of the head, which is useful in basic grooming tasks.

PNF UE D1F (shoulder flexion, adduction, external rotation) with the elbow straight or extending promotes overhead reaching across the midline of the body, which is important for the patient with unilateral neglect of one side of the body (see Fig. 10–7B).

PNF UE D1F (shoulder flexion, adduction, external rotation) with the elbow flexing promotes reaching to the mouth or opposite shoulder, which is useful for many BADLs such as feeding and grooming.

PNF UE D1 Thrust (shoulder flexion, adduction with elbow extension and forearm pronation) promotes forward reaching, which is useful in bringing the hand in front of the body to protect the face with the elbow extended (see Fig. 10–10A).

PNF UE D1 Reverse Thrust (shoulder extension, abduction with elbow flexion and forearm supination) promotes scapula adduction with shoulder extension, which is useful to bring the hand flexed and close to the body in a withdrawal pattern (see Fig. 10–10B) or pulling motion.

Bilateral patterns: Bilateral symmetrical and asymmetrical patterns combine to allow performance of many different functional tasks such as raking or shoveling snow, and sports-related activities such as paddling a canoe.

Motor control goal. Controlled mobility, static-dynamic control.

Indications. Weakness, impaired motor control of UE muscles (for example, in the patient with ataxia).

Functional outcomes. The patient is able to move the upper limbs in all directions needed for UE function; the patient independently performs basic activities of daily living (BADLs) such as bathing, grooming, dressing and feeding.

Grasp Training Activities

Training activities for the grasp component of functional activities are task dependent, shaped by the size, weight, shape, and use of the object to be grasped.

- Practice is directed toward everyday objects with varying sizes, shapes, weights and textures—for example, grasping a cup or a ball (Fig. 16–6).
- Practice is directed toward different functional tasks—for example, drinking from a cup or mug, eating with a spoon or fork, and so on.
- The grasp component is initially isolated from reaching—for example, the object to be grasped is positioned close to the patient's body, with the UE supported on a table top.

The therapist may need to guide the patient's movements initially and provide verbal cues for the movements desired, such as "Open your hand and grasp this object." Initial pre-positioning of the limb may be necessary; for example, supination may need to be combined with an open hand to facilitate function.

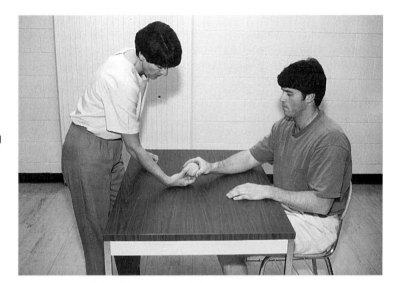

Figure 16–6. Sitting: grasping a ball—active movements.

Reach and Grasp Training Activities

Training activities are progressed to include activities that involve both reach and grasp components.

* The object is positioned away from the patient's body. The patient must reach toward the object and grasp the object; for example, the patient must pick up an object and reposition it, pick up an object and throw it, or pick up an object and manipulate it.
* Practice is directed toward transporting an object; for example, the patient must pick up an object and move it toward the body.
* The patient must bring an object to the mouth as needed for eating or drinking (Fig. 16–7A and B).
* The patient must bring an object to the head as needed for combing the hair or washing the face.

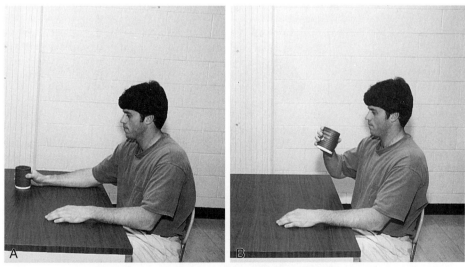

Figure 16–7A and B. Sitting: reach and grasp exercise using a cup—active movements.

Resistive Patterns

Hand opening with a reach component can be promoted by using the PNF UE D2F or D1E patterns. Resistance is directed to train and strengthen the wrist and finger extensors. Hand closing with a reach component can be promoted by using the PNF UE D1F and D2E patterns. Resistance is directed to train and strengthen wrist and finger flexors.

Bimanual Tasks

Training activities that involve simultaneous use of both UEs (bimanual tasks) should be introduced as soon as possible. The patient is instructed to:

- Grasp a wand or cane and raise it to the forward horizontal position, overhead, or out to the side (cane exercises); the range can be varied to increase difficulty
- Catch and throw a ball: the size and weight of the ball can be varied to increase or decrease difficulty; for example, the patient can progress from a kickball to a weighted medicine ball)
- Pick up an object (for example, a plate or box) with both hands and reposition it; size and weight can be varied to increase difficulty
- Pour a liquid from one cup to another (Fig. 16–8)
- Use a knife and fork to cut up food

Reach and Grasp Activities with Trunk Movements

Training activities involve simultaneous use of UE reach and grasp components with trunk movements, as in the following activities:

- In sitting position, the patient must bend forward and pick up an object off the floor (this requires trunk flexion and extension with reach and grasp.
- In sitting or standing, the patient must turn and reach to one side or behind to grasp an object (this requires trunk rotation with reach and grasp.
- In standing, the patient must stoop and pick up an object off the floor (this requires trunk and LE flexion and extension with reach and grasp).

Comments

Rehabilitation of upper limb function requires repetition and practice of functional tasks. The therapist can assist in re-establishing desired patterns through optimal positioning and structuring the practice of the desired movement patterns. The patient should be instructed in ways to reduce or eliminate undesired or unnecessary movement components. A direct, hands-on approach (using guided and/or facilitated movements) should be lim-

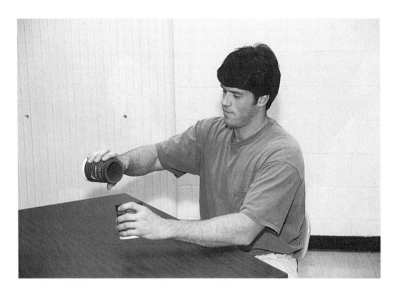

Figure 16–8. Sitting: pouring from one cup to another—active movements.

ited to early training. The focus should be on active movements and active learning. Upper limb tasks involve complex combinations of movements and necessitate training using a variety of movement combinations. Early practice of daily life tasks and situations is important to ensure desired functional outcomes.

Motor control goal. Controlled mobility and skill.

Indications. Impaired motor control of UE—for example, in the patient with weakness, ataxia, and/or abnormal synergistic patterns.

Functional outcomes. The patient is able to use the upper limb for daily function. The patient independently performs basic activities of daily living (BADLs) such as bathing, grooming, dressing, and feeding, and instrumental activities of daily living (IADLs) such as writing, meal preparation, housekeeping tasks, money management, and so on.

Clinical Decision Making: Application to Functional Training

This portion of the manual focuses on practice activities for clinical problem solving with emphasis on functional training. It provides an opportunity to apply content from Sections I and II to specific clinical problems and case-study examples. It is divided into two segments, with sequential introduction of more comprehensive clinical management problems as the segments progress.

This section is designed in workbook format. The learner is provided progressively more challenging units of information about clinical problems and is asked to make critical decisions about how to address the problems or needs of the patient presented. A variety of clinical examples are offered at levels representing the complexity of challenge inherent in clinical practice. More examples may be offered than is necessary for the learner to become skillful with the specific level of decision making. As the levels of practice required will differ from learner to learner, the number of applications required to gain mastery will also vary.

CLINICAL DECISION MAKING

Within the context of the clinical applications, practice activities are designed to promote clinical decision-making skills. The learner is encouraged to place considerable emphasis on developing and practicing these skills, as they provide the bases on which effective, comprehensive, and cost-efficient treatment can be systematically planned. This process of clinical decision making, also called clinical reasoning, refers to the thinking, problem analysis, and decision making that provide the foundation for sound clinical practice. Focusing attention on the interrelated steps inherent in clinical decision making will assist the learner in establishing an effective model for selection of interventions, analysis of treatment decisions, exploration of alternative treatment options, assessment of results, and development of treatment outcomes compatible with the needs of the individual patient. The steps comprising the foundation for clinical decision making include: (1) collection of patient data, (2) data analysis and formulation of a problem list, (3) identification of outcomes and priorities, (4) development of treatment intervention(s), (5) implementation of treatment, and (6) assessment of patient response and outcomes of treatment.

Feedback is a critical feature in promoting learning of any new task or activity. This is particularly true in development of decision-making skills to address specific clinical problems, as several options are likely available to confront a single problem. Decision making will require logical selection of the best treatment option(s), how and why several options might be combined to facilitate a desired outcome, and how these interventions should be sequenced. The number of *practice repetitions* as well as the *type and amount of feedback* required for acquisition of decision-making skills will vary among learners. This process will be highly influenced by the individual's preferred learning style and optimum mode of feedback. The learner is encouraged to proceed at an *individual pace* and to obtain *feedback at intervals* compatible with a *preferred learning style.* Input on responses can be obtained by: (1) referring back to specific content areas in Sections I and II of this laboratory manual, (2) consulting the suggested readings provided at the end of the manual, (3) reviewing the questions for review, references, and supplemental reading lists in O'Sullivan, and Schmitz,[1] (4) individual or group interaction with peers, (5) classroom discussions and case presentations with course faculty, and (6) consulting Appendix A for suggested answers to the clinical problems. Please note that the answers provided in Appendix A represent only one possible solution to a given problem. Because of the variety of treatment options available, the selection of an alternative position, activity, or technique may be equally effective in accomplishing a desired outcome. These situations clearly warrant feedback from colleagues or instructors.

Consideration of the sample clinical problems presented here should be addressed with recognition that patient management has, in many respects, entered a new and challenging phase for physical therapists. Fundamental changes within the health care system have created a cost-conscious environment requiring therapists to provide more efficient care in less time. The frequency of visits for most patients as well as the overall duration of treatment has been reduced. The length of stay for inpatient services has been reduced for most diagnoses in almost all settings. The proliferation of managed-care plans designed to control medical expenditures has placed restrictions on the patient's choice of health care providers (typically, care is available only through preferred providers affiliated with the program). In addition to constraints imposed by these changes, therapists must also address such issues as prior authorization (approval from the managed-care plan to establish the course of treatment), case managers (individuals who function to monitor and assess treatment strategies for specific diagnoses), diagnostic "pathways of care" (diagnosis-driven allocation of services), and capitation (contractual agreements with set fee schedules for services provided).

These combined influences have confronted therapists with the critical need to optimize the available treatments to achieve desired outcomes in a shorter time. Well-honed clinical decision-making skills are perhaps the therapist's greatest ally in this atmosphere of rapid change. They allow selection of the optimum treatment intervention to achieve the desired outcome in the most efficient and cost-effective manner. These skills also permit the therapist to make logical decisions about optimizing intensity of treatment strategies with emphasis on functional training and outcomes. Emphasis on function assists in preparing the patient for safe discharge or transition to the next level of care. Therapists have also placed a priority on earlier use of adjunctive (supportive) treatments to achieve desired outcomes within established time constraints. Although adjunctive treatments are time-honored components of treatment, they have taken on more important roles as earlier interventions to help achieve the desired response to treatment. For example, greater emphasis is placed on early education with a shift in selected treatment responsibilities to the patient and family, physical therapist assistants, and home health aides. Focus has also been directed toward effective use of home exercise programs and patient involvement in formal group exercise programs.

Skill in clinical decision making also assists the therapist with integration of information from an expanding knowledge base. New theories of motor control have required therapists to confront critical decisions about how these theories might be integrated into clinical practice. For example, the systems theory has provided new information about how the central nervous system (CNS) controls movement. This information has challenged therapists to design rehabilitation interventions based on experience and new understanding of CNS function, together with knowledge of specific task requirements and the implications of different environmental contexts.

The most logical model for developing strategies to improve motor control and motor learning appears to rely on incorporating useful aspects of traditional rehabilitation approaches with new information about the ways the brain controls movement. New information from the neuroscience literature has called into question some components of traditional therapeutic interventions. For example, there is now considerable evidence that the CNS demonstrates a high level of flexibility and does not function in a rigid, top-down hierarchical manner, as was once believed. This early assumption of a hierarchical organization within the CNS provided the foundation for many physical therapy treatment interventions. It led to the notion that brain injury resulted in abnormal movement because of loss of inhibitory control normally imposed by higher centers. This "released" lower centers to function without the modulating influence from higher center control. Owing to this loss of inhibition, movements then became automatic, stereotypical, and more primitive, with marked abnormalities of tone. It was further assumed that function would follow a predictable, sequential pattern of recovery that modeled the progression of normal human motor development.

The systems theory presents the concept of a distributed mode of motor control with units of the CNS organized around specific task demands. Highly skilled or complex tasks may involve the entire CNS; only portions of the CNS may be needed for simple tasks. Normal motor control appears to be achieved through integrated action of CNS systems. Theoretical understanding of the CNS is incomplete, evolving, and changing. However, our current knowledge base strongly suggests approaching treatment with focus on *integrated function*.

Motor learning theory has also provided new and important considerations for treatment. Motor learning theory suggests that changes in the CNS can be inferred through *changes in motor behaviors*. Improvements in motor behavior such as improved control or timing are dependent on **practice** of the desired outcome together with appropriate feedback. This information has directed attention to new and effective strategies for facilitating motor learning. It has also presented the therapist with a variety of areas for clinical decision making leading to effective integration of both *practice* and *feedback* into a specific treatment plan with consideration to the individual learning needs of the patient.

TERMINOLOGY

The acquisition of skill in clinical decision making and treatment interventions should be accompanied by a developing understanding of the appropriate terminology to document patient status and communicate findings. Although this has always been a professional responsibility for physical therapists, consistent and accurate verbal communication and written documentation takes on greater implications in an era of cost containment. It allows the therapist to provide justification for treatment provided, provides data on patient response to treatment or changes in functional status, supports additional requests for treatment, and assists with establishing an open line of communication with the insurance company case manager. As the reader may already be aware, common terminology among physical therapists, other disciplines, and insurance providers offers several important benefits. Use of common terms facilitates communication both among physical therapists as well as with the disciplines and third-party payment agencies with whom we collaborate and interact. It typically allows for greater accuracy in reporting patient data owing to an understanding of the exact nature of a standard meaning. It may also speed communication by allowing a distinct explanation to be conveyed by a single word or phrase by virtue of a commonly accepted definition.

In many ways, terminology provides a historical chronicle to our profession. As older theories and forms of treatment have been replaced by new theories and interventions, new terminology has been introduced. Older terms may be considered less descriptive or even obsolete. Although the evolution is a slow process, language within the health fields will continue to evolve as new research, technological advances, and treatment interventions are introduced.

From a more global perspective, to facilitate communication among health organizations in various countries around the world, the World Health Organization (WHO) has advocated the use of common terminology. The WHO's *International Classification of Impairments, Disabilities, and Handicaps* (ICIDH) provides a systematic framework for identification and classification of clinical observations.[9] Unique to the recommendations of the WHO is movement away from the traditional biomedical model, which lends itself to describing patients on the basis of disease characteristics. The use of such descriptors is nonspecific, precludes quantification, and, perhaps most importantly, does not acknowledge the dignity of the patient as an individual functioning within the context of specific psychological, cultural, and social influences.

The notion of a uniform definition of terms, is critical to the widespread exchange of ideas and scientific findings. The work of Guccione,[10] Nagi,[11] and Schenkman and Butler[12] provides excellent references for further understanding the need for, and development of, terminology based on a uniform conceptual framework. Several terms are of particular importance within this developing framework and will be described here. These terms include: **impairment** (direct, indirect and composite), **disability,** and **handicap.** These specific terms are uniquely important because of their common and frequent use in describing dysfunction. **Direct impairments** are the result of pathology or disease state and include any deviations from normal physiologic, anatomic, or psychologic function.[9] Examples include direct manifestations of a disease state or insult such as diminished range of motion (ROM) or strength, sensory loss, impairments in motor planning, or trunk rigidity or instability. Impairments may or may not be permanent.

Schenkman and Butler[12] suggest a further delineation within the definition of impairment and have expanded it to differentiate among direct (defined above), indirect, and composite effects of pathology. **Indirect impairments** are those occurring *not* from the specific insult but from sequelae (secondary complications) of the insult. Indirect impairments might include respiratory involvement, contractures, renal calculi, and deep venous thrombosis. Indirect impairments occur in systems other than the one affected by the primary insult. They are frequently associated with prolonged inactivity, inadequate positioning, or lack of regular physical therapy or other rehabilitation intervention. **Composite impairments** are those with multiple underlying origins. These include both direct impairments (from the specific lesion) and indirect impairments. Abnormal endurance and balance deficits are examples of composite impairments.[12] Two other terms provided uniform definitions are **disability** and **handicap. Disability** refers to an inability to complete a functional task within parameters typically considered reasonable or normal for that individual. Disability results from impairments and is categorized as either physical, mental, social, or emotional.[9,11] **Handicap** encompasses the social disadvantages imposed by impairment or disability. It is exemplified by the inability to fulfill a social, family, or employment role normally ascribed to an individual.[10,11]

Nagi's model [10,11,13,14] varies somewhat from the terminology proposed by the ICIDH. This model incorporates four terms: **disease, impairment, functional limitation,** and **disability.** The definitions of diseased and impairment are consistent with the ICIDH model. However, **functional limitation** is defined as the inability to perform a task, expectations of usual role responsibilities, or typical daily activities as a result of impairment. Disability includes overall patterns of behavior associated with the presence of long-term impairments imposed by functional limitations.

The Functional Independence Measure (FIM[SM]) instrument* is an assessment scale of functional status that provides standard terminology for describing performance.[15] The FIM instrument (Figure 1) is a component of the Uniform Data Set for Medical Rehabilitation (UDS[MR][SM]). Function is scored using a seven-point scale, ranging from seven (7), which represents complete independence, to one (1), which indicates total assistance is

---

*FIM[SM] is a service mark of the Uniform Data System for Medical Rehabilitation, a division of U B Foundation Activities, Inc.

UDS$_{MR}$^{SM} FIM^{SM} Instrument

	ADMISSION*	DISCHARGE*	GOAL
SELF-CARE			
A. Eating			
B. Grooming			
C. Bathing			
D. Dressing - Upper			
E. Dressing - Lower			
F. Toileting			
SPHINCTER CONTROL			
G. Bladder			
H. Bowel			
TRANSFERS			
I. Bed, Chair, Whichair			
J. Toilet			
K. Tub, Shower			
LOCOMOTION	W-Walk C-wheelChair B-Both		
L. Walk/Wheelchair			
M. Stairs			
COMMUNICATION	A-Auditory V-Visual B-Both		
N. Comprehension			
O. Expression			
SOCIAL COGNITION	V-Vocal N-Nonvocal B-Both		
P. Social Interaction			
Q. Problem Solving			
R. Memory			

* Leave no blanks. Enter 1 if not testable due to risk.

FIM LEVELS

No Helper

7 Complete Independence (Timely, Safely)

6 Modified Independence (Device)

Helper - Modified Dependence

5 Supervision (Subject = 100%)

4 Minimal Assistance (Subject = 75% or more)

3 Moderate Assistance (Subject = 50% or more)

Helper - Complete Dependence

2 Maximal Assistance (Subject = 25% or more)

1 Total Assistance or not testable (Subject less than 25%)

Figure 17–1. The Functional Independence Measure (FIM^{SM}) instrument scores function using a seven-point scale based on percentage(s) of active participation from patient. (From the Uniform Data System for Medical Rehabilitation, a division of UB Foundation Activities, Inc. [UDS$_{MR}$^{SM}]. Copyright 1996. Guide for the Uniform Data Set for Medical Rehabilitation [including the FIM^{SM} instrument], Version 5.0. Buffalo, NY: State University of New York at Buffalo; 1996, with permission).

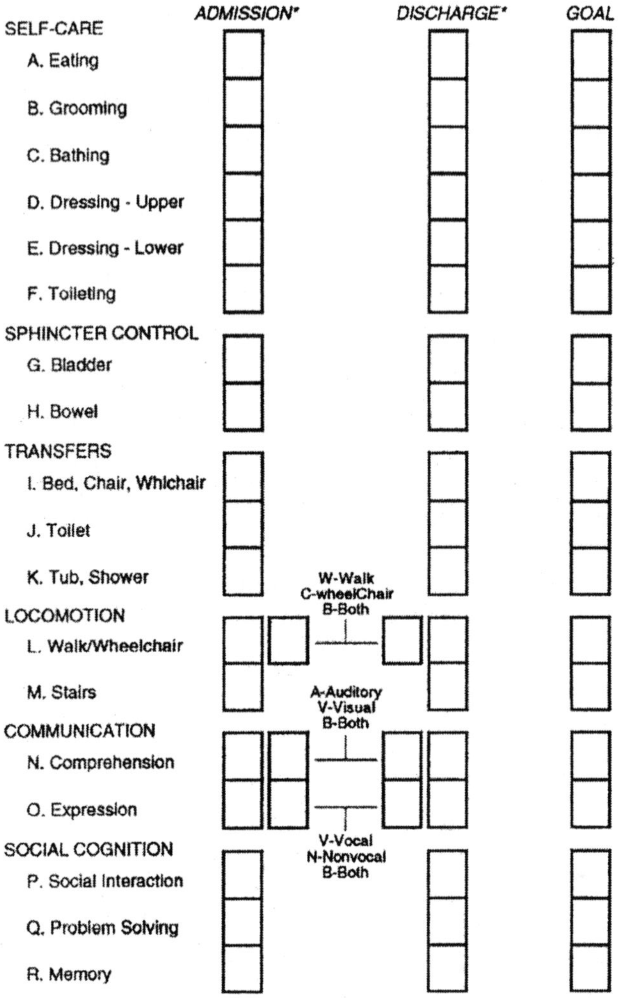

needed. The majority of intervening scores are defined by percentage of capability. For example, minimal contact assistance (level 4) represents a level of performance at which the patient accomplishes 75 percent of the task.

LITERATURE RESOURCES

The suggested readings listed at the end of this manual address key elements of specific treatment interventions, clinical decision making and use of common terminology in health care. The list represents only a small segment of the literature available in these content areas. The readings have been selected on the basis of both topic focus as well as their collective scope and breadth of content coverage.

The suggested readings included have several intended uses for the learner. The readings represent the work of key authors and will provide the learner with additional information on both the conceptual framework and practical application of the content areas. The suggested readings will also direct the interested learner on a guided course of additional study. Many of the suggested readings have a carefully constructed reference list to assist in further exploration of an area of interest. The readings can also serve the learner well as a focus for discussion between or among learning colleagues. This may be particularly useful during the early stages of learning, when decisions may be somewhat tentative. Combining progression through this clinical applications section together with consulting the literature and participation in discussion groups offers the inherent opportunity for feedback. Importantly, it will allow decision analysis in practice activities among learning colleagues with consideration of a larger theoretical framework on which a technique might be based. This will provide both *immediate feedback and knowledge of results.*

Clinical Decision Making: Focus on Clinical Problems

This initial section focuses on individual clinical problems as a precursor to more comprehensive case studies. It presents a series of problems involving different patients and allows the learner to make critical decisions on a possible treatment option. Focus is placed on selection, application, and justification (outcomes) for treatment using **functional training** activities.

Directions: For each of the following clinical problems, identify the **position/activity, technique, manual contacts,** and **goal** of the intervention selected to address the deficit. Inherent in this process is selecting the optimum treatment intervention. Practice activities should include developing a list of all the possible options for addressing a problem. The rationale for selection of a treatment option should be identified together with justification for it being the best possible course of action.

Note that some of the clinical problems also include guiding questions. These guiding questions are intended to direct the learner's attention to a specific aspect of the patient problem or treatment (for example, modifying an intervention in response to an unexpected outcome or patient's response, altering a treatment to make it of greater or lesser challenge, use of cognitive input, consideration of reflex influence, and so forth). Note also that this first section addresses developing treatment decisions to specific clinical problems. Details regarding patient history, medical status, or treatment interventions have been *intentionally omitted* to allow focus on this initial phase of decision making.

Remember that *practice* is at the heart of all learning and that mastery—*independent performance with relatively few errors*—is the goal of practice. However, practice requires appropriate and guided support until independence is achieved. Structured practice, within the context of these clinical problems, must be accompanied by consistent, supportive *feedback*. This will include reinforcement of correct practice as well as corrective feedback for errors produced.

CLINICAL PROBLEM 1

▼ A 27-year-old patient presents with *generalized weakness and low tone* following brain injury secondary to a motor vehicle accident. The intention of treatment is to facilitate active movement in rolling as a component of the initial progression. To date, isometric contractions of moderate holding capability have been achieved in the trunk muscles using the sidelying position. Midrange, and, inconsistently, full-range trunk movement has been accomplished with dynamic verbal commands and guided movements (using the technique of hold-relax active movement). Upper extremity movements are weak and uncoordinated. The focus is now on facilitating active movement from supine to sidelying position, working toward independent rolling.

Guiding Questions

1. Identify the position/activity, technique, manual contacts, and outcome (goal) of the intervention selected to address the clinical problem.

2. How many times should the selected technique be practiced with this patient? What would be used as a marker that sufficient practice has occurred?

3. What modifications in both *upper* and *lower extremity* positioning could be used to make this activity less challenging and more successful for the patient?

CLINICAL PROBLEM 2

▼ A 24-year-old patient presents with ***diminished ankle control*** secondary to a bi-malleolar fracture sustained during a fall from the parallel bars while practicing gymnastics. The fracture sites are stable and healed. Full weight bearing in upright postures is *not permitted;* weight bearing *to tolerance* during mat activities is encouraged. You are currently working on lower trunk activities and directing attention to other problems sustained in the fall. You have successfully progressed through hooklying, lower trunk rotation, holding, and have recently been focusing on controlled mobility activities using active techniques. A portion of your goal for the next component of treatment is to select an activity that allows for (1) early weight bearing through the foot and ankle without the body-weight demands of a fully upright posture, and (2) use of resisted techniques to recruit foot and ankle musculature.

Guiding Questions

1. Identify the position/activity, technique, manual contacts, and outcome (goal) of the intervention selected to address the clinical problem.

2. Provide a justification for your selection of hand placement. What specific advantage did this hand placement provide?

3. Describe application of the technique you selected. Consideration should be given to therapist position, type of contraction, and verbal cues.

CLINICAL PROBLEM 3

▼ You are continuing treatment for the same 24-year-old patient presented in Clinical Problem 2 with ***diminished ankle control.*** Response to the treatment activity described above has been good. You are ready to continue progressive weight-bearing challenges during mat activities for the affected ankle. The primary goals for your next segment of treatment are to focus on dynamic control while incorporating progressive stabilization and weight-bearing demands.

Guiding Questions

1. Identify the position/activity, technique, manual contacts, and outcome (goal) of the intervention selected to address the clinical problem.

2. What is the purpose of your manual contacts during the initial application of this treatment intervention?

3. The upper extremities can provide varying elements of stabilization during treatment activities. Contrast the upper extremity positioning you would use during *initial training* versus *later training* as control progresses.

4. During early use of this activity, you notice the patient is demonstrating initial difficulty in maintaining a level pelvis. How might you address this problem?

5. In planning for this segment of treatment, which lower extremity would be the initial support limb? What movement demands would you place on the free limb as control develops? What is the purpose of these movements?

CLINICAL PROBLEM 4

▼ A 64-year-old patient with a right above-knee amputation displays **diminished range of motion** at the hip owing to hip flexor tightness. The amputation was performed 3 years ago secondary to a long-standing history of peripheral vascular disease. Four weeks ago the patient underwent bilateral cataract removal. The patient had been ambulatory using a prosthesis for functional distances prior to the eye surgery. However, the recent surgical intervention together with the temporary visual impairment prevented participation in functional activities during the recovery period. Current passive hip flexion range of motion is 20 to 100 degrees.

Guiding Question

1. Identify the position/activity, technique, manual contacts, and outcome (goal) of the intervention selected to address the clinical problem.

CLINICAL PROBLEM 5

▼ This problem refers to the same 64-year-old patient with a right above-knee amputation presented in Clinical Problem 4 above. Muscle tightness must always be considered with reference to its potential influence on both sides of a joint. With tightness in the hip flexors, one might reasonably expect reduction in strength of the opposing muscle. This might occur because of an inability of the hip extensors to move into their full range (secondary to flexor tightness) combined with the effects of an overall reduction in activity imposed by the surgery. The hip flexor tightness has now been diminished by the intervention selected above. Assume the selection for a treatment activity is within the *controlled mobility* stage of motor control. Identify the position/activity, technique, manual contacts, and goal of an intervention for addressing **hip extensor weakness.**

Guiding Questions

1. Identify the position/activity, technique, manual contacts, and outcome (goal) of the intervention selected to address the clinical problem.

2. What is the general, overall outcome of treatment for the controlled mobility stage of motor control?

3. What implications do the strength of the hip extensor muscles have for a patient with an above-knee amputation using a quadrilateral socket?

4. How can the technique selected be made either more challenging or less challenging for this patient?

5. Consider that a decision was made to apply both quick stretches and resistance during the hip extension exercises. What are the inherent benefits of each? How would they be applied within the context of treatment for this patient?

CLINICAL PROBLEM 6

▼ A 78-year-old patient with Parkinson's disease has been experiencing *diminished rotational movements of the trunk* that interfere with movement transitions and functional skills. The recent focus of treatment has been on facilitating controlled mobility in rolling. Within the past two treatments, moderate success has been achieved in accomplishing log rolling; tracking resistance appears particularly useful in facilitating movement for this patient. The next outcome (goal) of treatment for this patient is to promote segmental upper and lower trunk rotation.

Guiding Questions

1. Identify the position/activity, technique, manual contacts, and outcome (goal) of the intervention selected to address the clinical problem.

2. What verbal input might be provided to the patient to facilitate the desired response for the treatment goal?

3. What is tracking resistance? How can it be used for this patient to promote upper and lower trunk rotation?

4. In addition to tracking resistance, what other sensory stimulation technique might be used?

CLINICAL PROBLEM 7

▼ Both this problem (7) and problem 8 refer to the same 78-year-old individual with Parkinson's disease described in Clinical Problem 6. Assume the patient has been responsive to your treatment and is now relaxed and can actively move in the pattern. How can you alter the selection of your technique from Clinical Problem 6 to promote increased controlled mobility function?

Guiding Questions

1. Identify the position/activity, technique, manual contacts, and outcome (goal) of the intervention selected to address the clinical problem.

2. Would the progression of activity for upper and lower trunk rotation include movement through *increments* or *decrements* of range? What is the major distinguishing

factor between normal and abnormal responses during activities within the controlled mobility stage of motor control?

3. Assume that during application of your technique you note that the patient demonstrates difficulty in completing the contraction in the shortened range. How would you alter the technique you selected to address this problem?

CLINICAL PROBLEM 8

▼ This problem refers to the same 78-year-old patient with Parkinson's disease described in Clinical Problems 6 and 7. The focus of treatment remains on the problem of **diminished rotational movements of the trunk.** Assume that moderate success has been achieved in facilitating controlled mobility in rolling. Although work will continue on promoting improved performance in upper and lower trunk rotation, performance is now sufficiently satisfactory to begin facilitating a higher level of coordinated movement in the trunk. The next outcome (goal) of treatment for this patient is progression to the *skill level* for trunk control.

Guiding Questions

1. Identify the position/activity, technique, manual contacts, and outcome (goal) of the intervention selected to address the clinical problem.

2. With the patient on a mat table, how would the therapist be positioned for promoting the skill level of control for the trunk? What verbal cues or commands might be used to optimize a response?

3. Could the upper extremities be incorporated within the treatment technique? Explain why it might promote or detract from a plan of progression for this patient.

CLINICAL PROBLEM 9

▼ An 85-year-old patient presents with a long-standing, structural, idiopathic scoliosis. The primary curve is right thoracic and measures 70 degrees. Compensatory curves in the opposite direction have developed above and below the primary curve. The patient lives in a rural community 35 miles away with a 75-year-old cousin who is in generally good health and is very involved in the patient's care. The physician requested a month-long stay at the extended care facility in which you practice owing to recurrent complaints from the patient about a **decrease in functional capabilities.** Specifically, the patient has noted an overall reduction in endurance level, greater "swing to the side" of the longer lower extremity while walking, and some slight discomfort in the small joints of the upper extremities following activity. The patient has also indicated reduced function in household and yard activities (for example, difficulty reaching and moving objects while cooking, gardening, cleaning or doing laundry, slight difficulty with some dressing activities, and increased difficulty getting in and out of the bathtub). Clinical signs include: shoulders and pelvis are not level, prominent elevated scapulae, asymmetric waist curves, poor posture, deformity of the back (prominent rib hump on forward bending, trunk rotation with rib prominence), and a standing leg-length discrepancy of 1 inch (2.5 cm) while wearing an already elevated shoe. Both of the patient's shoes are badly worn. Ambulation is accomplished using the elevated shoe with minimal assist of one person (FIM level = 4). The patient just recently changed from using a standard cane to a small-based quadruped cane purchased at a local hardware store. The notion of surgery or bracing has long ago been rejected and the primary concern is for improved function.

The patient is extremely cooperative, well motivated, and a good history source. It appears that compliance will be high. Although a 30-day inpatient stay was requested, the managed-care company has only approved an 8-day stay.

Guiding Questions

1. Although more than one approach will be drawn from, which of the traditional treatment approaches provides the most logical overall perspective for physical therapy intervention with this patient? Provide a rationale for your answer.

2. Would you include a functional assessment in your plan for gathering information about this patient? What would be the purpose? How will the results of the functional assessment be used?

3. Given the immediate focus on improved function for this patient together with the limited time period available to accomplish the outcome, what strategies would you use to make changes in the patient's overall approach to functional tasks?

4. As the patient's therapist, you felt very strongly about the importance of an interdisciplinary, on-site home assessment. However, when you requested approval for the cost of transportation from the managed-care company, it was denied. What would be the purpose of doing an on-site home assessment for this patient? Why was it a priority? Given that an on-site visit will not be feasible, how will you address the objectives you hoped to accomplish during the home assessment?

CLINICAL PROBLEM 10

▼   A 30-year-old patient sustained a pelvic fracture 6 weeks ago secondary to a motor vehicle accident. Management included bed rest and traction; the fracture is now healed and stable and there are no restrictions on weight bearing. Because of the prolonged bed rest and immobility, a sequential progression was required through the initial rolling activities in supine and sidelying and prone activities. The focus of intervention is now on the problems of **weakness and instability of the lower trunk, weak hip musculature** (especially the abductors and adductors), **and diminished lower trunk rotation.** In addition, the patient is extremely anxious about moving the pelvis or adjacent areas associated with fear of eliciting pain. Weight bearing through the feet and ankles (even in supine position with the upper body supported) *still elicits pain.* The patient has **great difficulty initiating pelvic movement.**

Identify a treatment sequence for this patient that incorporates four combinations of position/activity and techniques. The first two should address the patient's apprehension about initiating movement; the second two should focus on the problems of weakness and instability.

Guiding Questions for the First Position/Activity

1. Identify the position/activity, technique, manual contacts, and outcome (goal) of the first intervention selected to address the problem of *apprehension* about initiating movement.

2. What instructions are provided to the patient during application of the selected technique to address the apprehension about initiating movement? Is the patient actively involved in attempting to elicit a contraction during movement?

3. What options are available for positioning the patient's upper extremities in the first selected position? What would be a logical starting position for this patient? Identify positioning of the therapist for application of the selected position/activity and technique.

Guiding Questions for the Second Position/Activity

1. Identify the position/activity, technique, manual contacts, and outcome (goal) of the second intervention selected to address the problem of *apprehension* about initiating movement.

2. Considering the goal(s) of the intervention, how would you "grade" or modulate the quality of your verbal input to the patient during treatment to help allay anxiety about initiating pelvic movement?

3. Describe the optimal quality of movement you would attempt to elicit to achieve the selected outcome (for example, fast versus slow, or high effort versus low effort). What type of movement would be sought (for example, passive, active, resistive)? Identify the sequence or progression you would use.

Guiding Questions for the Third Position/Activity

1. Identify the position/activity, technique, manual contacts, and outcome (goal) of the first intervention selected to address the problem of *weakness and instability*.

2. What type of movement or contraction would be sought (for example, passive, active, or resistive) to address the weakness and instability? Identify the sequence (order) in which the movements or contractions would be used.

3. Describe how you would apply this technique (your response should address positioning of the therapist as well as the sequence of desired movements or contractions).

4. What type of sensory input might be added to the selected technique to enhance the isotonic contraction? Would a high- or a low-threshold input be most appropriate? At what point in the sequence of isotonic movement would the sensory input be applied? When would the sensory input be eliminated? Provide justification for your response.

5. What type of verbal input would be used with this technique? What would be your goal in selection and use of verbal commands?

Guiding Questions for the Fourth Position/Activity

1. Identify the position/activity, technique, manual contacts, and outcome (goal) of the second intervention selected to address the problem of *weakness and instability*.

2. Describe how you would apply resistance with this technique to improve the strength and stability of the lower trunk pelvis. In what direction(s) would it be applied?

3. For techniques that involve holding together with changing direction(s) of resistance, transitional verbal commands to the patient are required just prior to, and during, the change in direction. Identify which transitional verbal command(s) you would incorporate. Why are they critical to achieving the outcomes (goals) of the technique?

CLINICAL PROBLEM 11

▼ A 36-year-old patient with multiple sclerosis demonstrates **difficulty with maintaining a steady position in unsupported sitting.** (Postural tremors are evident in weight bearing, antigravity postures.) In supported sitting, a forward head and functional kyphosis are evident.

Guiding Questions

1. Identify the position/activity, technique, manual contacts, and outcome (goal) of the intervention selected to address the clinical problem.

2. Describe how the patient should be placed in *modified pivot prone* position. What benefits or treatment implications might this position have for the clinical problem identified?

3. Assume the selected treatment intervention achieved control in the uppermost segment of the trunk. Which area would be addressed next?

4. How would the treatment selected for this problem be made either more or less challenging for a patient?

5. What term is used to describe a pattern of movement that includes the prone position while lifting the head, arms, upper trunk, and legs off the mat in a total extension pattern? What might be the potential benefits and contraindications for use of this pattern of movement?

CLINICAL PROBLEM 12

▼ A 64-year-old patient with marked hemiparesis secondary to a left middle cerebral infarct presents with **diminished head and upper trunk control.** Response to rolling activities is satisfactory, with good initiation of movement. However, movements are not well controlled, well coordinated, or sustained. Activities in sitting position have been unsuccessful because of the patient's inability to hold the posture (lack of isometric postural control).

Guiding Questions

1. Identify the position/activity, technique, manual contacts, and outcome (goal) of the intervention selected to address the clinical problem.

2. What are the general indications for use of sensory stimulation techniques? What general considerations influence the effectiveness of patient response to these techniques?

If incorporated as a component of treatment, when should they be used and how is a determination made to phase them out?

3. Assume a decision has been made to use *quick stretch* and *joint approximation* with this patient to facilitate head and upper trunk control. Describe how each would be applied and what response would be expected during treatment.

CLINICAL PROBLEM 13

▼ A 68-year-old patient underwent elective surgery for a total hip replacement on the right 2 weeks ago and a second total hip replacement on the left 6 days ago. The patient has a long-standing history of osteoarthritis. The original plan for surgical intervention included a 6-month interval between the respective total hip repairs. However, shortly after the first surgery, the patient fell en route to the bathroom. A decision was made to replace the second hip immediately. The patient's insurance plan precludes the additional days in the hospital that you, the physician, and social worker have all advocated for. And, to date, only four outpatient physical therapy visits have been approved (one per week for 4 weeks). The patient is well motivated, compliant with treatment, and has an extremely supportive spouse. You have decided to approach the problem with a detailed home exercise program. Among several stability problems you address with your plan is **bilateral weakness of the gluteus medius muscles.** Your current mat program has been focusing on lower trunk activities. You have worked on controlled mobility using a variety of resisted techniques in hooklying. You have progressed to bridging activities using active movements and active holding. You have just introduced resisted techniques on the active holding. Your only precaution for mat activities is to avoid hip flexion beyond 90 degrees for both lower extremities.

Guiding Questions

1. Identify the position/activity, technique, manual contacts, and outcome (goal) of the intervention selected to address the clinical problem.

2. What implications for sensory stimulation are provided by the intervention selected?

3. What *precautions* and *information* might you provide the patient and spouse regarding this treatment activity?

CLINICAL PROBLEM 14

▼ You have been working with a 32-year-old patient who sustained a midshaft fracture of the humerus following a fall during a motorcycle race. The humerus has healed well with nonoperative treatment; the radial nerve is intact. Following removal of the cast, your initial treatment emphasis was on promoting range of motion at the elbow and radial ulnar joints. Therapeutic exercise was initiated using guided movements (active-assistive movement), focusing on accuracy and avoidance of compensatory movements, promoting early learning, and reducing anxiety about movement. Work has now progressed to active exercise in gravity-resisted postures using upper extremity PNF patterns. However, a problem immediately identified is **lack of consistent strength of isotonic contraction of the biceps throughout the flexion range of movement.**

Guiding Questions

1. Identify the position/activity, technique, manual contacts, and outcome (goal) of the intervention selected to address the clinical problem.

2. Describe application of the technique selected to address the problem identified. What neuromuscular response does this technique elicit?

3. What can be added to this technique to further promote desired response? What advantage(s) would this addition provide?

CLINICAL PROBLEM 15

▼   An 86-year-old patient was admitted to the hospital 3 days ago for severe lower back and buttock pain originating in the sacroiliac joint. The pain subsides with rest in the supine position and is exacerbated with trunk rotation and prolonged sitting. The medical assessment indicates a long-standing history of ankylosing spondylitis. There are three adult, supportive children living close-by. Until recently, the patient lived independently in a small apartment; each child shared the responsibilities for daily care of their parent on a rotating basis. However, owing to the patient's diminished functional capabilities and increased care needs, together with greater time demands placed on the children by their own families and careers, continuation of care in the patient's home seems unrealistic. In a recent case conference, a difficult decision was made to seek alternate placement for the patient in an extended care facility. The family was notified by the social service department that a bed was not immediately available in any of the local facilities. Placement could take up to 2 or 3 months. The family had been informed several months ago that medical benefits from their parent's retirement package were recently assumed by a managed-care company. The company allows a maximum of 5 days hospitalization for low back pain. The only immediate option for continued care is to take the parent into one of the children's homes pending placement in an extended care facility. The family is extremely anxious about the potential difficulties in providing appropriate care at home. At the team conference a decision was made to provide assistance and support to the family by educating them in the needed aspects of care. One of your immediate concerns is to instruct the family members in *safe movement transitions from supine to sitting.* You plan to practice with the family members *prior* to working with the patient.

Guiding Questions

1. Identify the position/activity, technique, description of movement transition/manual contacts and goal (outcome) of the intervention selected to address the clinical problem.

2. Time with the family will be limited. In order to optimize the contact, *feedback* (essential for learning) must be carefully organized and integrated into your plan. Describe the type(s) of feedback will you use.

3. What strategies could be used to optimize effectiveness of the feedback?

CLINICAL PROBLEM 16

▼ An 8-year-old patient presents with a diagnosis of bilateral Legg-Calvé-Perthes disease. The child's mother reports a history of painful limping and radiating pain down the inner aspect of the thigh toward the knee. The discomfort was aggravated by ambulation and relieved with bed rest. A walker was used for ambulation; the child relied heavily on the assistive device, using a forward, flexed posture. Following the diagnosis, a plastic abduction orthosis was used to maintain each femoral head within its respective acetabulum. The abduction brace was required for 18 months. During the course of wearing the orthosis, ambulation was accomplished using bilateral axillary crutches or a walker. Having worn the brace for 15 months, the child sustained a fall while attempting to get to the basement level of the home. The fall resulted in a midshaft fracture of the right femur and a minimally displaced fracture of the right radial head (landing on an outstretched hand with elbow extended). It is now 10 weeks after the fall.

The cast for the right femur was removed 3 weeks ago. The abduction brace has also been removed and the femoral heads have healed without deformity. Upright weight bearing is not permitted; however, initial weight bearing is allowed during mat activities. There are no restrictions on upper extremity activities. Physical therapy was initiated 3 weeks ago. Recent treatment has included a progression from initial activities (rolling and sidelying) through sitting activities. Response to manual perturbations in sitting (on a stationary surface) has been satisfactory, with appropriate compensatory responses evident. Treatment is now directed toward **diminished balance responses** and gradually increasing challenges to **stabilizing postural muscles (static control work)** on a mobile support surface. Ten days ago sitting activities were initiated using a curved-bottom equilibrium board placed on the floor. Work on the equilibrium board has progressed from balanced (centered) sitting to patient-initiated active weight shifts, tilting the board in varying directions (stimulation of balance responses). Prior to last week, although the child has been cooperative, you encountered some considerable difficulty maintaining interest in activities leading up to completion of sitting activities. However, the equilibrium board was met with abundant enthusiasm; use of the Swiss ball will be initiated today. Your plan is to overlap continuation of balance training with **advanced stabilization** activities. Your first activity should address use of the equilibrium board; the second activity, using the Swiss ball.

Guiding Questions

1. For use of the *equilibrium board:* Identify the position/activity, technique, manual contacts and outcome (goal) of the intervention selected to address the clinical problem.

2. The *curved-shape* and *dome-shape* bottoms of equilibrium boards have specific clinical uses. Differentiate between the two types of boards based on movements allowed and type of patient information guiding selection.

3. Differentiate between patient-initiated challenges to balance (active weight shifts on equilibrium board) and therapist-initiated challenges (manually tilting the board) on the bases of type(s) of adjustments to balance promoted. Which of the two type(s) would you include in treatment for this child?

4. For use of the *Swiss ball:* Identify the position/activity, technique, manual contacts and outcome (goal) of the intervention selected to address the clinical problem.

5. Identify your initial directions to the patient once seated on the ball (i.e., what would you ask the patient to focus on?).

6. In general, completion of what functional activity is considered prerequisite for progression to Swiss ball activities?

7. With the child safely seated on the ball, you notice quickly that a slouched posture has been assumed. How would you address this problem and promote an upright sitting posture? What type of sensory input will be provided?

CLINICAL PROBLEM 17

▼   Assume treatment intervention continues for the above 8-year-old patient with Legg-Calvé-Perthes disease. You have been focusing on holding activities (static control work) using the Swiss ball and dynamic balance control using an equilibrium board. A progression has also been made to a dome-bottom board. The focus of treatment is now on *controlled mobility* to further **promote dynamic balance control** using the Swiss ball.

Guiding Questions

1. Identify the position/activity, technique, manual contacts, and outcome (goal) of the intervention selected to address the clinical problem.

2. In working toward controlled mobility, identify your initial activities on the Swiss ball.

3. What additional activities could be used to challenge dynamic postural control while sitting on the ball?

CLINICAL PROBLEM 18

▼   A 72-year-old patient with a right hemiparesis secondary to a stroke has recently progressed to work in the sitting position. Isolated movements are available in both the right upper and lower extremity. To date, activities have included holding, holding with UE weight bearing on an extended elbow, holding in side-sitting position, holding in modified pivot prone position, weight shifts with extended upper extremity support, weight shifts with a large ball (upper extremities supported), and weight shift with upper trunk rotation. This last activity was used in combination with slow reversals (SRs) and slow reversal-hold (SRH). Your current goal of treatment is to continue work in sitting position and to provide progressive dynamic challenges to postural control and stabilization. The plan is to continue work on a stable mat surface using greater involvement of the upper extremities to **promote dynamic balance control.**

Guiding Questions

1. Identify two (unilateral) upper extremity PNF patterns to promote dynamic postural control. Describe the patterns of movement for each.

2. What general guidelines were used to select the patterns?

3. What options are available for application of resistance using the selected patterns? What advantage does use of resistance provide?

4. How would you emphasize or focus on motor learning during use of the PNF patterns?

CLINICAL PROBLEM 19

▼   A 32-year-old patient presents following a traumatic injury to the right wrist, shoulder, and scapula. The injury was sustained during a fall from a ladder while the patient was painting a ceiling. Extensive soft tissue injury was incurred at the shoulder with a nondisplaced partial fracture of the body of the scapula. In addition, a right Colles fracture was sustained in the fall. The shoulder and scapula were treated with a short course of immobilization, anti-inflammatory agents, and analgesics. The right wrist was casted. Both the fracture sites are now healed. The cast has been removed from the wrist and replaced with a plastic supportive splint. Weight bearing through the wrist is contraindicated owing to pain and limitation in range of motion. Among several related problems, you plan to address the ***instability and diminished postural holding capability at the upper trunk and shoulder.*** Your assessment of the shoulder and scapula indicate weakness and marked reduction in stability of the right shoulder and scapula; however, there is no evidence of scapular winging. Pain has diminished in the shoulder region and range of motion is within normal limits. To initiate treatment, you decide to select a position that will protect the wrist but allow focus on the shoulder and scapula.

Guiding Questions

1. Identify the position/activity, technique, manual contacts, and outcome (goal) of the intervention selected to address the clinical problem.

2. What variation to the treatment you selected could increase the proprioceptive loading of shoulder abductor stabilizers, with specific emphasis on the rotator cuff muscles?

3. Assume the initial assessment identified winging of the scapula (vertebral border of scapula greater than 1 inch—2.5 cm—off the thorax). This would be indicative of weakness of which muscle? Would this finding have altered your selection of a position/activity? Provide a rationale for your response. If your answer included a modification in position/activity, how would you change the one you selected?

4. The *stability* stage of motor control refers to the ability to maintain a steady weight-bearing, antigravity posture. This stage of motor control is used to facilitate **tonic holding** and **co-contraction.** Define each of these terms.

5. Identify the verbal commands you would use for the technique(s) selected.

CLINICAL PROBLEM 20

▼   A 28-year-old patient with Guillain-Barré syndrome is making slow, steady gains since initiation of treatment 6 weeks ago. Mat activities have progressed from initial work in sidelying and rolling through completion of lower trunk activities. A transition has now been made to sitting position. To date, sitting activities have included weight shifting, active reaching, weight shifts (rocking) with extended upper extremity support and weight shifts with both upper extremities supported on a large Swiss ball. Resisted techniques for the trunk have included slow reversals (SRs) and slow reversal-hold (SRH). The current focus of treatment is now on ***diminished upper trunk antigravity control.*** This problem is exacerbated during *dynamic activities* of the upper extremities. You plan to continue work in sitting using a stable mat surface with greater involvement of the upper extremities to increase dynamic challenges to postural control and stabilization.

Guiding Questions

1. Identify two PNF trunk patterns to address the decreased upper trunk antigravity control. Describe the pattern of movement for each.

2. What are the advantages of using PNF patterns?

3. During application of the patterns you decide to direct the patient's attention to accuracy of the arm movements. Why did you elect this approach as opposed to attention directed toward the trunk?

4. What general guidelines were used to select the patterns?

5. How will you determine the appropriate level of resistance? Identify therapist positioning for each of the two patterns selected.

6. How would you modify the use of selected pattern if adequate stabilization is lacking?

CLINICAL PROBLEM 21

▼ A 9-year-old patient presents with *decreased range of motion in both ankles.* A diagnosis of flexible flat feet has been made. On weight bearing the heels are everted, with the forefoot appearing pronated and abducted. In non-weight-bearing positions the feet look relatively normal in alignment. The patient reports symptoms have recently become more persistent and include pain, burning, and easy fatigability. With the heel inverted, passive dorsiflexion for both ankles is limited secondary to heel-cord tightness. The mother reports the child's father has a similar condition, which required surgery; a hereditary component is suspected. The referral indicated concern over excessive stretching and damage to the medial ligaments of the foot and ankle with growth in the presence of heel-cord tightness. The plan is to fit the patient with bilateral orthoses once maximum gains in ankle range of motion are achieved. Identify two treatment interventions to address the problem of diminished ankle range of motion. Include one *mat activity* to address limitations imposed by the soleus muscle (Clinical Problem 21) and one *upright activity* that addresses tightness of both the soleus and gastrocnemius (Clinical Problem 22).

Guiding Questions

1. Identify the position/activity, technique, manual contacts, and outcome (goal) of the intervention selected to address the clinical problem.

2. Identify both the positioning of the patient and therapist for this activity.

3. During initial training you notice the young patient has difficulty attending to all components of the activity simultaneously. How might you assist and make the activity less challenging while still maintaining the selected position?

4. What verbal input would be provided to the patient during the activity?

5. During the initial phase of treatment for the diminished ankle motion, which facilitation technique is inherently accessible within the position selected? Which receptors would be influenced? What response would you anticipate? How could the response be enhanced?

CLINICAL PROBLEM 22

▼ You continue to work with the 9-year-old patient described in Clinical Problem 21 who presents with *decreased range of motion in both ankles.* Your current focus is on planning one *upright activity* that addresses *tightness of both the soleus and gastrocnemius.*

Guiding Questions

1. Identify the position/activity, technique, manual contacts, and outcome (goal) of the intervention selected to address limitations imposed by both the soleus and the gastrocnemius.

2. Identify the patient positioning for this activity.

3. How could you use this position/activity to work in a progression of ankle dorsiflexion range of motion (that is, how could you modify the position to gradually increase the dorsiflexion range)?

4. What verbal input would be provided to the patient during the activity?

5. Which facilitation technique is inherently accessible within the upright position selected? How could the response be enhanced? As treatment progresses, how might the position be modified to allow greater focus of this facilitation influence on a single lower extremity as opposed to both?

CLINICAL PROBLEM 23

▼ A 54-year-old firefighter sustained a left intertrochanteric femur fracture after becoming trapped between floors of a burning building when a portion of the floor gave way. The protective clothing and relatively rapid rescue by co-workers prevented any significant thermal injuries. The patient enters the physical therapy department ambulating with a standard, aluminum adjustable cane on the right. You notice immediately that the patient is pressing downward forcefully with the hand on the cane while walking and using a Trendelenburg gait pattern. One of your early emphases of treatment will be on the problem of *hip abductor weakness.*

The patient's insurance company has authorized six outpatient visits. Following your initial assessment, you and the patient discuss your plan of care and possible options for the best utilization of the allotted visits. You come to a mutual agreement that the best approach would be to see the patient once per week for 6 weeks. You also agree to institute a home exercise program designed to focus on the same treatment sequence you will address during the physical therapy visits.

Assume you have completed instruction in three mat (floor) exercises for the patient to use independently at home. You now plan to add two additional exercises to be performed in standing position. For Clinical Problem 23, select a standing activity to address the hip abductor weakness. For Clinical Problem 24, recommend an advanced stabilization activity in standing to address the problem.

Guiding Questions

1. Identify the position/activity, technique, manual contacts, and outcome (goal) of the intervention selected to address the clinical problem.

2. Describe patient performance to accomplish the intervention selected. How could the intervention be modified to make it more challenging?

3. Which facilitation techniques might you consider using for the support limb? Identify the stimulus, response, and technique.

4. Which facilitation techniques might you consider using for the dynamic limb? Identify the stimulus, response, and technique.

CLINICAL PROBLEM 24

▼   This problem refers to the same 54-year-old firefighter described in Clinical Problem 23. Recommend an advanced stabilization activity in standing to address the problem of *hip abductor weakness.*

Guiding Questions

1. For the *advanced stabilization activity* in standing position to address hip abductor weakness: Identify the position/activity, technique, manual contacts, and outcome (goal) of the intervention selected.

2. Describe patient performance to accomplish the intervention selected. If the patient were experiencing difficulty accomplishing the activity, how would you modify your intervention to make it less challenging and allow the patient greater success?

3. As a component of the home exercise program, what directions would you give the patient for this activity? Would you have the activity begin with the weaker limb or the stronger limb?

CLINICAL PROBLEM 25

▼   A 38-year-old patient involved in an automobile accident sustained an injury to the low back. The diagnosis of nerve-root compression owing to probable disk protrusion was made. Conservative management, which included bedrest, traction, and medication (analgesics, anti-inflammatory agents, and muscle relaxants), was initially recommended. However, the pain was unrelieved by complete bedrest and the patient continued to experience recurrent episodes of severe pain and sciatica. A decision was made to perform a laminectomy when marked lower extremity muscle weakness persisted and neurologic deficits progressed despite the complete bedrest.

The patient has been ambulatory for the past 2 weeks. Gait activities are accomplished using bilateral Loftstrand crutches with a two-point gait pattern. You have continued with mat activities and recently overlapped them with advanced stabilization activities in standing position. Your current focus of treatment is on the problem of *bilateral quadriceps weakness and preparation for stair-climbing activities.* Plan a treatment activity in standing to address these two areas of intervention.

1. Identify the position/activity, technique, manual contacts, and outcome (goal) of the intervention selected to address the clinical problem.

2. Describe patient performance to accomplish selected intervention. If the patient were experiencing lower back discomfort during the activity, what modification would you make?

3. Assume the patient is having difficulty sliding the trunk against the wall. How could you change the activity to facilitate sliding against the wall?

4. How could the activity you selected be further modified to place greater focus on recruiting the vastus medialis oblique (VMO)?

5. As you begin to consider the next phase of treatment for this patient, how could the activity be modified to increase the overall challenge as control improves?

CLINICAL PROBLEM 26

▼   A very gregarious 21-year-old patient with Down's syndrome (trisomy 21) sustained a right ankle injury while playing volleyball. Following a jump to hit the ball, the patient's balance was disturbed by contact with another player. The patient attempted to break the fall with outstretched arms but landed with most of the body weight on an inverted ankle. The patient is moderately retarded but clearly able to understand and act on one- and two-level commands. ("Pick up the ball and put it on the mat" is an example of a two-level directive because it includes two components: (1) pick up the ball, and (2) put it on the mat; each of these two directives taken separately would constitute a one-level command).

The injury occurred several hours ago. The patient arrives in a wheelchair from the emergency room with both parents. The ankle is visibly swollen, and warm to the touch. The emergency room notes indicate there are no fractures. The patient came to physical therapy for a single visit. The family is without medical insurance; the parents are essentially indigent. The hospital intake coordinator was against sending the patient to physical therapy because of the unlikely possibility of reimbursement for service; however, the emergency room physician successfully advocated on behalf of the patient.

You have been requested to train the patient in crutch walking (non-weight-bearing on the right leg); elevation, icing, and Ace bandage wrapping to reduce the swelling; and gentle, active range-of-motion exercises (ankle pumps). Your time with the patient is very limited and you want to optimize learning. As a component of your plan, you decide to carefully organize and integrate feedback and practice into the treatment session.

Guiding Questions

1. Identify your very first strategy to promote motor learning. (That is, what information will you give the patient prior to beginning actual instruction ?)

2. Identify the practice schedule you will use. What are the characteristic features of the type of practice you selected? Why is the type of practice selected appropriate for this patient?

3. The patient's learning will also depend heavily on the feedback you provide. How will you approach this aspect of your plan? What type of environmental influences will you consider?

4. What strategies would you use to optimize the influence of your relatively short treatment intervention with the patient?

CLINICAL PROBLEM 27

▼ A young married couple with a 3-month-old infant are referred to you from the Pediatric Clinic. The couple is extremely distraught over the relative **hypersensitivity, irritability, and high arousal levels** demonstrated by the child. Although the parents have been seeking additional information about the source of the problem, no diagnosis has been made. The parents are feeling enormously ineffective and somewhat guilty about their inability to comfort the child. They have done considerable reading and have learned that physical therapists are knowledgeable about handling techniques to calm the child.

Guiding Question

1. Identify two separate handling interventions (exteroceptive stimulation techniques) to assist the parents in addressing the child's hypersensitivity, irritability, and high arousal levels. Your description should include the stimulus, the receptors activated, desired response, and technique for application.

CLINICAL PROBLEM 28

▼ A 42-year-old patient sustained an incomplete spinal injury at the C7 level. The injury occurred as the result of a fall from a scaffold while the patient was working. To date, your mat program has progressed to completion of activities and techniques in the quadruped (all-fours) position. The next goal you have established with the patient is work on **movement transitions from quadruped into kneeling** (kneel-standing).

Guiding Questions

1. Describe how you would approach this next focus of treatment. Include both *patient movement sequence* and *therapist participation* in the movement transition. What motor control goals are promoted with this activity?

2. Compare and contrast the general characteristics of the *quadruped* position (prone kneeling) with those of *kneeling* (kneel-standing).

CLINICAL PROBLEM 29

▼ You are continuing work with the 42-year-old patient described above who sustained an incomplete spinal injury at the C7 level. The patient is now in the kneeling position, bearing weight on both knees and legs with the head and trunk held upright and the hips extended. The next goal of treatment is to **promote stability** in this posture. Identify two separate interventions that would assist in achieving this goal.

Guiding Questions for First Intervention

1. For intervention #1 to *promote stability:* Identify the position/activity, technique, manual contacts, and outcome (goal) of the intervention selected.

2. Describe how you would apply resistance to promote stability in kneeling using this technique.

3. How could you alter the kneeling position if, during initial training, the patient required additional support?

Guiding Questions for Second Intervention

1. For intervention #2 to *promote stability:* Identify the position/activity, technique, manual contacts, and outcome (goal) of the intervention selected.

2. What verbal input would you provide the patient to achieve the desired response?

3. How might simultaneous proprioceptive loading and contraction of the lateral hip muscles be accomplished during this activity?

CLINICAL PROBLEM 30

▼ You are continuing work with the same 42-year-old patient described above who sustained an incomplete spinal injury at the C7 level. Mat activities continue to progress in the kneeling position. A satisfactory level of stability has been achieved and you are ready to help the patient progress to the next phase of the mat sequence. Your goal of treatment is to **promote controlled mobility** in this posture. Identify two separate interventions that would assist in achieving this goal.

Guiding Questions for First Intervention

1. For intervention #1 to *promote controlled mobility:* Identify the position/activity, technique, manual contacts, and outcome (goal) of the intervention selected.

2. Describe application of the selected intervention to promote controlled mobility. Include a description of both patient and therapist positioning.

3. Identify the verbal commands you would use to accomplish the technique.

Guiding Questions for Second Intervention

1. For intervention #2 to *promote controlled mobility:* Identify the position/activity, technique, manual contacts, and outcome (goal) of the intervention selected.

2. Identify your approach for application of resistance together with the verbal commands you selected.

3. Describe application of the selected intervention to promote controlled mobility. Include a description of both patient and therapist positioning.

Part
18

Clinical Decision Making: Focus on Case Studies

This portion of the manual provides activities designed to promote clinical decision-making skills within the context of case studies. The foundational steps comprising the theoretical framework for clinical decision making include: (1) collection of patient data, (2) data analysis and formulation of a problem list, (3) identification of outcomes and priorities, (4) development of treatment intervention(s), (5) implementation of treatment, and (6) assessment of patient response and outcomes of treatment. In addressing the case-study examples, the learner is provided an opportunity to practice application of this theoretical framework by analyzing data from assessment procedures, establishing and prioritizing a problem list, formulating goals of treatment and functional outcomes of physical therapy intervention, and developing a plan of care designed to achieve appropriate functional outcomes. Inherent in this process is:

- Integration of information from assessment procedures (objective tests and measures) to establish goals and functional outcomes
- Inclusion of the patient, family, and practitioners of other disciplines involved in the patient's care in determining goals and functional outcomes
- Determination of a time frame to achieve goals and expected outcomes based on imposed constraints such as payment source, health status, financial resources, social support, community resources, and so on
- Prioritization of goals and functional outcomes
- Development of a plan of care to achieve goals and functional outcomes consistent with knowledge of the patient's prognosis, impairment, and disability
- Involvement of the patient, family, and home-based care providers in a plan of care to promote independence and self-management or assisted management
- Decision making regarding effectiveness of the plan of care based on achievement of functional outcomes

The first three case studies place heavy emphasis on application of the decision-making process to patient care. These cases provide guiding questions, strategies, and practice in making decisions along a continuum from selecting assessment procedures to developing a plan of care. Case 4 assumes a transitional format between the first three and the last seven cases. Guiding questions and considerations are significantly reduced but not eliminated completely. Readers with previous experience in clinical decision making may prefer to begin this section with Case Study 4; the decision-making practice activities in the first three case studies can be bypassed. In cases 5 through 10, practice activities specific to the clinical decision-making process are eliminated. These cases focus on clinical information pertinent to the diagnosis and allow independent practice of decision-making skills through application of content from Sections I and II of this manual. The decision-making questions in these cases 5 through 10 use a template format that addresses the characteristic sequence used by physical therapists in determining a plan of care. This format includes establishing a prioritized problem list from the case data, determining the patient asset list, formulating goals and outcomes of treatment, establishing a plan of care consistent with the goals and outcomes identified, and providing a rationale for the decision making inherent to treatment planning.

In case studies 4 through 7 the format of the questions is designed to focus attention first on establishing a physical therapy plan of care and then toward justification (rationale) for the treatment selected. Practice activities are directed toward each of these areas separately. This is actually an artificial separation to place early emphasis on specific portions of the decision-making process. Physical therapists, however, engage in decision making that requires addressing these two areas at the same time. Questions 8 through 10 require consideration of these areas concurrently.

Feedback remains a critical feature in promoting learning during practice of clinical decision-making skills within the context of the case-study examples. The learner is again encouraged to proceed at an individual pace and to obtain feedback at intervals compatible with a preferred learning style. Input on responses can be obtained by: (1) referring back to specific content areas in Sections I and II of this manual, (2) consulting the suggested readings provided at the end of the manual, (3) reviewing the content in O'Sullivan and Schmitz[1] (when applicable, suggested chapters for review appear at the beginning of each case study); (4) interacting with peers, both as individuals and in a group; (5) participating in classroom discussions and case presentations with course faculty, and (6) consulting Appendix B for suggested answers to questions posed within the case studies. Please note that the answers provided in Appendix B represent *only one solution to a given problem.* Because of the variety of treatment options available; expansion of our knowledge base; substantial changes in the health care system; the increased focus on cost containment, which creates demands for accountability; and the health care environment's volatile potential for continued change will all influence and shape how physical therapy practice achieves desired patient outcomes in the context of an unpredictable future. These fluctuating influences clearly warrant feedback from colleagues and instructors to achieve optimum patient outcomes.

▼

Case Study 1: **SPINAL CORD INJURY**

Suggested Chapters for Review
Traumatic Spinal Cord Injury
Clinical Decision Making: Planning Effective Treatments
Influence of Values on Patient Care

In O'Sullivan, SB and Schmitz, TJ (eds): *Physical Rehabilitation: Assessment and Treatment,* ed.3. FA Davis, Philadelphia.

─────────

▼ Two weeks ago, a 32-year-old man fell asleep at the wheel of a large moving van during an overnight trip. The van hit a telephone pole, causing the vehicle to roll over onto its side. The driver sustained a T4-T5 spinal fracture dislocation together with chest, facial, and upper extremity contusions. He did not lose consciousness. He was admitted to the hospital in spinal shock with total loss of sensation and muscle function below the level of the lesion. He was immediately placed on high doses of methylprednisolone (a corticosteroid) in an attempt to improve neurologic recovery. Twenty-four hours after hospital admission, he underwent surgery for a decompression laminectomy with removal of bone fragments and Harrington rod placement. Postoperatively he was placed in a bivalved, plastic body jacket to be worn for 8 to 10 weeks.

Since the injury occurred out of the patient's home state, following the 2 weeks of acute care, he was transferred to a rehabilitation facility approximately 10 miles from his home. He was diagnosed with a *complete* transection of the spinal cord.

1. Given this limited information about the patient, what key muscles would you expect the patient to have intact?

Nursing admission note to rehabilitation facility. The patient was transferred from the acute-care setting via an interstate ambulance service. He was placed in a standard hospital bed. Physical examination revealed an average-sized man approximately 6 feet tall in no acute distress. He weighed 170 pounds, blood pressure was 140/96, and his oral temperature was 98.6°F. An external urinary catheter was in place. He was unable to turn himself in bed, and the skin on both heels and both elbows was dry and reddened. He was placed immediately on a turning program using a log-rolling technique. He voiced concerns and apprehension about the rehabilitation program as well as his prognosis.

Social history. The patient has been married for 6 years and is the father of 3-year-old twin boys. He comes from a large, supportive family, whose members all live in the same community. His wife is 31 years old and works part-time with the family moving company. They both consider their marriage "the best decision of our lives." The couple owns a modest two-bedroom home in a local suburb. They are enormously proud of owning a home and having their own business. Both the patient and his wife completed an associate's degree in business management at a local community college. Medical coverage is provided by a health maintenance organization (HMO) policy. The couple has expressed considerable concern over the amount of coverage which will be provided by their current plan.

2. This question asks you to momentarily divert your attention from the acute phase of care to the end of the subacute phase. Column A presents a list of selected functional capabilities typically addressed during rehabilitation management of individuals with spinal cord injury. In Column B below, you are asked to identify the expected outcome for each of the functional capabilities listed. This will require you to think toward the future. The *outcomes of physical therapy* (long-term goals) are the level of function you expect for this patient at the very end of your planned interventions. Although every patient will be different, your answers should be based on the typical or expected functional accomplishments of individuals with lesions at the same or similar level. The outcome for the specific functional capability should address the level of assistance and/or equipment needs you anticipate required for this patient. In other words, what is the highest level of function a patient with a T4-T5 level lesion would likely achieve (independence, moderate assistance, and so on) for each functional capability? What equipment (wheelchair, adaptive equipment, and so on) is needed for the patient to accomplish each functional capability?

Column A: Functional Capabilities	Column B: Outcomes of Physical Therapy (Long-Term Goals): Assistance or Equipment Required
Activities of daily living	
Standing	
Locomotion	
Housekeeping	
Curb climbing in wheelchair	
Wheelchair sports	

Physical examination (brief examination by admitting physician). The patient was cooperative and alert, appeared approximately his stated age, and was accompanied by his wife. Muscle strength in the upper extremities (UEs) was within the good range. No active motion elicited below the level of the lesion. Sensation intact for all modalities above the level of the lesion; absent for all modalities below lesion. Cranial nerves intact. Absent deep tendon reflexes in the lower extremities (LEs). Patient is incontinent of urine and will require a bowel program. Past medical history is unremarkable. Medically cleared for participation in physical therapy with use of the plastic body jacket (to be worn when out of bed). Radiographic findings have established stability of the fracture site. Rehabilitation program can be initiated; straight-leg lifts of more than 60 degrees and hip flexion beyond 90 degrees are to be avoided. Request made for physical therapy to perform a detailed assessment and initiate a plan of care.

3. You have been asked to assume treatment responsibilities for this patient. Prior to seeing the patient, you develop a plan for the initial assessment. In formulating this plan you consider the following assessment procedures:

Respiratory assessment (function of respiratory muscles, chest expansion, breathing pattern, cough, and vital capacity)
Skin assessment
Manual muscle test and (MMT) range of motion (ROM) assessment
Cardiovascular endurance
Sensory assessment
Assessment of tone and deep tendon reflexes
Functional assessment
Presence of sacral sparing

Directions: For each assessment under consideration, check "yes" if you would include this item in your initial assessment; check "no" if it is not an appropriate component of your initial assessment and you would rule it out. For each assessment to which you responded "yes," indicate how you would approach the assessment (include what data or information you need to obtain and the tests or measures you would use to collect the needed patient information). For each item to which you responded "no," indicate your rationale for ruling out the assessment.

Yes: Indicate the approach, including data or information needed, and the test(s) or measures required.

No: Indicate the rationale for ruling out the assessment.

AREAS OF ASSESSMENT

Respiratory Assessment

1. Function of respiratory muscles

   Yes___   No___

   Approach or Rationale:

2. Chest expansion

   Yes___   No___

   Approach or Rationale:

3. Breathing pattern

   Yes___   No___

   Approach or Rationale:

4. Cough

    Yes___ No___

    Approach or Rationale:

5. Vital capacity

    Yes___ No___

    Approach or Rationale:

Skin Assessment

    Yes___ No___

    Approach or Rationale:

Manual Muscle Test (MMT) and Range of Motion (ROM) Assessment

    Yes___ No___

    Approach or Rationale:

Cardiovascular Endurance

    Yes___ No___

    Approach or Rationale:

Functional Assessment

    Yes___ No___

    Approach or Rationale:

Sensory Assessment

Yes___   No___

Approach or Rationale:

Assessment of the Tone and Deep Tendon Reflexes

Yes___   No___

Approach or Rationale:

Sacral Sparing

Yes___   No___

Approach or Rationale:

4. Assume for a moment you are now planning to execute your initial assessment. You will be working with the same group of assessment procedures identified above. However, assessment time is limited today because the patient has an appointment with the urologist. You anticipate you will have time to complete *only four (4) assessment procedures*. This will require making some decisions about the priority of each assessment. To guide your thinking in prioritizing the list, consider the following questions:

• Will any assessments add more to the clinical data base of information than others?
• Will any assessments add to or detract from the correctness of the diagnosis?
• Is data from one assessment more crucial than another?
• Will data from any assessment contribute to preventing a secondary complication?

Consider the list of assessment procedures presented earlier:

Respiratory assessment (function of respiratory muscles, chest expansion, breathing
   pattern, cough, and vital capacity)
Skin assessment
Manual muscle test (MMT) and range of motion (ROM) assessment
Cardiovascular endurance
Sensory assessment
Assessment of tone and deep tendon reflexes
Functional assessment
Presence of sacral sparing

Directions: From the list presented above, identify the four assessments you would place as *highest priorities* for this patient. You are not required to prioritize among the four procedures selected—you are asked only to identify and list the four highest. After you select and list a high-priority assessment, identify the rationale for placing it among your choices.

PRIORITIES FOR INITIATING PATIENT ASSESSMENT

Priority 1.

Rationale for selection:

Priority 2.

Rationale for selection:

Priority 3.

Rationale for selection:

Priority 4.

Rationale for selection:

Assume that on the following day, you were able to complete your initial assessment and develop your problem list. Among the items on the list were the following findings (this is a partial list of findings):

- Decreased chest expansion (3/4 of an inch—2 cm—measured at the xiphoid process)
- Dependent in skin inspection: FIM level* = 2; patient unaware of importance of skin inspection
- Tightness in heel cords (0–10 degrees)
- Dependent in bed mobility (rolling, FIM level = 3; supine-to-sit transfers, FIM level = 2)
- Proximal upper extremity muscles all graded as "good" using MMT with modified positions
- Postural hypotension (tolerance: 4–6 minutes with head of bed elevated to 30 degrees).

For each of the patient problems identified above, indicate your projected outcome of treatment (short-term goal) together with the treatment procedure you would use to accomplish the outcome. Your outcome(s) for specific treatment procedures should, as often as possible, *incorporate quantitative (measurable) data.* This will not be possible with every outcome of treatment. However, use of quantitative data improves accuracy in monitoring patient status, assists in establishing efficacy of treatment, and provides a common language of interpretation. In addition, reimbursement agencies increasingly call for these types of data both to justify the type of treatment and the number of visits allocated.

---

*The FIM level is measured from 1 to 7 using the Functional Independence Measure scale (FIM^{SM} instrument). FIM^{SM} is a service mark of the Uniform Data System for Medical Rehabilitation, a division of U B Foundation Activities, Inc.

Recall the scoring system comprising the FIM^{SM} Instrument presented earlier, in Part 17. The scoring system is summarized below. Note that each numeric value has a specific definition. By virtue of these definitions, a given score always represents the same relative level of function. Note that quantitative values may be used to identify *current patient status* as well as *projected functional outcome* level at the end of treatment intervention.

The Functional Independence Measure (FIM^{SM})*: Summary of Scoring System

7	Complete Independence (timely, safely) ⎤	NO HELPER
6	Modified Independence (device) ⎦	
5	Supervision (Subject = 100%) ⎤	HELPER—MODIFIED
4	Minimal Assistance (Subject = 75% or more) ⎬	DEPENDENCE
3	Moderate Assistance (Subject = 50% or more) ⎦	
2	Maximal Assistance (Subject = 25% or more) ⎤	HELPER—COMPLETE
1	Total Assistance (Subject less than 25%) ⎦	DEPENDENCE

*FIM^{SM} is a service mark of the Uniform Data System for Medical Rehabilitation, a division of UB Foundation Activities, Inc.

---

5. ***Directions:*** For each of the clinical problems identified below, indicate your projected outcome (short-term goal) of treatment together with the treatment procedure(s) you would use to accomplish the outcome.

Clinical Problem:

Decreased chest expansion (3/4 inch—2 cm—measured at the xiphoid process).

Outcome of Treatment (Short-Term Goal):

Treatment:

Clinical Problem:

Dependent in skin inspection: FIM level = 2; patient unaware of importance of skin inspection.

Outcome of Treatment (Short-Term Goal):

Treatment:

Clinical Problem:

Tightness in heel cords (0–10 degrees).

Outcome of Treatment (Short-Term Goal):

Treatment:

Clinical Problem:

Dependent in bed mobility (positional changes): FIM level = 2.

Outcome of Treatment (Short-Term Goal):

Treatment:

Clinical Problem:

Proximal upper extremity muscles all graded as "good" using MMT with modified positions.

Outcome of Treatment (Short-Term Goal):

Treatment:

Clinical Problem:

Postural hypotension (tolerance: 4–6 minutes with head of bed elevated to 30 degrees).

Outcome of Treatment (Short-Term Goal):

Treatment:

This is the 4th day of hospitalization for the patient. When you arrive at the hospital that morning, you find a message on your voice mail from the patient's wife requesting a meeting at your earliest convenience. She has indicated that your advice is needed and that the matter is urgent. The message also advises that she will be at the hospital by 7:30 A.M. After collecting your voice mail messages, you call the patient's floor and learn that the patient's wife has already arrived. You decide not to delay speaking with the couple since you have meetings and patients scheduled for most of the morning and there would not be another opportunity.

When you arrive at the patient's room, both he and his wife are visibly distraught. It appears that the wife has been crying. The social worker has just left. The couple takes turns explaining the problem: as one's emotions run too high to continue speaking, the other takes over. When a decision was made to open the family moving company, they opted for an HMO health care plan. Since the family was young and unlikely to have any major medical needs in the near future, the HMO plan seemed a good choice. The HMO plan provided lower costs, preventative care, checkups, immunizations, and screenings for early detection. There were no claim forms, and the fixed co-payments for prescriptions were low. The disadvantages of the HMO plan were restricted access to physicians, hospitals, and treatments; services subject to approval by a case manager and review board; preauthorization for hospital care; and geographic limits of care.

After multiple attempts to reach the case manager, the wife finally received a phone call from the HMO last night. She has been told that the HMO provides for *only 30 days of inpatient rehabilitation.* Preauthorization is needed for any equipment purchases. She has also been informed that acute hospital stays in out-of-state locations are generally approved for only 1 week. Since her husband has stayed for 2 weeks and the HMO was not notified until 3 days after the injury, reimbursement is in question for the acute hospitalization. The patient and his wife are concerned that if uncovered medical costs exceed their small savings and if state medical assistance is their only option for help, they risk losing both their home and moving business.

As the couple is speaking, you begin to mentally sort through the information in an effort to come to the best decision about how to respond. As you begin this decision-making process, you also begin to think about the vast array of things that need to be accomplished prior to the patient's return home. Flashing before you on the face of a 30-day calendar page are thoughts of mat activities; bed mobility and transfer skills; therapeutic exercise; activities-of-daily-living (ADL) skills; bowel and bladder training; the need for occupational therapy, psychologic, and social service interventions; family counseling; equipment orders; and home and community assessment. You want to make the best decision about how to respond. You are feeling overwhelmed both by the emotional context of the situation and the limitations imposed on rehabilitation services.

Reflect for several minutes on the situation just described by the couple. In the space below you will be asked to describe how you would respond to the couple's request for advice. This will likely take some additional, careful thought. Perhaps you feel ill-prepared to speak to the magnitude of the problem. You will certainly not be able to resolve such a multifaceted problem on the spot. Your thoughts can be guided by considering the interrelated steps that comprise the clinical decision-making process. There may be gaps in your data base that require communication with other care providers or the HMO case manager. Consider for a moment the questions posed under each of the steps of the process:

   a. *Step 1: Collect data.* Do you have sufficient information to define the couple's problem? Can you identify resources available to address the problem? Do you have adequate subjective and objective data?

   b. *Step 2: Analyze data and identify problems.* Begin to organize and analyze the available data (sometimes it is helpful to do this on paper until the clinical decision-making process becomes more automatic for you). Recall that therapeutic decisions must be based on a thorough understanding of the problems identified, the needs of the patient, and the resources available. Next, generate an asset list. This follows from the data analysis and focuses on optimizing inherent strengths in the situation. These areas should be supported and emphasized during the rehabilitation process. This approach will provide the patient a greater opportunity for successful use of available hospital days as well as improve the patient's motivation and compliance.

   c. *Step 3: Set outcomes (goals) and priorities.* Determine a goal for addressing the problem. What are your greatest concerns about the situation? What do you want to see happen? What will make you feel that you are making progress? How will you involve the patient in the decision-making process? Do you need to set more than one goal to address the problem? How will these be prioritized?

   d. *Step 4: Formulate a plan.* What interventions or activities will be required to meet the outcomes (goals)?

   e. *Step 5: Implement the plan.* How will you carry out the plan? How will you optimize its effectiveness? How will you explain the plan to the patient? How will it influence the problem identified by the couple?

   f. *Step 6: Evaluate the outcome.* Given the uncertainties and constraining variables inherent to the problem, how will you determine the effectiveness of your plan?

6. **Directions:** In the space provided on the next page, describe how you would respond to the couple's request for advice.

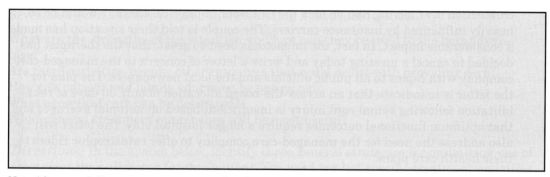

Note: After completing your response, proceed to the next activity. You will obtain feedback on your response by comparing it to three possible responses in item 7 below.

7. ***Directions:*** You will now be asked to consider your response to the situation by comparing it with three alternative approaches. The three options are listed below as *Decision 1, Decision 2,* and *Decision 3.* Assess each decision separately and contrast it with your own. As you consider each decision, remember that an appropriate, understanding response might take several forms.

For each decision-option, you are asked to: (1) Decide if the *response is compatible with your own decision making* about responding to the couple's request for advice. (2) Provide justification for your decision about the response. That is, identify the aspects of the response (option) that caused you to accept it as compatible or reject it as incompatible with your own decision making. This might include issues of professional behavior, type of information provided by the therapist, problem-solving skills demonstrated, therapist/patient interaction, types of behaviors which promote healing versus those that detract, and so on.

a. *Decision 1.* The therapist decides to conceal any compassion for, and empathy with the couple. The logic of this decision is to minimize the couple's tendency to dwell on the situation and cause them to view it as a less ominous problem. Humor is interjected to distract attention away from the problem. Although the therapist is in contact with this HMO regularly, the therapist is honest with the couple and admits shortcomings in knowing how flexible the policies are with allocations for rehabilitation. The therapist indicates a lack of urgency about the situation and promises to speak to the case manager next week in their regular bimonthly telephone conference. Further explanation is provided about how difficult it is to remember the rules and regulations of every managed-care company. The therapist leaves on a positive note by suggesting that this information should not alter the plan for rehabilitation intervention.

Is the response compatible with your own decision making?

Yes___   No___

Justification for your decision about response:

b. *Decision 2.* The therapist begins by expressing personal unhappiness with the situation the couple is facing. The therapist continues by indicating considerable impatience and constant anger with the whole managed-care system. Feelings of personal and professional frustration are expressed related to functioning within time limitations imposed by insurance companies. In addition, the therapist expresses

You plan to begin your initial assessment of the patient today. You have already gathered considerable demographic data, relevant history, and information on chief complaints from the medical record, interview with the wife and children, and the family case conference. You begin to mentally sort through the list of potential areas of assessment you will need to address with this patient. Although the assessment list is lengthy, you anticipate limited patient tolerance and plan to complete six assessment procedures on the initial visit. Your list includes the following assessments:

List of Assessment Procedures:

1. Motor control—muscle tone, reflexes and reactions, voluntary movement patterns, motor planning ability
2. Coordination
3. Balance
4. Perception
5. Functional assessment—rolling, supine-to-sit transfers, sit-to-stand transfers

6. Skin condition and edema
7. Sensation
8. Joint mobility—range of motion (ROM), joint play, soft-tissue compliance
9. Endurance/cardiorespiratory status
10. Gait
11. Mental status
12. Environmental assessment and equipment needs for discharge
13. Communication ability

Prioritizing Assessments

Prioritizing decisions can be guided by using the same interrelated steps in the clinical decision-making process described earlier. Consider for a moment the steps in the process as they might relate to prioritizing assessments. How would you begin to apply this model for establishing priorities? First, recall the six steps in the process: (1) collect data, (2) analyze data, (3) set outcomes (goals) and priorities, (4) formulate a plan, (5) implement the plan, and (6) evaluate the outcome. We will now implement this process to guide thinking about establishing priorities. Each step in the process will be addressed individually. In the next section the clinical decision-making process is applied to prioritizing patient assessment procedures.

Stroke: Application of Clinical Decision-Making Process to Prioritizing Assessment Procedures

Step 1: Collect data.

1. Do you have sufficient information to define the problem?

   Yes___ No___

2. Can you identify resources available to address the problem?

   Yes___ No___

3. Do you have adequate subjective and objective data?

   Yes___ No___

1. *Do you have sufficient information to define the problem?* Yes. Your problem is, *which data are the most important or most critical* to collect first? Your academic background has provided you with knowledge of the etiology and clinical manifestations following stroke. This information will guide your decisions. Although each patient will present unique needs and problems, your knowledge base provides strong leads on the types of data that typically need to be collected following a neurologic insult of this type. Although the list of assessments was provided earlier, you would likely have developed a very similar list working independently.

2. *Can you identify resources available to address the problem?* Yes. You have two major resources at your disposal: (1) Your knowledge base allows you to consider the typical etiology, pathophysiology, symptomatology, and sequelae of stroke. (2) Your studies have also provided information on the various tests and measures available to physical therapists to gather patient data.

   Your academic background on stroke together with your knowledge of assessment procedures are your best resources to address the problem. This combination of information provides the foundation for selection of assessments appropriate to the typical clinical manifestations. Consideration of clinical features and assessments simultaneously allows one to select those needed and rule out others.

3. *Do you have adequate subjective and objective data?* Yes. You have a sound knowledge of the clinical picture of stroke. You are able to determine the assessment procedures most applicable. You are able to perform the assessments, document findings, and interpret results.

   Step 2: Analyze data and identify problems.

1. Do patients with stroke typically present with problems of coordination?

   Yes___ No___

2. Are changes in functional abilities typical after stroke?

   Yes___ No___

Begin to organize and analyze the available data to make decisions about all the different assessments that need to be included. This is where you make connections between the clinical manifestations typically seen and all of the assessments potentially needed to address the clinical problems. Although this has already been done for you in this example, this step is where you actually generate your entire list of assessments. The total group of assessments assists with formulation of both a problem and asset list. The list is generated from your combined knowledge of the signs and symptoms of stroke and physical therapy assessment procedures. Now, consider asking yourself a series of questions about the clinical manifestations:

1. *Do patients with stroke typically present with problems of coordination?* Incoordination can result from cerebellar or basal ganglia involvement, from proprioceptive losses, or motor weakness. Since these are potential clinical manifestations, your answer is "yes" and coordination is added to the list as a needed assessment.
2. *Are changes in functional abilities typical after stroke?* Again your answer is "yes." Functional skills following stroke are typically impaired or absent and vary considerably from patient to patient. A functional assessment is added to the list.

Your mental list of questions should continue until you have exhausted all of the features of the diagnosis. Note, however, that your initial assessment may expand after contact with the patient because of specific needs that are unique to the individual.

Step 3: Set outcomes (goals) and priorities.

Determine a goal for addressing the problem. What are your greatest concerns about the situation? What do you want to see happen?

- Your *outcome (goal)* is to collect the most important or critical data first.
- Your *priority* is to accomplish those assessments first which might provide data that influences (or provides an explanation for) data obtained from subsequent tests or measures.
- Your *greatest concern* is addressing and valuing the patient's needs by applying your knowledge and skill in an effective, efficient manner.
- *What you want to see happen* is the organization of available data sufficient to allow establishing an order to the assessments.

Step 4: Formulate a plan.

What interventions or activities will be required to meet the outcome (goal)?

This is where you select those assessments required to meet your outcome (goal). There are two critical questions you need to ask yourself to assist in this decision-making process: (1) Will the results of an assessment potentially affect data collection or interpretation of results from subsequent measures? (2) Will the results of any assessment potentially affect the validity of subsequent measures?

These questions should be posed for each test or measure. Any item with a "yes" response will be added to the high-priority list. The assessments with the greatest impact on the largest number of subsequent tests will be moved to the top of the list.

Step 5: Implement the plan.

How will you carry out the plan? How will you optimize its effectiveness?

The plan will be carried out in the order identified by your decision-making process. The effectiveness of assessment procedures is enhanced by careful adherence to standardized protocols for execution and documentation. Any deviations from the protocol should be indicated.

Step 6: Evaluate the outcome.

How will you determine the effectiveness of your plan?

Feedback on your initial plan can be addressed by assessing your own decision making. Consider asking yourself the following questions: (1) During the course of the patient assessment did critical tests or measures come to mind that were not among the priorities? (2) How were they overlooked? (3) What information was missing in the decision-making process? (4) Is documentation complete? (5) Were all components of the assessment completed? (6) Were all required deviations from standardized protocols or positions documented with a rationale? (7) Are findings consistent or compatible with those of other disciplines working with the patient?

6. **Directions:** From the list of assessment procedures identified above and repeated below, select six (6) that you feel are the most important for this patient. Once you have identified those six assessments, prioritize your list. Imposing a priority order on the assessment list requires decisions about which is the very most important, the second most important, and so on. This will provide the order in which data will be collected (priority 1 will represent the most important, priority 2 the second most important, and so forth).

   For each assessment selected, you are asked to indicate your *rationale* for its high placement (priority 1, 2, 3, 4, 5, or 6), the *specific information you need to gather*, and whether *collaborative input* from other disciplines is warranted.

List of Assessment Procedures:

1. Motor control—muscle tone, reflexes and reactions, voluntary movement patterns, motor planning ability
2. Coordination
3. Balance
4. Perception
5. Functional assessment—rolling, supine-to-sit transfers, sit-to-stand transfers
6. Skin condition and edema
7. Sensation
8. Joint mobility—range of motion (ROM), joint play, soft-tissue compliance
9. Endurance/cardiorespiratory status
10. Gait
11. Mental status
12. Environmental assessment and equipment needs for discharge
13. Communication ability

Carefully consider the list of assessments. In the spaces provided below, indicate the *six most important initial assessments* for this patient. You need not prioritize them at this point; you only need to generate a list.

Generate a list of the 6 most important assessments:

1.	2.	3.
4.	5.	6.

7. **Directions:** Now, consider your list of the six most important assessments and prioritize your list below (1 being the most important, 2 the second most important, and so forth).

Prioritize the list of the 6 most important assessments:

1.	2.	3.
4.	5.	6.

8. **Directions:** In the spaces provided below, enter your prioritized list of assessments (priority 1, 2, 3, 4, 5, or 6), your rationale for its high placement, needed information from the assessment, and whether collaborative input is warranted.

Priority 1:   *Needed information:*

Rationale: *Collaborative input:*

Priority 2:   *Needed information:*

Rationale: *Collaborative input:*

Priority 3:   *Needed information:*

Rationale: *Collaborative input:*

Priority 4:   *Needed information:*

Rationale: *Collaborative input:*

Priority 5:   *Needed information:*

Rationale: *Collaborative input:*

Priority 6:   *Needed information:*

Rationale: *Collaborative input:*

9. This next question asks that you *move forward approximately 2 weeks* in time. Assume you have completed a detailed assessment that generated a lengthy list of clinical problems. Based on your assessment, you developed the initial aspects of the treatment plan. There is growing support from the family to have the patient transferred to the rehabilitation facility. The patient's wife is also reconsidering this option. She is not dissatisfied with the care, but is concerned about the emotional impact on her husband of being surrounded by patients with acute problems who progress quickly and leave the hospital. No definite decisions have been made and you will continue care as long as he remains in the acute facility.

    Your treatment plan has largely focused on a mat progression. Clear evidence of improvement has been noted. The patient is independent (FIM level = 7) in both rolling and assuming prone-on-elbows position. Assuming and maintaining quadruped, hooklying, and bridging require moderate assistance (FIM level = 3). Sitting balance is poor (FIM level = 2) because of *decreased trunk stability*. Tonal imbalances and impaired voluntary control render the patient unable to hold an antigravity posture.

    Focus your attention *only on the problem of decreased trunk stability in sitting position*. You have begun to plan your selection of techniques for use in the sitting position. A potential list of techniques you are considering includes:

1. Alternating Isometrics	5. Slow Reversals
2. Rhythmic Initiation	6. Placing and Holding (hold after positioning)
3. Hold-Relax	7. Agonist Reversals
4. Rhythmic Stabilization	

You now need to make decisions about the *optimal technique(s)* to achieve the desired outcomes. The decision-making process follows the same interrelated steps. The steps are briefly summarized in the box below.

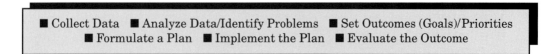

■ Collect Data   ■ Analyze Data/Identify Problems   ■ Set Outcomes (Goals)/Priorities
■ Formulate a Plan   ■ Implement the Plan   ■ Evaluate the Outcome

Application of Decision-Making Process to Selection of Treatment

Techniques to Address Decreased Trunk Stability

- *Collect Data:* Your data are the entire list of possible treatment techniques you selected for consideration (use the list of seven techniques above, even though it may not include choices you would have made).
- *Analyze Data / Identify Problems:* Identify the *features* (type of contraction, application, motor control goal) and *indications* of techniques appropriate to address decreased trunk stability in sitting. This step can be facilitated by asking yourself the following questions:
  1. What should the techniques selected be emphasizing to achieve the outcome? Repetitions of movement? Increasing range of motion? Weight bearing, holding in antigravity postures?
  2. Which clinical problems are the techniques under consideration designed to address? Tonal imbalances? Decreased mobility? Changing movement direction?
  3. What is the motor control goal associated with the technique? Mobility? Stability? Skill?
- *Set Outcomes (Goals) / Priorities:* At this step in the process, the features of and indications for each technique on the list are compared to those needed for the individual patient. Techniques that are compatible with the desired patient outcomes (goals) remain on the list of treatment options, others are ruled out.
- *Formulate a Plan:* This is the point where a final list of techniques is developed. It is also the point where the techniques are sequenced to achieve the optimum results. In sequencing treatment techniques consideration should be given to the following questions: (1) Do the techniques represent any logical progression in terms of increasing difficulty within the position? (2) Does one technique require difficult prerequisite skills than another? (3) How many joints or body segments are involved? (4) Do the types of contractions involved represent incremental levels of challenge? (5) Is weight bearing on or through a joint required?
- *Implement the plan:* Describe the application of treatment techniques within context of treatment plan.
- *Evaluate the outcome (goal):* Assess patient response to selected techniques. Were techniques successful at achieving identified outcomes of treatment (short-term goals)?

10. ***Directions:*** You will now be asked to make some clinical decisions about the list of treatment techniques identified earlier. The clinical problem you are addressing is *decreased trunk stability in sitting position*. First, identify the features needed (type of contraction, application, motor control goal) and the indications for techniques appropriate to address decreased trunk stability. Next, identify the features and indications for each technique under consideration. Compare what you *need* with what each technique *will provide*. Comparing the indications and features needed to address de-

creased trunk stability with those of each technique under consideration, the therapist can make decisions about whether to include the technique in treatment or rule it out.

LIST OF TREATMENT TECHNIQUES

1. Alternating Isometrics
2. Rhythmic Initiation
3. Hold-Relax
4. Rhythmic Stabilization
5. Slow Reversals
6. Placing and Holding (hold after positioning)
7. Agonist Reversals

In the space provided below, identify the features of and indications for techniques appropriate to address *decreased trunk stability in sitting position.*

The features of the techniques needed are:

Indications for these techniques are:

11. **Directions:** In the spaces provided below (pp. 224–227) identify the features and indications of each technique. Compare this information with what you need (listed above). Determine the individual technique's compatibility with the needs you have established. If it is compatible, include the technique in treatment. If not, rule it out.

Alternating Isometrics

Application:

Indications:

Contraction:

Compatible with needs:

Yes___ No___

Include / Rule out:

Rhythmic Initiation

Application:

Indications:

Contraction:

Compatible with needs:

Yes___ No___

Include / Rule out:

Hold-Relax

Application:

Indications:

Contraction:

Compatible with needs:

Yes___ No___

Include / Rule out:

Rhythmic Stabilization

Application:

Indications:

Contraction:

Compatible with needs:
Yes___ No___

Include / Rule out:

Slow Reversals

Application:

Indications:

Contraction:

Compatible with needs:
Yes___ No___

Include / Rule out:

Placing and Holding

Application:

Indications:

Contraction:

Compatible with needs:
Yes___ No___

Include / Rule out:

Agonist Reversals

Application:

Indications:

Contraction:

Compatible with needs:
Yes___ No___

Include / Rule out:

This is the beginning of the 3rd week of treatment for the patient in the acute-care hospital. At a family conference today, you learn that the family has decided to admit the patient to the rehabilitation facility approximately 30 miles away. His wife will take temporary lodging near the facility. The patient was discharged at the end of the day.

▼
Case Study 3: RHEUMATOID ARTHRITIS

Suggested Chapter for Review
Arthritis and Functional Assessment

In O'Sullivan, SB and Schmitz, TJ (eds): *Physical Rehabilitation:
Assessment and Treatment,* ed. 3. FA Davis, Philadelphia.

▼ A new outpatient has scheduled an appointment at your clinic today. She has a long-standing history of rheumatoid arthritis. The patient referral came from the hospital rheumatology clinic, where she was seen yesterday. The patient is a 91-year-old woman who lives in an adjacent rural community. She is in town for 4 weeks visiting with her grandchildren and great-grandchildren. Physical therapy services are not available in her community. Consequently, she has decided to take advantage of the availability of outpatient care while she is on vacation. This is the beginning of the 1st week of her stay in the area. She arrives at the clinic ambulating slowly but unassisted except for an ill-fitting standard wooden cane with a worn suction tip.

Social history. The patient has been a widow for 22 years. She lives on a working livestock farm that she and her husband started shortly after they were married. She employs a staff of six people to run the farm. However, she oversees all day-to-day operations. She and her husband met while in graduate school. She holds a doctoral degree in English literature. Her husband completed his degree in forestry. She has four living children; one child recently died from cancer at the age of 61. She reports, "It's a loss I will never get over." She is very proud of her life accomplishments, which include raising her family, assisting her husband in establishing and running the farm, her career as a freelance writer (for which she has gained some considerable recognition) and her instrumental role in founding a small, thriving community college in her home town. She reports her favorite activities are maintaining her husband's farm, riding her bicycle, reading, fishing, and growing vegetables. She wants to give up none of these activities. She comes from a very close, supportive family. Two siblings—a brother aged 83, and a sister aged 86—came to live with her after they had lost their spouses. She is accompanied today by her brother, who has offered to be of any help he can in facilitating his sister's improvement.

Presenting problem. The patient presents with ***pain and instability in her right knee,*** secondary to "flare-ups" of rheumatoid arthritis. The knee problem has affected her walking endurance and interfered with functional activities. She also complains of increasing difficulty getting going in the morning. Lately, it seems the "bad knee days" are more frequent than the "good knee days." She indicates that the symptoms are alleviated by aspirin. She has never been seen by a physical therapist before today.

History of chief complaint. The patient reports "a very difficult pain" in the right knee. She recalls the knee has been larger than the left for some time now. However, the knee was asymptomatic until 2 months ago, when she sustained a fall while riding a bicycle. At the time of the fall, the patient felt a "terrible pulling" in her knee. Following the fall, the knee became red and swollen and she remained non-weight bearing for several days. After about a week of rest, the knee seemed quite back to normal and she resumed her regular activities. However, she then noticed the knee felt a little unstable. She began using her husband's cane only for outdoor activities, including her twice-daily inspection of the farm. Within the past 2 weeks, she has found it necessary to use the cane indoors as well. She has given these painful episodes little thought because of the known arthritic involvement. Her assumption was that the fall exacerbated the rheumatoid arthritis and the symptoms would gradually disappear.

PHYSICAL THERAPY ASSESSMENT

Your assessment findings are consistent with long-standing rheumatoid arthritis. The involvement presents as bilateral, with clinical manifestations in all extremities. This patient presents with greater involvement in the lower versus the upper extremities. The knees and ankles demonstrate the greatest manifestations, which are greater on the right than on the left.

Review of Systems

Cough. Effective; nonproductive.

Vision. Intact with corrective lens.

Respiratory rate. 14 breaths per minute.

Coordination. Within normal limits.

Lung sounds. Within normal limits.

Skin condition. Intact; unremarkable.

Blood pressure. 130/80.

Sensation. Intact.

Functional Assessment

The patient is independent in all areas of **basic activities of daily living (BADL),** with the exception of stair climbing. She uses a foot-over-foot reciprocal pattern; this is a labor-intensive pattern that creates additional pain in the right knee; she requires the use of a cane, and minimal assistance of one person (FIM level = 4). She will not attempt stair climbing unassisted. The patient requires minimal assistance of one person (FIM level = 4) for **instrumental activities of daily living (IADL).** This is influenced by pain, knee instability, and low tolerance for ambulatory activities. There is no history of cardiac involvement.

Range of Motion (ROM) Assessment: Lower Extremities

Range of Motion (Degrees)		Right	Left
Hip:	Flexion	0–100	0–110
	Extension	0–0	0–0
	Abduction	0–25	0–25
	Adduction	0–20	0–20
	External rotation	0–10	0–15
	Internal rotation	0–10	0–20
Knee:	Flexion	5–110*	0–115
Ankle:	Dorsiflexion	0–0	0–10
	Plantar flexion	0–20	0–25
	Inversion	0–20	0–30
	Eversion	0–0	0–10

*Last 10 degrees of flexion elicit pain.

Patient's report of pain (with right knee flexion) using the Pain Scale below (PS = 6):

Pain Scale (PS)

(0 = none)   0   1   2   3   4   5   6   7   8   9   10   (10 = worst)

---

1. During the course of the initial assessment, the patient again mentions her difficulty participating in activity during the early part of the day. She states the joints of her legs feel "rusty" and hard to move. How would you respond to these comments?

Strength Assessment: Lower Extremities

Strength (MMT)		Right	Left
Hip:	Flexion	G	G
	Extension	G	G
	Abduction	G−	G
	Adduction	G−	G
	External rotation	G−	G
	Internal rotation	G−	G
Knee:	Flexion	F	G−
	Extension	F	G−
Ankle:	Dorsiflexion	F	G−
	Plantarflexion	F	G−
	Inversion	F−	G−
	Eversion	F−	G−

Standing: Weight-Bearing Assessment

Right lower extremity (LE). Hip: Excessive adduction (20 degrees). **Knee:** Moderate distension of the joint secondary to chronic synovitis; genu valgum (25 degrees); Collateral ligament damage and laxity. **Ankle:** Excessive subtalar pronation (15 degrees). *Note:* During non-weight-bearing assessment, relative neutral alignment is achieved at the hip and ankle; genu valgum is reduced to 10 degrees.

Left lower extremity (LE). Hip: Alignment within normal limits. **Knee:** Slight distension of the joint secondary to chronic synovitis. **Ankle:** Alignment within normal limits.

Upper Extremity Assessment

The upper extremities are less involved than the lower extremities. The patient reports some morning stiffness in the shoulders and elbows that quickly subsides. She denies pain or discomfort of the upper extremities; she reports that her arms "are fine" and do not limit her activities in any way. Strength throughout the upper extremities is generally within the good range. **Shoulders:** ROM is generally within functional limits with tightness, crepitus, and pain (PS = 7) bilaterally at the extremes (end range) of motion. **Elbows:** ROM on the right: 10–130 degrees; ROM on the left: 15–135 degrees; slight inflammation evident bilaterally. **Wrist:** ROM within functional limits; excess volar subluxation of 10 degrees bilaterally. **Fingers:** ROM within functional limits; minimal soft-tissue swelling and ulnar drift at the MCP joints.

Additional Findings

Shoes: The patient's shoes are badly worn; there is a noticeable bulging on the lateral side of the right shoe with excessive medial wear. The patient is aware that she needs supportive shoes, but she is uncertain about shoe requirements and wants your recommendations.

Gait: Excessive dependence on poorly fitted standard cane. Patient denies any episodes of knee buckling; decreased time in stance on right; uneven step length.

Patient Outcomes (Goals): Better tolerance for walking—improve function, decrease "bad knee days." Keep as active as possible and occasionally ride her bicycle.

Insurance Coverage: The patient has been allocated eight outpatient visits by the insurance company. She has been told this is the maximum coverage allowed because of the preexisting nature of the problem. However, the patient states that she will do "whatever it takes to get better." She has further indicated that some personal savings could be used for physical therapy if additional treatments are warranted. The patient has expressed willingness to come for treatment every day of the vacation, if it will help.

Formulating the Plan of Care

Once the overall outcome of treatment has been established and discussed with the patient, selection of treatment interventions to achieve improved function must be determined. Physical therapists have a wide variety of activities and techniques available. It is important to identify all possible treatment alternatives, to carefully weigh those options, and to decide on those interventions that have the best probability of success for the individual patient. Inherent in this process is a commitment to life-long learning, keeping abreast of recent professional literature, and being knowledgeable about new treatment options. An integrated treatment approach, based on functional training and outcomes, provides multiple treatment options and is often the one with the greatest chance for success.

2. ***Directions:*** Attention will now be directed toward application of your decision-making skills to *determine the plan of care* for the patient. Once again, the decision-making process follows the same interrelated steps. Mentally review the steps.

Review of Key Questions Guiding Decision Analysis

3. ***Directions:*** The key questions posed earlier under the various steps of the process are designed to help guide your decision-making process. They assist the therapist in analyzing the database, identifying the problems, synthesizing material, and formulating conclusions. They help guide choices when multiple options are available and assist integration of pertinent variables with consideration to desired patient outcomes.

   Prior to initiating treatment planning, fill in the missing steps of the decision-making process in the spaces below *after the roman numerals* II, III, IV, and VI. Then, after each step in the decision-making process below, identify the *key question(s)* you will ask yourself at each step in the decision-making process as you develop the plan of care. In the space provided, *fill in these questions after each step in the process.* Recall that all questions associated with an individual step may not be applicable to every situation in which the decision-making process is used.

I. Collect data   *Key question(s):*

II.   *Key question(s):*

III.   *Key question(s):*

IV.   *Key question(s):*

V. Implement the plan   *Key question(s):*

VI.   *Key question(s):*

Having reviewed the decision-making process, you are now ready to integrate information from the various steps in the clinical decision-making process to generate a problem list (clinical decision-making step 2, using data from step 1), develop a list of treatment outcomes (short-term goals) for step 3, and formulate a plan (step 4). If you feel prepared for this challenge, progress directly to *Question 4.* If you feel that more guidance would be beneficial before working with this many variables, follow the directions immediately below in the boxed area entitled **Determining Plan of Care** before you continue. When you feel comfortable to begin practicing with integrating the steps, proceed to the directions immediately following the box in *Question 4.*

Determining Plan of Care

It is certainly not unusual to feel a little overwhelmed while practicing application of newly acquired knowledge and skills. And, at the same time, maintaining your greatest concern of addressing the patient's needs. You are to be commended on your self-assessment skills, which caused you to pause and work through this material before proceeding. Continued practice will help develop the needed skills to integrate the steps in the decision-making process.

   Directions: Go back and read the case information several times. After reading the case, complete the following activities. Refer back to the case information as needed. Write down your answers so they can be considered (or reconsidered) as you progress through the following practice activities:

1. *Examine data.* First, focus only on reviewing the data collected during the initial assessment. Consider each piece of data one at a time. Begin to think about which items constitute abnormal findings. Among the abnormal findings, determine the items that contribute to limiting the patient's function.

2. *Develop a problem list.* Again, consider each piece of data as a single entity and determine its relative importance for achieving improved patient function (high, medium, low, or change would not be expected). This will guide development of a problem list. Remember that *all patient problems are not amenable to change.* In fact, attempting to change a safe, habit pattern may reduce rather than promote improved function; multiple factors must be considered here, including the patient's age, diagnosis and level of involvement, use of assistive device, and so on. To guide establishing your priorities here, consider asking yourself the following questions: What are the patient's greatest concerns? What are your greatest concerns? Would resolving a specific patient problem first contribute to improvement in more than one area of function? Keep the issue of priorities in your mind as you progress; you will be required to prioritize the problem list shortly.

3. *Set functional outcomes (goals) and priorities.* Consider each piece of data that you can expect to change and subsequently contribute to improved function. This information will provide the bases for formulating functional outcomes (i.e., the level of function you expect the patient to achieve as the result of physical therapy intervention). Remember that *multiple impairments* may contribute to a *single disability* or, conversely, a *single impairment* may contribute to *more than one disability*.

4. *Formulate a plan.* Determine how you will achieve each functional outcome. First, identify all possible treatment alternatives; consider the potential of each treatment alternative to contribute to resolution of the problem. Select those with the greatest probability of achieving desired patient outcomes. If needed, review the section in Case Study II entitled "Application of Decision-Making Process to Selection of Treatment Techniques to Address Decreased Trunk Stability."

   When you feel sufficient practice has been achieved, move onto Question 4.

4. **Directions:** Assume you are responsible for this patient's care. You have completed the initial assessment and are about to document your findings as a problem list, establish outcomes of treatment (short-term goals), and plan treatment intervention. Many therapists use a format for assessment that includes columns or spaces for *clinical problems, outcomes of treatment* (short-term goals—STGs), *treatment intervention,* and projected number of visits to achieve outcomes (this last area will be addressed shortly). These four areas of physical therapy documentation are requirements for Medicare reimbursement. As often as possible, the outcomes of treatment should be stated *in functional terms.*

In the space provided below, formulate a *problem list* for this patient (as you develop the problem list, you should begin to considered the relative importance of each problem in addressing the patient's needs; you will be asked to prioritize this list shortly). For each problem identified, indicate the *outcome of treatment* (short-term goal) to be achieved. Finally, indicate your *treatment* intervention or strategy to achieve the outcome. *Note:* The list of *patient problems* and *outcomes of treatment* (short-term goals) should be as concise as possible, using only common abbreviations. They should also include all available quantitative data. This would exclude, however, extensive listings of decreases in ROM or strength. In these situations a more global statement should be used such as "decreased LE ROM" or "decreased LE strength." The reader can then refer to the detailed goniometric or MMT assessment. When decreases in ROM or strength are isolated to a select few joints or muscles, the values *are* typically included in the problem list. In the space below, first develop your **Clinical Problem List:**

Clinical Problem List:

5. **Directions:** In the spaces below, take each of your clinical problems *individually* and enter it after the designation **Clinical Problem** (one problem per cell). For each clinical problem, identify the **Outcome of Treatment** (short-term goal), and the proposed **Treatment** to achieve the outcome. *Be certain to include any required consultations with other disciplines in your plan.*

Clinical Problem 1:　　　*Outcome of Treatment (STG):*　　　*Treatment:*

Clinical Problem 2:　　　*Outcome of Treatment (STG):*　　　*Treatment:*

Clinical Problem 3:　　　*Outcome of Treatment (STG):*　　　*Treatment:*

Clinical Problem 4:　　　*Outcome of Treatment (STG):*　　　*Treatment:*

Clinical Problem 5:   *Outcome of Treatment (STG):*   *Treatment:*

Clinical Problem 6:   *Outcome of Treatment (STG):*   *Treatment:*

Clinical Problem 7:   *Outcome of Treatment (STG):*   *Treatment:*

Clinical Problem 8:   *Outcome of Treatment (STG):*   *Treatment:*

Clinical Problem 9:   *Outcome of Treatment (STG):*   *Treatment:*

Clinical Problem 10:   *Outcome of Treatment (STG):*   *Treatment:*

Clinical Problem 11:   *Outcome of Treatment (STG):*   *Treatment:*

Clinical Problem 12:   *Outcome of Treatment (STG):*   *Treatment:*

Clinical Problem 13:   *Outcome of Treatment (STG):*   *Treatment:*

Priorities for Initiating Treatment

Your next consideration is determining the priorities in approaching treatment. It is important to note that an artificial separation has been made here of the component steps in formulating a plan of care. In order to present information in smaller, sequential units with greater detail, identifying *priorities* has been separated from developing a *problem list, establishing outcomes,* and determining a *treatment plan.* These four items are logically considered in sequence or concurrently.

Your attention is now directed toward determining the priorities of the patient problems and organizing your approach to treatment. Now that you have completed your clinical problem list, identified functional outcomes, and treatment to accomplish the outcomes, you should establish a priority order. Assume for a moment you are now planning to begin your treatment for this patient. Consider the same group of clinical problems you identified above. Which of the clinical problems constitute a priority for treatment intervention? This will require making some decisions about the urgency of each problem. To guide your thinking in prioritizing the problem list, ask yourself the following questions: (1) Is early intervention for one problem more crucial than another? (2) Will priority placement of a problem make a difference in preventing further joint damage or pain? (3) Will resolution of a specific problem add more to improved function than another? (4) Will addressing any single problem contribute to minimizing or eliminating another problem? (5) Is it possible to select treatment that may influence more than a single problem?

6. **Directions:** Consider the list of clinical problems you identified earlier. From that list, determine the six problems you would place as your initial priorities. In the spaces below, list the problems in prioritized order (1 = most important, 2 = next most important, and so on).

Priority List of Clinical Problems:

1.   2.   3.

4.   5.   6.

---

7. **Directions:** In the space below, identify your general treatment approach or strategies for this patient together with the rationale for your decision making in prioritizing the problem list.

General treatment or strategy:

Rationale for priorities:

Determining Projected Number of Visits to Accomplish Outcomes

In a highly cost-conscious environment, therapists are often required to provide an estimate of the number of visits required to achieve the desired outcomes. Managed-care companies place specific constraints on the number of visits allowed for a given problem or diagnosis. In order to achieve patient outcomes within the established time frame, the therapist is challenged to select the most useful treatments, apply treatment in an efficient and cost-effective manner, increase intensity of treatment with an emphasis on function, shift responsibility for care to the patient earlier, and incorporate creative ancillary measures (patient education materials, community resources, group exercise programs, and so on) to accomplish outcomes.

Initially, determining the projected number of visits to accomplish outcomes appears a daunting task. This skill will improve with additional clinical exposure. However, you already have the foundational knowledge and skill to address this issue. A good way to initially approach this determination is to consider it from a more global perspective. For example, quickly peruse Column A and B in the table below. Compare example 1 from Column A with example 1 from Column B, then 2 with 2, and 3 with 3. Decide if the approximate time to accomplish each outcome would be different or approximately the same.

Column A	Column B
1. Gait training with crutches: 24-year-old patient with a fractured tibia following a fall from a trampoline.	1. Gait training with quadruped cane: 67-year-old patient with (R) hemiplegia using a new ankle/foot orthosis.
2. Teach use of constant passive motion unit: 68-year-old patient with a total knee replacement.	2. Improve trunk stability: 51-year-old patient with multiple sclerosis.
3. Increase ROM in (R) wrist following uncomplicated fracture of radius: 29-year-old well-motivated patient.	3. Increase ROM in (R) wrist following uncomplicated fracture of radius: 39-year-old well-motivated patient.

Granted, these examples are very straightforward. Examples 1 and 2 in Column A would take relatively less time to accomplish compared to examples 1 and 2 in Column B. For the third example in each column, the number of visits required would likely be similar.

Most frequently, therapists are asked to determine the length of time required to accomplish more discrete components of treatment. For this patient with rheumatoid arthritis, you have a lengthy list of patient education items you want to incorporate into your plan of care (signs and symptom of the disease, joint conservation techniques, home exercise program, and so on). Your past experience tells you it typically takes three visits to accomplish all these activities. If your past experience is not well developed yet, an experienced colleague will be a good resource as you begin making projections about required number of visits. Now, with the "three-visit average" in mind, consider asking yourself the following guiding questions: (1) Is there anything different or unusual about this patient's situation? (2) What unique resources are available? (3) Is the patient's cognitive status intact? (4) What is the patient's motivation level? (5) Are there any potential complicating factors? (6) Is the patient medically stable? (7) Is the patient compliant?

8. ***Directions:*** For each of the clinical problems, outcomes of treatment (short-term goals) and treatments identified below, enter the number of visits you project are needed to accomplish the outcome for this patient. Your answer should be placed after the designation **Projected Number of Visits.** Provide a rationale for your response using the guiding questions above. Then consider the availability of the *eight visits* approved by the insurance company. Are these sufficient? Would you recommend additional treatment at the patient's private expense? How many times per week would you suggest she come in? How would you distribute the visits over the month?

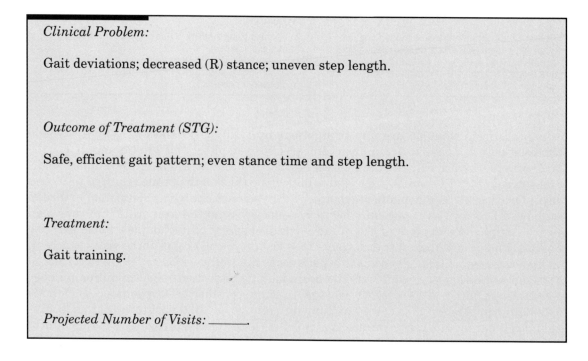

Clinical Problem:

Joint swelling (multiple areas); morning stiffness; MCP ulnar drift volar subluxation.

Outcome of Treatment (STG):

Decrease biomechanical stress on all affected joints.

Treatment:

Patient education; joint conservation techniques.

Projected Number of Visits: _____

Clinical Problem:

Gait deviations; decreased (R) stance; uneven step length.

Outcome of Treatment (STG):

Safe, efficient gait pattern; even stance time and step length.

Treatment:

Gait training.

Projected Number of Visits: _____.

Clinical Problem:

Ill-fitting/worn cane.

Outcome of Treatment (STG):

Correct use of well-fitted cane.

Treatment:

Provide new cane; patient education; gait training.

Projected Number of Visits: _____.

Clinical Problem:

Stair climbing (FIM level = 4).

Outcome of Treatment (STG):

Stair climbing (FIM level = 6).

Treatment:

Stair climbing training using standard cane; appropriate LE sequence.

Projected Number of Visits: _____.

Rationale for Projected Number of Visits

There are a number of unique aspects to this case that influence the number of visits required. The patient asset list includes: intact cognitive function, high motivation level, high patient compliance, stable medical status, absence of complicating factors to achieving outcomes, and a supportive family member willing to assist with care. The asset list provides sufficient support to accomplish the required treatment well within the allocated time frame. For example, the patient's cognitive status allows expanded use of written or videotaped patient education materials. Family support is available for any assistance needed with the home exercises. Motivation and compliance levels will ensure practice to accomplish learning the information needed (joint conservation techniques, gait training, and stair-climbing activities). Each of these items will contribute to maximizing the effectiveness of patient visits.

9. **Directions:** Consider the eight visits approved. Answer the following questions relative to this time allocation. (a) Are the eight visits approved sufficient? (b) Would you recommend additional treatment at private expense? (c) How many times per week would you suggest the patient schedule physical therapy? (d) How would you distribute the visits over the month?

PROGRESSION TO APPLICATION OF CONTENT

Case study 4 is the next in the series. It uses a *transitional approach* between the guided-question format in cases 1, 2, and 3 and the independent clinical decision-making process you will practice in cases 5 through 10. Several guided reminders about the decision-making process are included in case study 4; however, these are kept to a minimum. The remainder of the cases (5 through 10) are presented without guiding questions or activities; these cases provide an opportunity for independent practice of clinical decision-making skills through application of content. In cases 5 through 10, only the relevant data needed to establish functional outcomes and develop the plan of care are presented. The decision-making questions use a template of standardized questions that address the characteristic sequence used by physical therapists in determining a plan of care. This format includes (1) establishing a prioritized clinical problem list from the case data, (2) determining the patient asset list, (3) formulating goals and outcomes of treatment, (4) establishing a plan of care consistent with those outcomes (goals) and (5) providing a rationale for the decision making inherent in treatment planning. The format of the remaining cases will address independent practice along the same continuum of clinical decision-making steps used in previous case-study exercises: selection of pertinent data from assessment findings, analysis of these findings and development of a problem list, establishing outcomes (goals) and priorities, and development of treatment interventions. *Feedback* remains a high priority in working through the case studies. Below is a summary of grading scales and definitions used in cases 5 through 10.

Summary of Grading Scales Used in Case Studies 5–10

Balance

- Normal: Patient is able to maintain position with therapist maximally disturbing balance.
- Good: Patient is able to maintain position with moderate disturbance from therapist.
- Fair: Patient is able to maintain position for short periods of time unsupported.
- Poor: Patient attempts to maintain position but requires assistance from another person.
- No balance: Patient is unable to maintain position.

Pain Scale (PS)

(0 = none)   0   1   2   3   4   5   6   7   8   9   10   (10 = worst)

The Functional Independence Measure (FIM^SM)*: Summary of Scoring System

7 Complete Independence (timely, safely)	}	NO HELPER
6 Modified Independence (device)		
5 Supervision (Subject = 100%)	}	HELPER–MODIFIED
4 Minimal Assistance (Subject = 75%+)		DEPENDENCE
3 Moderate Assistance (Subject = 50%+)		
2 Maximal Assistance (Subject = 25%+)	}	HELPER—COMPLETE
1 Total Assistance (Subject = less than 25%)		DEPENDENCE

*FIM^SM is a service mark of the Uniform Data System for Medical Rehabilitation, a division of UB Foundation Activities, Inc.

Sensation

1. Intact—normal, accurate

2. Decreased—delayed response
3. Exaggerated—increased sensitivity

4. Inaccurate—inappropriate perception of stimulus
5. Absent—no response
6. Inconsistent or ambiguous

Review of Definitions

Direct impairments are the result of pathology or disease state and include any deviations from normal physiologic, anatomic, or psychologic function (1). Examples include direct manifestations of a disease state or insult such as diminished range of motion or strength, sensory loss, impairments in motor planning, or trunk rigidity or instability. Impairments may or may not be permanent.

Indirect impairments are those occurring *not* from the specific insult but from sequelae (secondary complications) of the insult. Indirect impairments might include decreased vital capacity, atrophy and weakness, contractures, decubitus ulcers, renal calculi, and deep venous thrombosis. Indirect impairments occur in systems *other than* that affected by the primary insult. These indirect impairments are frequently associated with prolonged inactivity, inadequate positioning, or lack of regular physical therapy or other rehabilitation intervention.

Composite impairments are those with multiple underlying origins. These include both direct (from the specific lesion), and indirect impairments. Abnormal endurance and balance deficits are examples of composite impairments (4).

Functional disability refers to an inability to complete a functional task within parameters typically considered reasonable or normal for that individual. Disability results from impairments, which are categorized as either physical, mental, social, or emotional in nature. (1, 3).

▼
Case Study 4: CONSTRUCTION ACCIDENT (TRAUMA)

▼ A 32-year-old patient presents following extensive trauma from a work-related accident. The patient is a foreman for a large construction firm. He has been with the company for the past 10 years. The accident occurred during a routine inspection of a construction site. A scaffold hoisting the patient to the top floor of the building gave way, causing a fall of approximately 100 feet. The patient was brought to the emergency room unconscious and remained in a coma for 3 days. Life-support interventions began immediately. As the coma subsided, the patient remained in a confused, agitated state for 4 days, when cognitive function began to slowly clear.

The patient sustained a severe cerebral contusion and multiple fractures. The fracture sites include: the mandible, the left femoral head and acetabulum, pelvis, left ankle (undisplaced bimalleolar; displaced talus), three left ribs, and the left humerus. A left pneumothorax was also sustained. The patient has been on numerous different analgesics, antibiotics, and expectorants.

Past medical history. Essentially unremarkable. Physical examination revealed intact cranial nerves with sensory deficits of the left upper extremity. No sensory deficits were noted for touch, vibration, pain, or position of the right upper extremity or either lower extremity. The patient was cooperative; he indicated that he expected complete recovery and was anxious to be able to do things for himself. He also reported a history of sporadic low back pain, which he treated with heat and rest. The pain was typically brought on by prolonged sitting. He reported the position as foreman required at least 1 day per week of office work to meet with clients and complete paper work. These were usually the days he experienced low back pain.

Social history. The patient has been married for 6 years and has two children, 2 and 4 years of age. The family lives in a suburban four-bedroom home. The patient's wife is a dental hygienist. She recently took a leave of absence from her position to care for her husband. This was not the original plan, as several close relatives had offered assistance upon the patient's return home. The promised help never materialized; this has caused some considerable dissention within the family and placed strain on the marriage. Most of the patient's financial needs are being met through workman's compensation.

Course of management. Orthopedic intervention included internal wiring of the mandible, prosthetic replacement of both the femoral head and acetabulum on the left, reduction of the fracture dislocation of the left talus with casting, and casting of the left humerus. The pelvis and rib fractures were nondisplaced and stable; they were treated with bed rest. The patient returned home non-weight bearing after an 11-day hospitalization and was monitored as an outpatient through the orthopedic clinic. He received home-care physical therapy three times per week.

It is now 47 days after the accident. The orthopedic surgeon has requested more intensive physical therapy. The patient is to begin treatment today as an outpatient four times per week. Transportation is provided through the worker's compensation benefits. The ankle and upper extremity casts were removed yesterday. The patient arrived at the outpatient department unaccompanied, using a standard wheelchair. He has been cleared for all weight-bearing mat activities on both the left upper and lower extremity. Upright weight bearing (standing) to tolerance on the left can begin in 10 days.

PHYSICAL THERAPY ASSESSMENT

Review of Systems

Vision. Intact.

Blood pressure. 120/75.

Skin condition. Intact; no breaks in skin noted; areas under cast dry and flaky.

Temperature. 97.5°F.

Coordination. (R) upper and lower extremities—within normal limits; (L) deferred.

Weight-bearing status. Non-weight bearing (L) lower extremity.

Cognitive Function

The patient demonstrates goal-directed behavior but is dependent on external input or direction. He is able to follow simple directions consistently and shows carryover for re-learned tasks such as self-care. Responses may be incorrect due to memory problems, but they are within the context of the functional task at hand. Past memories show more depth and detail than recent memory.

Respiratory Assessment

Respiratory Rate: 14 breaths per minute. **Depth:** Shallow; decreased lung expansion and chest wall movement; circumferential chest measurement (difference between maximum exhalation and maximum inhalation) = 1 in. (2.5 cm). **Rhythm:** Regular. **Lung sounds:** Within normal limits (WNL). **Pulse (radial):** 70 beats per minute. **Cough:** Effective, nonproductive; elicits pain in left thoracic region.

Pain Assessment

Patient reports pain on motion of the left hip, ankle, and shoulder. **Left Hip:** PS = 5; **Left Ankle:** PS = 7; **Left Shoulder:** PS = 8; **Left Elbow:** PS = 7.

Sensation

Left upper extremity (UE): Deficits noted primarily along the radial three-quarters of the dorsum of the hand, dorsum of the thumb, dorsum of the index and middle fingers, and the distal radial half of the ring finger; Sharp/Dull: 2; Light Touch: 2; Temperature: 2; Proprioceptive Sensations: 2; Cortical Sensations: 2.

Functional Assessment

Bed mobility: *Rolling:* sidelying to right and left; FIM level = 7. *Movement transitions:* Supine-to-sit; FIM level = 4. *Bridging:* FIM level = 3. *Transfers:* Sit-to-stand: FIM level = 3 (non-weight bearing on [L] lower extremity). Stand-to-sit: FIM level = 3 (non-weight bearing on [L] lower extremity). Stand-pivot to wheelchair on right lower extremity: FIM level = 4. *Wheelchair mobility and use:* Mobility: independent in open areas: FIM level = 7.

Use (brakes, foot pedals, removable armrests, and so on): FIM = 7. *Activities of daily living:* Eating: FIM = 7; bathing: FIM = 4; dressing: FIM = 4.

Range of Motion Assessment: Upper and Lower Extremities

Goniometric Assessment (ROM): Lower Extremities			
Range of Motion (Degrees)		Right	Left
Hip:	Flexion	WFL*	0–100
	Extension	WFL	0–0
	Abduction	WFL	0–30
	Adduction	WFL	0–5
	External Rotation	WFL	0–25
	Internal Rotation	WFL	0–20
Knee:	Flexion	WFL	0–130
Ankle:	Dorsiflexion	WFL	0–5
	Plantar flexion	WFL	0–10
	Inversion	WFL	0–5
	Eversion	WFL	0–5

Goniometric Assessment (ROM): Upper Extremities			
Range of Motion (Degrees)		Right	Left
Shoulder:	Flexion	WFL*	0–120
	Extension	WFL	0–30
	Abduction	WFL	0–90
	External Rotation	WFL	0–50
	Internal Rotation	WFL	0–45
Elbow:	Flexion	WFL	0–100
Forearm:	Pronation	WFL	0–25
	Supination	WFL	0–30
Wrist:	Extension	WFL	0–55
	Flexion	WFL	0–60
	Radial Deviation	WFL	0–15
	Ulnar Deviation	WFL	0–20
Fingers:	Flexion†		

*WFL: Within functional limits.
†Finger flexion (mass grasp): Patient able to close hand approximately three-quarters through normal range of flexion; end ranges not available.

Strength Assessment: Lower Extremities

Manual Muscle Test (MMT)		Right	Left
Hip:	Flexion	WFL*	F−
	Extension	WFL	F−
	Abduction	WFL	F−
	Adduction	WFL	F−
	External rotation	WFL	F−
	Internal rotation	WFL	F−
Knee:	Flexion	WFL	G−
	Extension	WFL	F
Ankle:	Dorsiflexion	WFL	P
	Plantar flexion	WFL	F−
	Inversion	WFL	F−
	Eversion	WFL	F−

*WFL: Within functional limits.

Strength Assessment: Upper Extremities

Manual Muscle Test (MMT)		Right	Left
Shoulder:	Flexion	WFL*	F−
	Extension	WFL	F−
	Abduction	WFL	F−
	External rotation	WFL	F−
	Internal rotation	WFL	F−
Elbow:	Flexion	WFL	G−
Forearm:	Pronation	WFL	F−
	Supination	WFL	F−
Wrist:	Extension	WFL	G−
	Flexion	WFL	G−
	Radial deviation	WFL	G−
	Ulnar deviation	WFL	G−
Hand	Grip	WFL	F−†
	Pinch	WFL	F−

*WFL: Within functional limits.
†Left grip strength: MMT grade = F−.

Patient Goals

- Return to "normal."
- Eliminate pain.
- Return to work.
- Independence in ambulation and all functional skills.

Additional Findings

1. The patient complains of tightness and weakness of the low back muscles; tightness of the left hamstrings.
2. Decreased lower trunk rotation (toward right, 0–30 degrees; toward left, 0–25 degrees).
3. Low tolerance for sitting (approximately 20 minutes); difficulty shifting weight in sitting position to relieve pressure.
4. Weakness of trunk extensors (MMT = F+).
5. Tightness and swelling of the left hand and fingers.
6. Although ROM is within functional limits, tightness is evident at the extremes of range for all right lower extremity motions.

Step 1: Formulate a Problem List

Directions: In the space on the following page labeled **Prioritized Physical Therapy Problem List,** formulate and prioritize the physical therapy problem list. Your problem list should, as often as possible, include all available quantitative data. This will provide baseline data you can use to document patient progress and the effectiveness of selected treatment interventions. To guide your thinking in prioritizing the list, consider the following questions:

1. Is early intervention for one problem more crucial than another?
2. Will priority placement of a problem make a difference in preventing further joint damage or pain?
3. Will resolution of a specific problem add more to improved function than another?
4. Will addressing any single problem contribute to minimizing or eliminating another problem?
5. Is it possible to select treatment that may influence more than a single problem?

It is important to note that it is unlikely that your answers here will be in the exact order of suggested priority as presented in Appendix B. This is perfectly acceptable. However, certain categories of problems should always be at the top of your list. These include problems such as cognitive status, pain, communication skills, sensory and perceptual deficits, and functional status.

Prioritized Physical Therapy Problem List:

Step 2: Formulate an Asset List

Directions: In the space below labeled **Patient Asset List,** develop an asset list by identifying the patient's strengths. The asset list requires analysis of the assessment data to determine patient strengths and abilities. It should include all areas of available patient function that can be emphasized during treatment to motivate the patient, such as a functional task that requires only minimal assistance or supervision.

Patient Asset List:

Step 3: Establish Functional Outcomes of Physical Therapy (Long-Term Goals) and Outcomes of Treatment (Short-Term Goals)

Directions: In the space provided below, indicate the functional outcome(s) of physical therapy for this patient (long-term goals—LTGs). This is the desired level of function at completion of treatment intervention. Below the entry, indicate the outcomes of treatment (short-term, incremental goals—STGs) that will contribute to achieving the overall desired outcome of physical therapy intervention. Your outcomes of treatment are written with consideration to a smaller time frame. A common time frame for outcomes of treatment is 2 weeks. This 14-day time frame should be used in formulating your short-term goals (STGs). Your outcomes of treatment should address each of the clinical problems identified.

The outcomes of treatment should, as often as possible, incorporate quantitative (measurable) data. This includes data from the patient assessment (patient status at beginning of the 2-week interval) compared with quantitative changes expected at the end of the 2-week interval of treatment.

Outcome(s) of Physical Therapy (Long-Term Goals):

Outcomes of Treatment (Short-Term Goals):

Step 4: Formulate the Physical Therapy Plan of Care

Directions: Consider your list of *physical therapy problems* identified above in Step 1. From this list, select five (5) highly prioritized problems that require advanced therapeutic exercise intervention. Select problems you will address in your initial 2 weeks of treatment. *Assume that the immediate problems of pain, swelling of the left hand, sensory deficits, and reduced chest expansion have already been addressed.* For each problem, determine the appropriate starting point in treatment, given the information in the case.

- Select the *five (5) problems* that require advanced therapeutic exercise intervention.
- For each problem, *select three (3) advanced procedures* that can be performed at this time to address the problem.
- *Prioritize the treatment* by indicating the procedure you will start with (first intervention), and what the order of progression will be for the other two procedures (second and third intervention).
- For each of the three (3) procedures you have selected to address the problem, include a description of the *position, activity,* and *technique.* If you have selected a movement transition (supine-to-sit, sit-to-stand, and so forth) to address the problem, describe how the activity will be *taught* and how you will *assist* the activity. Your response should incorporate both patient and therapist positioning, hand placements, influence of gravity or body weight, and verbal directions to the patient.

Fill in the five (5) boxes below as follows:

1. Enter each of your five selected problems at the very top of each box after the label "Problem 1," "Problem 2," and so forth. (Enter one problem per box.)
2. For each of the five problems, enter your outcome of treatment (short-term goal) on the next line after the designation "*Outcome of Treatment (Short-Term Goal)*." (Enter one outcome per box.)

3. Then enter the three selected positions/activities or movement transitions below the appropriate labels: "*First Intervention*, Position/Activity (or Movement Transition)"; "*Second Intervention*, Position/Activity;" and so forth. (Three interventions should be listed per box, *in order of priority*.)
4. After the label "Technique," indicate your *selected technique* for each Position/Activity, or, for movement transitions, describe how the activity will be *taught* and how you will *assist* the activity.

Note: Be sure to list therapeutic exercise procedures in sequential order of intended use (1: First Intervention, 2: Second Intervention, and 3: Third Intervention). For each therapeutic exercise intervention include *position, activity,* and *technique;* and for each movement transition include *teaching strategy* and *method of assistance.*

Problem 1:

Outcome of Treatment (Short-Term Goal):

1. **First Intervention**
   Position/Activity
   (or Movement Transition):   Technique:

2. **Second Intervention**
   Position/Activity: Technique:

3. **Third Intervention**
   Position/Activity: Technique:

Problem 2:

Outcome of Treatment (Short-Term Goal):

1. **First Intervention**
   Position/Activity
   (or Movement Transition):   Technique:

2. **Second Intervention**
   Position/Activity: Technique:

3. **Third Intervention**
   Position/Activity: Technique:

Problem 3:

Outcome of Treatment (Short-Term Goal):

1. **First Intervention**
   Position/Activity
   (or Movement Transition):   Technique:

2. **Second Intervention**
   Position/Activity: Technique:

3. **Third Intervention**
   Position/Activity: Technique:

Problem 4:

Outcome of Treatment (Short-Term Goal):

1. **First Intervention**
   Position/Activity
   (or Movement Transition):   Technique:

2. **Second Intervention**
   Position/Activity: Technique:

3. **Third Intervention**
   Position/Activity: Technique:

Problem 5:

Outcome of Treatment (Short-Term Goal):

1. **First Intervention**
   Position/Activity
   (or Movement Transition):   Technique:

2. **Second Intervention**
   Position/Activity: Technique:

3. **Third Intervention**
   Position/Activity: Technique:

Step 5: Justification for Treatment Procedure or Movement Transition

Provide a rationale for your decision making in selection of procedures to address the five highly prioritized problems. Your rationale should address: biomechanical considerations (center of gravity, base of support, and so forth), and any needed equipment such as Theraband tubing or a Swiss ball, stage of motor control (mobility, stability, controlled mobility, or skill); and relevant motor control factors.

Directions: From the information you identified earlier, enter each of your five Outcomes of Treatment on the lines below labeled **Outcome of Treatment (Short-Term Goal) 1 through 5:** Enter one outcome of treatment per box, in the same numerical order as used earlier. Below each outcome, indicate the **Therapeutic Exercises** or **Movement Transitions** selected. This information should then be followed by your **Rationale for Selection** of the *therapeutic exercise* or *movement transition*. Next, indicate the **Techniques** selected, together with the motor control goals and indications.

Examples of *Rationale for Selection* of the therapeutic exercise or movement transition might include: alterations in base of support or center of gravity, demands on postural control and balance or specific limb segments, planes of movement required, types and combinations of muscle contractions required, proprioceptive input, influence of body weight and gravity, use and rationale for any needed equipment, and so on.

Techniques should include the *motor control goal* (mobility, stability, controlled mobility, or skill) and *indications* for use, such as active movement control, effective problem solving, inability to complete full range of movement, poor eccentric control, and so on.

Outcome of Treatment (Short-Term Goal) 1:

Therapeutic Exercise or Movement Transition:

Rationale for Selection:

Techniques (Motor Control Goal and Indications):

Outcome of Treatment (Short-Term Goal) 2:

Therapeutic Exercise or Movement Transition:

Rationale for Selection:

Techniques (Motor Control Goal and Indications):

Outcome of Treatment (Short-Term Goal) 3:

Therapeutic Exercise or Movement Transition:

Rationale for Selection:

Techniques (Motor Control Goal and Indications):

Outcome of Treatment (Short-Term Goal) 4:

Therapeutic Exercise or Movement Transition:

Rationale for Selection:

Techniques (Motor Control Goal and Indications):

Outcome of Treatment (Short-Term Goal) 5:

Therapeutic Exercise or Movement Transition:

Rationale for Selection:

Techniques (Motor Control Goal and Indications):

▼
Case Study 5: STROKE

Suggested Chapters for Review
Stroke
Assessment and Treatment Planning Strategies
for Perceptual Deficits
Neurogenic Disorders of Speech and Language

In O'Sullivan, SB and Schmitz, TJ (eds): *Physical Rehabilitation:
Assessment and Treatment,* ed.3. FA Davis, Philadelphia.

▼ The patient is a 52-year-old male executive who sustained a left cerebral vascular accident (CVA) secondary to a ruptured aneurysm of the left middle cerebral artery with resultant right hemiplegia. The stroke occurred eight days ago. He was transferred from the acute-care hospital to the rehabilitation facility late yesterday afternoon. The patient has been assigned to your caseload and you are in the process of planning your initial assessment.

Past medical history. The patient has a history of mild hypertension controlled by medication. His last physical exam (6 months ago) indicated a high cholesterol level of 240 mg/dL (dietary control has been recommended). He is approximately 20 pounds overweight and recently gave up smoking a pack of cigarettes per day. There is no family history of stroke. However, both of his parents were diagnosed with premature coronary artery disease.

Social history. The patient lives with his wife. They have three adult children. He has a master's degree in business administration. He advanced quickly through a series of promotions within a large advertising firm and now holds the position of vice president. He and his wife live in a new ranch-style home in a nearby suburb. His wife reports some "considerable distancing" has occurred between the couple owing to his demanding work schedule.

PHYSICAL THERAPY ASSESSMENT

Cognitive Function

There has been some marked return of intellectual function within the past 3 days. However, major deficit areas persist. The patient's verbal task performance is better than his performance of spatial perceptual tasks. He has difficulty with problem solving, new learning, and recognition. Language skills are dysarthric, although functional, with marked episodes of perseveration. Difficulty is also noted with interpretation of word definitions, multilevel tasks, and conceptual thoughts or ideas.

Range of Motion

Upper extremities (UEs). Within functional limits; right shoulder demonstrates pain and tightness in extremes of all ranges.

Lower extremities (LEs). Within functional limits (except [R] dorsiflexion); right dorsiflexion (0–5 degrees).

Sensation

Right UE (hemisensory loss). Sharp/Dull: 2; Light Touch: 2; Temperature: 4; Proprioceptive Sensations: 5; Cortical Sensations: 5.

Right LE (hemisensory loss). Sharp/Dull: 2; Light Touch: 4; Temperature: 4; Proprioceptive Sensations: 5; Cortical Sensations: 5. Patient reports pain in both right upper and lower extremities (PS = 7).

Assessment of Muscle Tone

Right UE. Moderate to severe tone increases in elbow flexors, shoulder adductors, and internal rotators. Consistent elbow flexor posturing in sitting.

Right LE. Moderate tone increases in hip extensors, knee extensors, and plantarflexors.

Motor Control Assessment

Right UE. Extensor synergy pattern present with effort (shoulder and elbow extension); no voluntary control of flexor synergy pattern evident; right upper extremity neglect (right upper extremity drops off lap or wheelchair armrest); no volitional movement outside of synergy.

Right LE. Both extensor and flexor synergy patterns present; extensor pattern dominant (extensor pattern only achieved with associated extensor pattern of right upper extremity); no volitional movement outside of synergy.

Left UE and LE. Full, active, isolated movement; good strength.

Trunk. Unable to sit unsupported; retracted right scapula with shoulder internal rotation and adduction; unable to extend trunk.

Coordination

Right UE and LE. Unable to test at this time.

Left UE and LE. Intact; within functional limits.

Posture

Sitting. Asymmetrical positioning—right hip and shoulder forward of the left; right shoulder droops down and forward; lateral flexion of right side of trunk; right upper extremity held in adducted, flexed posture; finger flexor hypertonicity; fair+ head control.

Standing. Not appropriate at this time.

Balance

Sitting. *Static:* Poor (FIM level* = 2); poor antigravity control; inability to hold posture. *Dynamic:* Poor⁻ (FIM level = 2).

---

*__Reminder:__ A summary of grading scales for balance, pain, the Functional Independence Measure (FIMˢᴹ), and sensation is located on pp. 240–241; a review of definitions (terminology) is on p. 241.

Endurance

Endurance. Fair; tolerates 30-minute treatment session.

Functional Assessment

Bed mobility. *Rolling:* requires moderate assistance; FIM level = 3; unable to assume sidelying to right or left; greater difficulty with attempts toward sound side; patient has difficulty keeping the affected UE forward to facilitate roll; unable to isolate upper and lower trunk movements. *Transfers:* Supine-to-sit: requires maximal assist; FIM level = 2. Sit-to-stand: FIM level = 2; stand-to-sit: FIM level = 2; stand-pivot to wheelchair: FIM level = 2. *Wheelchair mobility:* In unobstructed, open areas: FIM level = 3 (verbal cueing required). *Activities of daily living:* eating: FIM = 4 (once set up); bathing: FIM = 3; dressing: upper extremity/trunk: FIM level = 3; dressing: lower extremity/feet: FIM level = 2.

Step 1: Formulate a Problem List and Identify Terminology

Directions: In the space below labeled **Prioritized Physical Therapy Problem List** *formulate* and *prioritize* the physical therapy problem list. As you develop the problem list, indicate in the adjacent space the term that describes each problem (direct impairment, indirect impairment, composite impairment, or functional disability).

Prioritized Physical Therapy Problem List:	*Impairment / Functional Disability:*

Step 2: Formulate an Asset List

Directions: In the space below labeled **Patient Asset List,** identify the patient's strengths. The asset list should include areas of available patient functions that require reinforcement during treatment.

Patient Asset List:

Step 3: Establish Functional Outcomes of Physical Therapy (Long-Term Goals) and Outcomes of Treatment (Short-Term Goals)

Directions: In the space below, indicate the *functional outcome(s) of physical therapy* for this patient. This is the desired level of function at completion of treatment intervention. Below the entry, indicate each outcome of treatment (short-term, incremental goals) that will contribute to achieving the overall desired functional outcome (long-term goal) of physical therapy intervention. Assume you are writing your outcomes of treatment for a *2-week period* of treatment. Your outcomes of treatment should include each of the clinical problems you plan to address during the initial 2 weeks of treatment.

Outcome(s) of Physical Therapy (Long-Term Goals):

Outcomes of Treatment (Short-Term Goals):

Step 4: Formulate the Physical Therapy Plan of Care

Directions: Consider your list of physical therapy problems identified above in Step 1. From this list, select five (5) highly prioritized problems that require advanced therapeutic exercise intervention. Select problems you will address in your initial 2 weeks of treatment. For each problem, determine the appropriate starting point in treatment, given the information in the case.

- Select the *five (5) problems* that require advanced therapeutic exercise intervention.
- For each problem, *select three (3) advanced procedures* that can be performed at this time to address the problem.
- *Prioritize the treatment* by indicating the procedure you will start with (first intervention), and what the order of progression will be for the other two procedures (second and third intervention).
- For each of the three (3) procedures you have selected to address the problem, include a description of the *position, activity,* and *technique.* If you have selected a movement transition (supine-to-sit, sit-to-stand, and so forth) to address the problem, describe how the activity will be *taught* and how you will *assist* the activity. Your response should incorporate both patient and therapist positioning, hand placements, influence of gravity or body weight, and verbal directions to the patient.

Fill in the five (5) boxes below as follows:

1. Enter each of your five selected problems at the very top of each box after the label "*Problem 1*," "*Problem 2*," and so forth. (Enter one problem per box.)
2. For each of the five problems, enter your outcome of treatment (short-term goal) on the next line after the designation "*Outcome of Treatment (Short-Term Goal)*." (Enter one outcome per box.)
3. Then enter the three selected positions/activities or movement transitions below the appropriate labels: "*First Intervention*, Position/Activity (or Movement Transition)"; "*Second Intervention*, Position/Activity;" and so forth. (Three interventions should be listed per box, *in order of priority*.)
4. After the label "Technique," indicate your *selected technique* for each Position/Activity, or, for movement transitions, describe how the activity will be *taught* and how you will *assist* the activity.

Note: Be sure to list therapeutic exercise procedures in sequential order of intended use (1: First Intervention, 2: Second Intervention, and 3: Third Intervention). For each therapeutic exercise intervention include *position, activity,* and *technique;* and for each movement transition include *teaching strategy* and *method of assistance.*

Problem 1:

Outcome of Treatment (Short-Term Goal):

1. First Intervention
   Position/Activity
   (or Movement Transition):   Technique:

2. Second Intervention
   Position/Activity: Technique:

3. Third Intervention
   Position/Activity: Technique:

Problem 2:

Outcome of Treatment (Short-Term Goal):

1. First Intervention
   Position/Activity
   (or Movement Transition):   Technique:

2. Second Intervention
   Position/Activity: Technique:

3. Third Intervention
   Position/Activity: Technique:

Problem 3:

Outcome of Treatment (Short-Term Goal):

1. First Intervention
   Position/Activity
   (or Movement Transition):   Technique:

2. Second Intervention
   Position/Activity: Technique:

3. Third Intervention
   Position/Activity: Technique:

Problem 4:

Outcome of Treatment (Short-Term Goal):

1. First Intervention
   Position/Activity
   (or Movement Transition):   Technique:

2. Second Intervention
   Position/Activity: Technique:

3. Third Intervention
   Position/Activity: Technique:

Problem 5:

Outcome of Treatment (Short-Term Goal):

1. First Intervention
   Position/Activity
   (or Movement Transition):   Technique:

2. Second Intervention
   Position/Activity: Technique:

3. Third Intervention
   Position/Activity: Technique:

Step 5: Justification for Treatment Procedure or Movement Transition

Provide a rationale for your decision making in selection of procedures to address the five highly prioritized problems. Your rationale should address: biomechanical considerations (center of gravity, base of support, and so forth), and any needed equipment such as Theraband tubing or a Swiss ball, stage of motor control (mobility, stability, controlled mobility, or skill); and relevant motor control factors.

Directions: From the information you identified earlier, enter each of your five Outcomes of Treatment on the lines below labeled **Outcome of Treatment (Short-Term Goal) 1 through 5:** Enter one outcome of treatment per box, in the same numerical order as used earlier. Below each outcome, indicate the **Therapeutic Exercises** or **Movement Transitions** selected. This information should then be followed by your **Rationale for Selection** of the *therapeutic exercise* or *movement transition.* Next, indicate the **Techniques** selected, together with the motor control goals and indications.

Examples of *Rationale for Selection* of the therapeutic exercise or movement transition might include: alterations in base of support or center of gravity, demands on postural control and balance or specific limb segments, planes of movement required, types and combinations of muscle contractions required, proprioceptive input, influence of body weight and gravity, use and rationale for any needed equipment, and so on.

Techniques should include the *motor control goal* (mobility, stability, controlled mobility, or skill) and *indications* for use, such as active movement control, effective problem solving, inability to complete full range of movement, poor eccentric control, and so on.

Outcome of Treatment (Short-Term Goal) 1:

Therapeutic Exercise or Movement Transition:

Rationale for Selection:

Techniques (Motor Control Goal and Indications):

Outcome of Treatment (Short-Term Goal) 2:

Therapeutic Exercise or Movement Transition:

Rationale for Selection:

Techniques (Motor Control Goal and Indications):

Outcome of Treatment (Short-Term Goal) 3:

Therapeutic Exercise or Movement Transition:

Rationale for Selection:

Techniques (Motor Control Goal and Indications):

Problem 3:

Outcome of Treatment (Short-Term Goal):

1. First Intervention
   Position/Activity
   (or Movement Transition):   Technique:

2. Second Intervention
   Position/Activity: Technique:

3. Third Intervention
   Position/Activity: Technique:

Problem 4:

Outcome of Treatment (Short-Term Goal):

1. First Intervention
   Position/Activity
   (or Movement Transition):   Technique:

2. Second Intervention
   Position/Activity: Technique:

3. Third Intervention
   Position/Activity: Technique:

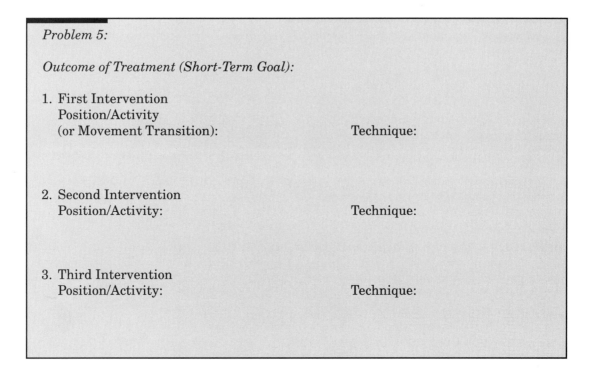

Step 5: Justification for Treatment Procedure or Movement Transition

Provide a rationale for your decision making in selection of procedures to address the five highly prioritized problems. Your rationale should address: biomechanical considerations (center of gravity, base of support, and so forth), and any needed equipment such as Theraband tubing or a Swiss ball, stage of motor control (mobility, stability, controlled mobility, or skill); and relevant motor control factors.

Directions: From the information you identified earlier, enter each of your five Outcomes of Treatment on the lines below labeled **Outcome of Treatment (Short-Term Goal) 1 through 5:** Enter one outcome of treatment per box, in the same numerical order as used earlier. Below each outcome, indicate the **Therapeutic Exercises** or **Movement Transitions** selected. This information should then be followed by your **Rationale for Selection** of the *therapeutic exercise* or *movement transition.* Next, indicate the **Techniques** selected, together with the motor control goals and indications.

Examples of *Rationale for Selection* of the therapeutic exercise or movement transition might include: alterations in base of support or center of gravity, demands on postural control and balance or specific limb segments, planes of movement required, types and combinations of muscle contractions required, proprioceptive input, influence of body weight and gravity, use and rationale for any needed equipment, and so on.

Techniques should include the *motor control goal* (mobility, stability, controlled mobility, or skill) and *indications* for use, such as active movement control, effective problem solving, inability to complete full range of movement, poor eccentric control, and so on.

Outcome of Treatment (Short-Term Goal) 1:

Therapeutic Exercise or Movement Transition:

Rationale for Selection:

Techniques (Motor Control Goal and Indications):

Outcome of Treatment (Short-Term Goal) 2:

Therapeutic Exercise or Movement Transition:

Rationale for Selection:

Techniques (Motor Control Goal and Indications):

Outcome of Treatment (Short-Term Goal) 3:

Therapeutic Exercise or Movement Transition:

Rationale for Selection:

Techniques (Motor Control Goal and Indications):

Outcome of Treatment (Short-Term Goal) 4:

Therapeutic Exercise or Movement Transition:

Rationale for Selection:

Techniques (Motor Control Goal and Indications):

Outcome of Treatment (Short-Term Goal) 5:

Therapeutic Exercise or Movement Transition:

Rationale for Selection:

Techniques (Motor Control Goal and Indications):

▼
Case Study 7: MULTIPLE SCLEROSIS

Suggested Chapter for Review
Multiple Sclerosis

In O'Sullivan, SB and Schmitz, TJ (eds): *Physical Rehabilitation:
Assessment and Treatment,* ed. 3. FA Davis, Philadelphia.

▼ A 37-year-old patient with a 6-year history of multiple sclerosis (MS) arrives for outpatient treatment today. The patient is well known to you. He has been admitted to the hospital twice over the past 3 years. He periodically returns to outpatient physical therapy to update his home program or when he notices changes in functional status or experiences difficulty accomplishing a particular task. The patient lives alone in an assisted-living apartment complex. He has a background in hospital administration and holds a part-time position at a hospital several blocks away.

Medical history. The onset of the multiple sclerosis began 6 years ago with severe, transient visual impairments that included blurred vision and bilateral upper field defects. The patient then experienced a remission of symptoms that lasted approximately a year. Following that initial year, symptoms have persisted somewhat unrelentingly, with greatest involvement in the lower extremities (LEs). He has long periods when his symptoms are relatively stable, but he has not experienced another true remission. He is able to functionally ambulate indoors on level surfaces using bilateral forearm crutches. A wheelchair is used for community and work-related activities.

Objective Findings

The patient indicated he has experienced a number of functional changes over recent weeks that are of major concern to him. These include:

1. During morning grooming activities (which he does standing), reaching for a towel or item from a shelf at eye level routinely throws him off balance.
2. He has also experienced difficulty sitting down. He recalls your teaching him an effective lowering technique, but lately he has just been plopping down hard into the chair without much control.
3. He can no longer get himself up from the floor to standing position. He often watches TV propped with pillows on the floor. He is no longer able to accomplish a floor to standing transfer.
4. Some noticeable increase in lower extremity spasticity levels has occurred. He feels as if the strength of the spasticity is actually pulling his legs together when he is walking; this has slowed down his speed and lowered his endurance. The lower trunk rotation activities he was taught to do in supine position are no longer effective in diminishing the spasticity.

Current Drug Management. Baclofen, 20 mg PO qid (four times daily); diazepam (Valium) 10 mg qid.

Social history. The patient has been divorced for 2 years. The marriage lasted 8 years. He has no children. Immediately following the divorce, he stayed with his parents for 18 months until an assisted-living apartment become available. He is the youngest of five children. His family is reasonably close-knit and he stays in touch with everyone. There is no family history of multiple sclerosis. He maintains a regular home exercise program

(HEP) of resistive UE strengthening and LE ROM and stretching exercises. He serves as the coordinator of a local MS information and support group. He drives using hand controls.

PHYSICAL THERAPY ASSESSMENT

Review of Systems

Cognitive status. Alert; oriented; memory intact.

Vision. Transient double vision.

Endurance. Fair to good; tolerance to activity is approximately 30 minutes (with some fluctuation) before rest is required.

Communication. Intact; with fatigue, speech assumes a dysarthric quality.

Range of Motion Assessment

Right dorsiflexion. 0–0 degrees.

Left dorsiflexion. 0–5 degrees.

All other joints. Range of motion within normal limits (WNL).

Assessment of Muscle Tone

Lower extremity (LE) involvement (bilateral). Severe extensor hypertonicity (slightly stronger on right) of quadriceps, adductors, and plantarflexors (posterior tibialis and gastrocnemius/soleus).

Motor Control Assessment

Diminished upright trunk and hip control; poor eccentric control (difficulty sitting down slowly); weakness and incoordination of postural extensors; diminished upright weight-shift control.

Gait Analysis

The patient is a functional indoor (household) ambulator using bilateral forearm crutches. He has not been able to climb stairs effectively for approximately 1 year.

Observational Analysis
1. Strong extensor and adductor spasticity, causing LEs to take on a scissoring-type pattern.
2. Overall decrease in speed of movement.
3. Diminished, awkward weight transfer.
4. Hip/pelvis (bilateral): Diminished lower trunk rotation; decreased pelvic rotation; uneven pelvis (elevated on right); hip hiking; diminished hip flexion.
5. Knee (bilateral): Diminished knee flexion; awkward, uncoordinated advancement of the tibia.
6. Foot/ankle: Heels do not touch the ground.

Sensation*

Lower extremities (LEs). Sharp/Dull: 1; Light Touch: 1; Temperature: 1; Proprioceptive Sensations: 4; Cortical Sensations: 1.

Upper extremities (UEs). Sharp/Dull: 1; Light Touch: 1; Temperature: 1; Proprioceptive Sensations: 1; Cortical Sensations: 1.

Strength Assessment

	Manual Muscle Test (MMT) Grades[†]		
Lower Extremities[‡]		Right	Left
Lower trunk:	Extensors	F	F
	Flexors	G	G
Hip:	Flexion	G	G
	Extension	F−	F
	Abduction	Unable to test—excessively high tone.	
	Adduction	Unable to test—excessively high tone.	
	External Rotation	F	F
	Internal Rotation	F	F+
Knee:	Flexion	Unable to test—excessively high tone.	
	Extension	Unable to test—excessively high tone.	
Ankle:	Dorsiflexion	Unable to test—excessively high tone.	
	Plantarflexion	Unable to test—excessively high tone.	
	Inversion	P+	P+
	Eversion	P+	P+

[†]*Note:* All MMT grades are approximate; hypertonicity prevented accurate testing using standard protocol.
[‡]Upper extremity strength: Within normal limits (WNL).

Coordination Assessment

Upper extremities. Bilateral low-frequency intention tremors; slight limb ataxia.

Lower extremities. Movements restricted by spasticity and spasms.

Balance*

Sitting. *Static:* Good+; able to maintain static position for unlimited period of time; minimal postural tremor evident. *Visual input:* Able to weight-shift to left and right 100% of limits of stability (LOS); *vision occluded:* Able to weight-shift to left and right 60% of limits of stability (LOS).

Sitting. *Dynamic:* Fair. *Visual input:* Able to weight-shift to left and right 50% of limits of stability (LOS) for approximately 10 minutes before postural tremors interfere with control; vision occluded: unable to maintain limits of stability (LOS).

Standing using parallel bars. *Static:* Good. (2) *Dynamic:* Fair−.

Reminder: A summary of grading scales for balance, pain, the Functional Independence Measure (FIMᔆᴹ), and sensation is located on pages 240–241; a review of definitions (terminlology) is on page 241.

Functional Assessment

Transfers. Floor-to-standing: FIM level = 3; the patient is independent in all basic activities of daily living—BADLs (FIM levels = 6 and 7), with the exception of floor-to-stand transfers; the patient is independent in approximately 85% of instrumental activities of daily living—IADLs (limitations imposed by fatigue and low ambulatory tolerance, patient's inability to climb stairs, and inaccessibility of some public buildings).

Step 1: Formulate a Problem List and Identify Terminology

Directions: In the space below labeled **Prioritized Physical Therapy Problem List,** *formulate* and *prioritize* the physical therapy problem list. Refer to the discussion of terminology included in the introductory material for this section of the text. As you develop the list, indicate the term that best describes the source of the individual problem (direct impairment, indirect impairment, composite impairment, or functional disability).

Prioritized Physical Therapy Problem List: *Impairment / Functional Disability:*

Step 2: Formulate an Asset List

Directions: In the space below labeled **Patient Asset List,** identify the patient's strengths. The asset list should include areas of available patient function that require reinforcement during treatment.

Patient Asset List:

Step 3: Establish Functional Outcomes of Physical Therapy (Long-Term Goals) and Outcomes of Treatment (Short-Term Goals)

Directions: In the space provided below, indicate the *functional outcome(s) of physical therapy* for this patient. This is the desired level of function at completion of treatment intervention. Below the entry, indicate each outcome of treatment (short-term, incremental goals) that will contribute to achieving the overall desired outcome of physical therapy intervention. Assume you are writing your outcomes of treatment for a *2-week period* of treatment. Your outcomes of treatment should include each of the patient problems you plan to address during the initial 2 weeks of treatment.

Outcome(s) of Physical Therapy (Long-Term Goals):

Outcomes of Treatment (Short-Term Goals):

Step 4: Formulate the Physical Therapy Plan of Care

Directions: Consider your list of physical therapy problems identified above in Step 1. From this list, select five (5) highly prioritized problems that require advanced therapeutic exercise intervention. Select problems you will address in your initial 2 weeks of treatment. For each problem, determine the appropriate starting point in treatment, given the information in the case.

- Select the *five (5) problems* that require advanced therapeutic exercise intervention.
- For each problem, *select three (3) advanced procedures* that can be performed at this time to address the problem.
- *Prioritize the treatment* by indicating the procedure you will start with (first intervention) and the order of progression for the other two procedures (second and third intervention).
- For each of the three (3) procedures you have selected to address the problem, include a description of the *position, activity,* and *technique.* If you have selected a movement transition (supine-to-sit, sit-to-stand, and so forth) to address the problem, describe how the activity will be *taught* and how you will *assist* the activity. Your response should incorporate both patient and therapist positioning, hand placements, influence of gravity or body weight, and verbal directions to the patient.

Fill in the five (5) boxes below as follows:

1. Enter each of your five selected problems at the very top of each box after the label *"Problem 1," "Problem 2,"* and so forth. (Enter one problem per box.)
2. For each of the five problems, enter your outcome of treatment (short-term goal) on the next line after the designation *"Outcome of Treatment (Short-Term Goal)."* (Enter one outcome per box.)
3. Then enter the three selected positions/activities or movement transitions below the label *"First Intervention, Position/Activity (or Movement Transition);" "Second Intervention, Position/Activity;"* and so forth. (Three interventions should be listed per box, *in order of priority.*)
4. After the label *"Technique,"* indicate your *selected technique* for each Position/Activity, or, for movement transitions, describe how the activity will be *taught* and how you will *assist* the activity.

Note: Be sure to list therapeutic exercise procedures in sequential order of intended use (1: First Intervention, 2: Second Intervention, and 3: Third Intervention). For each therapeutic exercise intervention include *position, activity,* and *technique;* and for each movement transition include *teaching strategy* and *method of assistance.*

Problem 1:

Outcome of Treatment (Short-Term Goal):

1. First Intervention
   Position/Activity
   (or Movement Transition):   Technique:

2. Second Intervention
   Position/Activity: Technique:

3. Third Intervention
   Position/Activity: Technique:

Problem 2:

Outcome of Treatment (Short-Term Goal):

1. First Intervention
   Position/Activity
   (or Movement Transition):   Technique:

2. Second Intervention
   Position/Activity: Technique:

3. Third Intervention
   Position/Activity: Technique:

Problem 3:

Outcome of Treatment (Short-Term Goal):

1. First Intervention
   Position/Activity
   (or Movement Transition):   Technique:

2. Second Intervention
   Position/Activity: Technique:

3. Third Intervention
   Position/Activity: Technique:

Problem 4:

Outcome of Treatment (Short-Term Goal):

1. First Intervention
   Position/Activity
   (or Movement Transition):   Technique:

2. Second Intervention
   Position/Activity: Technique:

3. Third Intervention
   Position/Activity: Technique:

Problem 5:

Outcome of Treatment (Short-Term Goal):

1. First Intervention
   Position/Activity
   (or Movement Transition):   Technique:

2. Second Intervention
   Position/Activity: Technique:

3. Third Intervention
   Position/Activity: Technique:

Step 5: Justification for Treatment Procedure or Movement Transition

Provide a rationale for your decision making in selection of procedures to address the five highly prioritized problems. Your rationale should address: biomechanical considerations (center of gravity, base of support, and so on), and any equipment needed such as Theraband tubing or a Swiss ball, stage of motor control (mobility, stability, controlled mobility, or skill); and relevant motor control factors.

Directions: From the information you identified earlier, enter each of your five Outcomes of Treatment on the lines below labeled **Outcome of Treatment (Short-Term Goal) 1 through 5:** Enter one outcome of treatment per box, in the same numerical order as used earlier. Below each outcome, indicate the **Therapeutic Exercises** or **Movement Transitions** selected to address the outcome of treatment. This information should then be followed by your **Rationale for Selection** of the *therapeutic exercise* or *movement transition*. Next, indicate the **Techniques** selected, together with the motor control goals and indications.

Examples of *Rationale for Selection* of the therapeutic exercise or movement transition might include: alterations in base of support or center of gravity, demands on postural control and balance or specific limb segments, planes of movement required, types and combinations of muscle contractions required, proprioceptive input, influence of body weight and gravity, use and rationale for any needed equipement, and so on.

Techniques (motor control goal and indications) should include the *motor control goal* (mobility, stability, controlled mobility, or skill); and *indications* for use, such as active movement control, effective problem solving, inability to complete full range of movement, poor eccentric control, and so on.

Outcome of Treatment (Short-Term Goal) 1:

Therapeutic Exercise or Movement Transition:

Rationale for Selection:

Techniques (Motor Control Goal and Indications):

Outcome of Treatment (Short-Term Goal) 2:

Therapeutic Exercise or Movement Transition:

Rationale for Selection:

Techniques (Motor Control Goal and Indications):

Outcome of Treatment (Short-Term Goal) 3:

Therapeutic Exercise or Movement Transition:

Rationale for Selection:

Techniques (Motor Control Goal and Indications):

Outcome of Treatment (Short-Term Goal) 4:

Therapeutic Exercise or Movement Transition:

Rationale for Selection:

Techniques (Motor Control Goal and Indications):

Functional Assessment

BADLs: Independent (FIM level = 7); **IADLs:** Independent (FIM level = 7).

Gait Analysis

Results of observational gait analysis (observed on both level and uneven surfaces): (1) Diminished forward pelvis and lower trunk rotation. (2) Diminished timing and sequencing of forward progression. (3) Decreased control of (limits of stability) LOS. (4) Decreased musculoskeletal responses necessary for balance. (5) Asymmetrical weight distribution.

Residual Limb Assessment

Essentially unremarkable. The limb was amputated through the middle third of the femur. Equal-length anterior and posterior skin flaps were used to close the incision. The scar is flexible, nonadherent, and placed at the distal end of the limb. Femoral pulse is strong and regular. The limb is conical without excess adipose tissue or dog ears. Phantom sensations have been experienced on a regular basis. For approximately 8 months following the amputation the patient experienced phantom pain, which gradually subsided.

Step 1: Formulate a Problem List and Identify Terminology

Directions: In the space below labeled **Prioritized Physical Therapy Problem List,** *formulate* and *prioritize* the clinical problem list. As you develop the list, indicate the uniform term that describes the individual problem (direct impairment, indirect impairment, composite impairment, or functional disability).

Prioritized Physical Therapy Problem List:	*Impairment/Functional Disability:*

Step 2: Formulate an Asset List

Directions: In the space below labeled **Patient Asset List,** identify the patient's strengths. The asset list should include areas of available patient function that require reinforcement during treatment.

Patient Asset List:

Step 3: Establish Functional Outcomes of Physical Therapy (Long-Term Goals) and Outcomes of Treatment (Short-Term Goals)

Directions: In the space provided below, indicate the *functional outcome*(s) *of physical therapy* for this patient. This is the desired level of function at completion of the treatment intervention. Below the entry, indicate each outcome of treatment (short-term, incremental goal) that will contribute to achieving the overall desired outcome of physical therapy intervention. Assume you are writing your outcomes of treatment for a *2-week period* of treatment. Your outcomes of treatment should include each of the clinical problems you plan to address during the initial 2 weeks of treatment.

For each outcome of treatment (short-term goal) identify the *projected number of visits* to accomplish the outcome (goal). In determining the projected number of visits, remember to ask yourself several important questions:

- Is there anything different or unusual about this patient situation?
- What unique resources are available?
- Is the patient's cognitive status intact?
- What is the patient's motivation level?
- Are there any potential complicating factors?
- Is the patient medically stable?
- Is the patient compliant?

For each of the outcomes of treatment (short-term goals) enter the number of visits you would project needed to accomplish the outcome for this patient. Your answer should be placed after the designation *Projected Number of Visits.* If you feel uncomfortable making decisions about projected number of visits at this point, move on and complete *Step 4: Formulate and Justify a Physical Therapy Plan of Care* and return to this question after decisions are made about the specific treatment interventions required.

Outcome(s) of Physical Therapy (Long-Term Goal):

Outcomes of Treatment (Short-Term Goals):   *Projected Number of Visits:*

Step 4: Formulate and Justify a Physical Therapy Plan of Care

Directions:

- From your list developed in Step 1, select *five (5) highly prioritized problems* that re-quire advanced therapeutic exercise intervention Select problems you will address in your initial two weeks of treatment. For each problem, determine the appropriate start-ing point in treatment, given the information in the case. In the boxes below, enter each of your five selected problems after the labels *"Problem 1" through "Problem 5."*
- For each of the five problems, enter your outcome of treatment (short-term goal) on the next line after the designation *"Outcome of Treatment (Short-Term Goal)."*
- For each problem, *select two (2) advanced treatment procedures* that can be performed at this time to address the problem. *Prioritize the treatment* by indicating the order of procedures (first intervention and second intervention). Enter this information below on the lines labeled *"First Intervention, Position / Activity (or Movement Transition)"* and *"Second Intervention, Position / Activity."* Immediately below this entry, include a description of the *position / activity* or *movement transition.* If you have selected a movement transition to address the problem, provide a description of how the activity will be *taught* and how you will *assist* the activity. Your response should incorporate both patient and therapist positioning, hand placements, influence of gravity or body weight, and verbal directions to the patient.
- Provide a rationale for you decision making in selection of procedures(s) to address the five highly prioritized problems. Justification for selection of the Position/Activity should be entered following the designation *"Rationale for Selection."*
- In the space labeled *"Technique,"* indicate your *selected technique(s)* for each Position/Activity or, for *movement transitions,* describe how the activity will be *taught* and how you will *assist* the activity.
- After the label *Motor Control Goals and Indications,* identify the *motor control goal* (mo-bility, stability, controlled mobility, or skill); and *indications* for the treatment selection.

Problem 1:

Outcome of Treatment (Short-Term Goal):

1. First Intervention
   Position/Activity (or Movement
   Transition):

   Technique:

   Rationale for Selection:

   Motor Control Goals and Indications:

2. Second Intervention
   Position/Activity:

   Technique:

   Rationale for Selection:

   Motor Control Goals and Indications:

Problem 2:

Outcome of Treatment (Short-Term Goal):

1. First Intervention
   Position/Activity (or Movement
   Transition):

   Technique:

   Rationale for Selection:

   Motor Control Goals and Indications:

2. Second Intervention
   Position/Activity:

   Technique:

   Rationale for Selection:

   Motor Control Goals and Indications:

Problem 3:

Outcome of Treatment (Short-Term Goal):

1. First Intervention
   Position/Activity (or Movement
   Transition):

   Technique:

   Rationale for Selection:

   Motor Control Goals and Indications:

2. Second Intervention
   Position/Activity:

   Technique:

   Rationale for Selection:

   Motor Control Goals and Indications:

Problem 4:

Outcome of Treatment (Short-Term Goal):

1. First Intervention
   Position/Activity (or Movement
   Transition):

   Technique:

   Rationale for Selection:

   Motor Control Goals and Indications:

2. Second Intervention
   Position/Activity:

   Technique:

   Rationale for Selection:

   Motor Control Goals and Indications:

Problem 5:

Outcome of Treatment (Short-Term Goal):

1. First Intervention
   Position/Activity (or Movement
   Transition):   Technique:

   Rationale for Selection: Motor Control Goals and Indications:

2. Second Intervention
   Position/Activity: Technique:

   Rationale for Selection: Motor Control Goals and Indications:

▼

Case Study 10: ACHILLES TENDON RUPTURE

▼ A 38-year-old patient ruptured her right Achilles tendon 2 months ago. The incident occurred while she was playing basketball on an indoor court during a routine practice before a scheduled game. The volleyball caught her unexpectedly off guard. As she suddenly jumped to hit the ball, she felt a sharp pain move up the back of her leg. She reports the pain started while the foot was still fixed to the floor. She immediately lost plantarflexion control and the foot/ankle began to swell. She also reported being able to palpate a gap in the tendon. The limb was packed in ice and she was transported via ambulance to the emergency room.

The tendon was surgically repaired and a non-weight-bearing cast was applied with the ankle in a plantarflexed position. The cast was in place for 7 weeks and removed 2 days ago. She is currently ambulating using crutches with weight bearing to tolerance. She reports that the current weakness of the muscles around the ankle are making the entire extremity feel very unstable. She is concerned about the potential for further injury.

The patient is a supervising nurse at a local hospital. During the period of casting she continued to work but reluctantly reduced her hours because of the increased energy expenditure required for walking with crutches and commuting. The injury has disrupted both her professional and leisure activities. She is very anxious about the impact of the injury on both her career and her favorite pastime. Past medical history is essentially unremarkable. She recalls being hospitalized only once before, for a childhood tonsillectomy.

PHYSICAL THERAPY ASSESSMENT

Patient Goals

- Restore ankle and foot to normal function as quickly as possible.
- Return to a full-time work schedule.
- Return to active participation in volleyball.

Range of Motion and Strength Assessment: Right Ankle

Goniometric Assessment (ROM) and Manual Muscle Test (MMT)		
Lower Extremity (R)	ROM	MMT
Ankle: Dorsiflexion	0–5	F–
Plantarflexion	0–10	F–
Inversion	0–10	F–
Eversion	0–5	F–

ROM and strength are within normal limits for all other extremities and trunk.

Balance Assessment

Upright balance: (1) Diminished limits of stability (LOS). (2) Reduced ankle excursion. (3) Impaired ankle excursion. (4) Diminished ankle strategies. (5) Increased dependence on hip strategies.

Functional Assessment

BADL: Independent (FIM level = 7). **IADL:** Independent (FIM level = 7).

Review of Systems

All findings negative:

- **Vital Signs:** WNL (within normal limits).
- **Sensation:** WNL
- **Posture:** WNL
- **Tolerance:** WNL
- **Coordination:** WNL

Step 1: Formulate a Problem List and Identify Terminology

Directions: In the space below labeled **Prioritized Physical Therapy Problem List,** *formulate* and *prioritize* the physical therapy problem list. As you develop the list, indicate the uniform term that describes the individual problem (direct impairment, indirect impairment, composite impairment, or functional disability).

Prioritized Physical Therapy Problem List: *Impairment/Functional Disability:*

Step 2: Formulate an Asset List

Directions: In the space below labeled **Patient Asset List,** identify the patient's strengths. The asset list should include areas of available patient function that require reinforcement during treatment.

Patient Asset List:

Step 3: Establish Functional Outcomes of Physical Therapy (Long-Term Goals) and Outcomes of Treatment (Short-Term Goals)

Directions: For each outcome of treatment (short-term goal) identify the *projected number of visits* to accomplish the outcome (goal). In determining the projected number of visits, remember to ask yourself several important questions:

- Is there anything different or unusual about this patient situation?
- What unique resources are available?
- Is the patient's cognitive status intact?
- What is the patient's motivation level?
- Are there any potential complicating factors?
- Is the patient medically stable?
- Is the patient compliant?

For each of the outcomes of treatment (short-term goals) enter the number of visits you would project needed to accomplish the outcome for this patient. Your answer should be placed after the designation *Projected Number of Visits*. If you feel uncomfortable making decisions about projected number of visits at this point, move on and complete *Step 4: Formulate and Justify a Physical Therapy Plan of Care* and return to this question after decisions are made about the specific treatment interventions required.

Outcome(s) of Physical Therapy (Long-Term Goal):

Outcomes of Treatment (Short-Term Goals):   *Projected Number of Visits:*

Step 4: Formulate and Justify a Physical Therapy Plan of Care

Directions:

- From your list developed in Step 1, select *four (4) highly prioritized problems* that require advanced therapeutic exercise intervention. Select problems you will address in your initial 2 weeks of treatment. For each problem, determine the appropriate starting point in treatment, given the information in the case. In the boxes below, enter each of your five selected problems after the labels *"Problem 1," "Problem 2," "Problem 3," "Problem 4."*
- For each of the five problems, enter your outcome of treatment (short-term goal) on the next line after the designation *"Outcome of Treatment (Short-Term Goal)."*
- For each problem, *select three (3) advanced treatment procedures* that can be performed at this time to address the problem. *Prioritize the treatment* by indicating the procedure you will start with (first intervention), and what the order of progression will be for the other procedures (second and third intervention). Enter this information below on the lines labeled *"First Intervention, Position / Activity (or Movement Transition);" "Second Intervention, Position / Activity;"* and *"Third Intervention, Position / Activity."* Immediately below this entry, include a description of the *position / activity or movement transition*. If you have selected a movement transition to address the problem, provide a description of how the activity will be *taught* and how you will *assist* the activity. Your response should incorporate both patient and therapist positioning, hand placements, influence of gravity or body weight, and verbal directions to the patient.
- Provide a rationale for you decision making in selection of procedures(s) to address the four highly prioritized problems. Justification for selection of the Position/Activity should be entered following the designation *"Rationale for Selection."*

- In the space labeled *"Technique,"* indicate your *selected technique(s)* for each Position/Activity or, for *movement transitions,* describe how the activity will be *taught* and how you will *assist* the activity.
- After the label *Motor Control Goals and Indications,* identify the *motor control goal* (mobility, stability, controlled mobility, or skill); and *indications* for the treatment selection.

Problem 1:

Outcome of Treatment (Short-Term Goal):

1. First Intervention   Technique:
   Position/Activity (or Movement
   Transition):

   Rationale for Selection: Motor Control Goals and Indications:

2. Second Intervention   Technique:
   Position/Activity:

   Rationale for Selection: Motor Control Goals and Indications:

Problem 2:

Outcome of Treatment (Short-Term Goal):

1. First Intervention
   Position/Activity (or Movement
   Transition):

   Technique:

   Rationale for Selection:

   Motor Control Goals and Indications:

2. Second Intervention
   Position/Activity:

   Technique:

   Rationale for Selection:

   Motor Control Goals and Indications:

Problem 3:

Outcome of Treatment (Short-Term Goal):

1. First Intervention
   Position/Activity (or Movement
   Transition):

   Technique:

   Rationale for Selection:

   Motor Control Goals and Indications:

2. Second Intervention
   Position/Activity:

   Technique:

   Rationale for Selection:

   Motor Control Goals and Indications:

Problem 4:

Outcome of Treatment (Short-Term Goal):

1. First Intervention
   Position/Activity (or Movement
   Transition):

   Technique:

   Rationale for Selection:

   Motor Control Goals and Indications:

2. Second Intervention
   Position/Activity:

   Technique:

   Rationale for Selection:

   Motor Control Goals and Indications:

APPENDIX A:

Suggested Answers to the Clinical Problems

Please note that the answers provided in Appendix A represent only one solution to a given problem in Part 17. Owing to the variety of treatment options available, the selection of an alternative *position, activity,* or *technique* may be equally effective in accomplishing a desired outcome. These situations clearly warrant feedback from colleagues or instructors.

CLINICAL PROBLEM 1

Guiding Questions

1. • Position/Activity: **Rolling supine to sidelying using PNF D1F extremity patterns.**
   • Technique: **Rhythmic Initiation (RI); Active Movement (AM).**
   • Manual Contacts:
     ○ Rhythmic initiation (RI): **The patient's upper limb is brought up and across the body in a D1F pattern and back down through the D1E pattern. Movement is first passive (PM), then active-assistive, (AAM), then resistive (RM). Active-assistive movement and resistive movement are unidirectional, emphasizing D1F. Movements in D1E are passive—the patient is not allowed to push back down to the side.**
     ○ Rolling with lower extremity D1F pattern: **The lower extremity (LE) is positioned in slight flexion over the therapist's knee. Manual contacts are on the dorsal/medial foot and thigh. Upper extremities (UEs) can be positioned in prayer position (hands clasped together in front of body).**
     ○ Rolling with simultaneous UE and LE D1F patterns: **In D1F patterns both the UE and LE move together up and across the body. The therapist can assist or resist one extremity while the other extremity moves actively.**
   • Outcome (Goal) of Selected Intervention: **Initiation of movement; progression to active movement. Mobility (AAM), progressing to controlled mobility (AM).**

2. *Duration of practice:* **Practice would continue until the patient is actively participating in the rolling activity.** *Marker of sufficient practice:* **Level of assistance and support would be systematically removed as the patient gradually achieves increasing active control.**

3. *Upper extremity:* **Placing the UEs in a prayer position (use of momentum)** *Lower extremity:* **Positioning the LE in hooklying..**

CLINICAL PROBLEM 2

Guiding Questions

1. • Position/Activity: **Bridging.**
   • Technique: **Slow reversals (SRs).**
   • Manual Contacts: **Knees.**
   • Outcome (Goal) of Selected Intervention: **Controlled mobility; promote more lower limb involvement, especially of foot and ankle muscles.**

2. *Justification for hand placement:* **Contacts at the knees increase the length of the lever arm with a subsequent change in the focus of muscle recruitment.** *Advantage:* **Recruits ankle and foot muscles (especially medial and lateral muscles) to shift the body from side to side.**

3. *Therapist position:* **In kneeling at the side of the patient.** *Type of contraction:* **Slow isotonic contractions of first agonist, then antagonist pattern using careful grading of resistance; side-to-side movements are progressed through increments of range; therapist alternates hand placement, first on one side of knees resisting as the knees pull away;**

then on the opposite side as the knees push back. *Verbal cues:* **Cues must be well-timed to facilitate smooth reversals of antagonists ("pull away" or "push back").**

CLINICAL PROBLEM 3

Guiding Questions

1. • Position/Activity: **Bridging; leg lifts (static-dynamic).**
   • Technique: **Guided movement transitions; progression from active-assistive (AAM) to active movements (AM).**
   • Manual Contacts: **Carefully graded assistance with focus on key elements. Optimum points of manual contact will be patient specific; may include static limb to promote stability, dynamic limb to promote stepping and free movement through space, or the pelvis to assist response to reduction in overall base of support (BOS) and shift in center of gravity.**
   • Outcome (Goal) of Selected Intervention: **Promote dynamic stability.**

2. *Purpose of manual contacts:* **To guide the movement with goal of reducing errors, facilitating early learning, and reducing anxiety.**

3. *Initial training:* **Support from UEs is maximized; shoulders can be abducted through partial range with elbows extended and forearms and hands resting on the mat.** *Later training:* **Support from UEs is reduced; shoulders can be gradually brought closer to the patient's trunk (gradually adducted), with progression to UEs crossed over chest or held in a prayer position.**

4. *Maintaining level pelvis:* **A wand can be placed across the patient's pelvis to provide a visual reminder to keep the pelvis level; tactile or verbal cueing can also be used.**

5. *Initial support:* **The stronger limb is generally used first for static support.** *Movement demands:* **The dynamic limb is constantly moving in a functional pattern.** *Purpose of movement:* **Movements imposed by dynamic limb further challenge static control.**

CLINICAL PROBLEM 4

Guiding Questions

1. • Position/Activity: **Supine; hip extension active movement, or PNF D1E pattern.**
   • Technique: **Hold-relax (HR); hold-relax active contraction (HRAC). HRAC is used after range of motion (ROM) has ben established with HR technique; active contraction into newly gained range of the agonist will serve to maintain the inhibitory effects through reciprocal inhibition).**
   • Manual Contacts: **One hand stabilizes the pelvis. The opposite hand on distal aspect of residual limb—on posterior surface to resist active movement in agonist pattern; on anterior surface to provide isometric resistance to tight hip flexors.**
   • Outcome (Goal) of Selected Intervention: **Increase ROM secondary to muscle tightness (hip flexor contraction).**

CLINICAL PROBLEM 5

Guiding Questions

1. • Position/Activity: **Bridging; pelvic elevation using padded stool or sandbags on the right, or using a small Swiss ball.**
   • Technique: **Slow reversals (SRs); slow reversal-hold (SRH) using padded stool or sandbags on the right; active movement using a Swiss ball.**
   • Manual Contacts: **Anterior and posterior pelvis.**
   • Outcome (Goal) of Selected Intervention: **Increase strength; ability to hold a posture**

while dynamic segments are free; smooth movement transitions between opposing muscle groups around hip.

2. *Overall outcome of treatment for controlled mobility:* **Promote smooth reversals of antagonists; develop proximal dynamic stability; develop steady holding of a posture and limb segments while dynamic segments are free to move.**

3. *Implications of hip extensor strength:* **Hip extensors required to provide strong contraction against posterior wall of socket to control prosthetic knee extension.**

4. *Options for increasing or decreasing challenge:*
   A. **From a supine position,** *reduce* or *increase* **the amount of support provided by the UEs in contact with the mat surface. Base of support (BOS) may progress from relatively full support of the UEs with the shoulders in approximately midrange of abduction, with arms, forearms, and hands fully in contact with the mat surface, to a reduced BOS. Upper extremities can be gradually returned to side of trunk (gradual adduction to decrease BOS provided by the UEs). A progression can be made to eliminating support by folding the UEs across the upper trunk. UEs may also be progressed from being held freely at the side of the trunk to movement toward full, unsupported shoulder flexion with UEs held above the patient's head.**
   B. **Alter the support provided by the intact LE by increasing or decreasing the amount of knee flexion; the intact LE may also be removed completely from contact with the supporting surface and progressed from a position of flexion to extension resulting in single-limb bridging (using the residual limb).**
   C. **If a bolster or foot stool is used to support the hip extension contraction on the amputated side, the height may be increased or decreased, or the supporting surface may be moved closer to or farther away from the patient's center of gravity.**
   D. **Use of a Swiss ball provides a moveable support surface and increased postural challenge to stabilizing muscles.**
   E. **Level of resistance may alter during application of slow reversals (SRs) and slow reversal-hold (SRH). Mechanical resistance (weights) can also be used.**

5. *Quick stretch:* **Facilitates or enhances a contraction and provides reciprocal innervation effects; a quick stretch could be applied to the hip extensors by tapping over the muscle belly or by applying a downward stretch on the manual contacts placed at the pelvis as the movement occurs toward hip extension. The quick stretch is usually applied at lengthened range to initiate contraction but can also be used to enhance a contraction where weakness is felt within a range of movement** *(repeated contractions).* *Resistance:* **Reinforces and maintains proprioceptive support of contraction and enhances kinesthetic awareness; it may provide overflow to other muscles. Resistance is inherent in techniques of slow reversal (SRs) and slow reversal-hold (SRH). It can also be applied through mechanical means.**

CLINICAL PROBLEM 6

Guiding Questions

1. • Position/Activity: **Sidelying, with LEs extremities extended in midline. The lower arm is positioned above the head; the uppermost arm can be flexed with the patient's hand resting on the pelvis or in a pants pocket if UE ROM limitations exist.**
   • Technique: **Rhythmic initiation (RI).**
   • Manual Contacts: **One hand is placed on the side of the trunk under the axilla or over the top of shoulder; the other hand is placed on pelvis. Manual contacts should avoid the arms or waist.**
   • Outcome (Goal) of Selected Intervention: **Mobility of trunk; promote muscle relaxation.**

2. *Verbal comments:* **"Relax, let me move you, back and forth" (passive movement). "Now move with me, back and forth" (active movements). "Now pull forward; push backward" (resisted movements).**

3. *Tracking resistance:* **Light resistance used to facilitate a movement response.** *For upper and lower trunk rotation:* **It can be used to promote smooth reversal of opposing muscles.**

4. *Sensory stimulation technique:* **A facilitatory quick stretch can be used to initiate the movement and should be carefully timed with verbal directions to the patient.**

CLINICAL PROBLEM 7

Guiding Questions

1. • Position/Activity: **Sidelying, upper trunk rotation (UTR), lower trunk rotation (LTR). The patient is positioned in sidelying and asked to move upper trunk and shoulder forward and back while keeping the lower trunk and pelvis stationary (UTR). The sequence is reversed for LTR with the lower trunk and pelvis moving forward and backward while the upper trunk and shoulder remain stationary.**
   • Technique: **Slow reversals (SRs).**
   • Manual Contacts: **Upper trunk, pelvis. One hand remains stationary on the segment to be stabilized; the other hand resists the movement first on the anterior aspect of the trunk and then is placed posteriorly to resist the opposite movement.**
   • Outcome (Goal) of Selected Intervention: **Controlled mobility (static-dynamic) of trunk.**

2. *Progression of activity:* **For controlled mobility, movements typically occur through** *increments of range* **(small to large); movements through** *decrements of range* **(large to small) are used for progression to stability control for patients with hyperkinesia.** *Distinguishing factor between responses:* **The major distinguishing factor between normal and abnormal responses is typically the degree to which rotation is incorporated into movement, a very large problem for many people with Parkinson's disease.**

3. *Alteration of technique:* **A hold (SRH) could be added in the shortened range. The hold is a momentary pause, held to a count of one; the antagonist movement is then facilitated. The hold can be added in one direction only or in both directions.**

CLINICAL PROBLEM 8

Guiding Questions

1. • Position/Activity: **Sidelying; trunk rotation.**
   • Technique: **Rhythmic initiation (RI). The patient is instructed to relax while the therapist passively moves each trunk segment in opposite directions (i.e., the lower trunk and pelvis move forward while the upper trunk and shoulder move backward). Movements are reversed and continued until the patient moves easily; the patient is then asked to actively participate in the movements.**
   • Manual Contacts: **Upper trunk and pelvis.**
   • Outcome (Goal) of Selected Intervention: **Skill-level control for trunk; smooth reversal of antagonists. Movements should look coordinated and flow in a continuous movement sequence.**

2. *Therapist position:* **Heel-sitting on the mat, in front of or behind the patient.** *Verbal commands:* **"Relax, let me move you, let me twist you; now let me twist you the other way. Now move with me, twist, now twist the other way."**

3. *Upper extremity involvement:* **Yes, the UEs could be incorporated; this could be accomplished by incorporating active reciprocal UE and/or LE movements; it would promote coordination of trunk movement with arm swing and stepping movement required for gait.** *Explanation:* **UE involvement would promote the plan for progression by calling up a more complete motor program.**

CLINICAL PROBLEM 9

Guiding Questions

1. *Most logical perspective:* **Compensatory training approach.** *Rationale:* **Changes in the structural deformities are not realistic; improved function is the desired outcome.**

2. *Include functional assessment:* **Yes.** *Purpose:* **Measures how the patient performs certain tasks, or fulfills certain roles in the various dimensions of living.** *How results will be*

used: **Provides baseline data to assist with setting function-oriented treatment outcomes; documents initial abilities and, when used periodically, indicates progress toward treatment outcomes; assists with determining needs for community services; assists with determining safety in performance of specific tasks; will help determine effectiveness of a specific intervention or piece of adaptive equipment in improving function, reducing energy cost, or protecting the joints.**

3. *Strategies to improve function:* **(a) The patient is made aware of areas of deficits (for example, excessive or improper use of small joints to perform an activity may result in increased pain and reduced endurance); (b) alternate ways to accomplish a task are considered, simplified, and adopted; (c) emphasis is placed on practice and relearning the alternate method to complete the task; repeated practice will promote consistency and habitual use of the new tactic; (d) the patient practices the functional skill in the environment(s) where function is expected to occur; (e) energy expenditures are monitored and energy conservation techniques are considered to ensure ability to complete all required tasks; and (f) the environment is adapted to facilitate relearning of skills, ease of movement, and optimal performance.**

4. *Purpose of visit:* **An on-site visit would allow assessment of degree of safety, level of function, and appropriateness of adaptive equipment in the specific environment in which the patient will be required to perform a task. This allows the therapist to make realistic recommendations regarding altering, coping with, or adapting specific or unusual environmental barriers and allows the therapist to recommend additional adaptive equipment unanticipated prior to the visit.** *Reason for priority:* **A home visit provides the unique opportunity to further assess and work with the patient in the actual environment in which the functional activities must be accomplished.** *Alternative approach:* **Plan several interviews with the patient and cousin to gather information about the home environment; guide and encourage the cousin to obtain specific information needed, such as the height and number of stairs, presence of railings and so forth. Suggest any available photographs of the home be brought to the next interview. Request that a mock floorplan be drawn depicting approximate dimensions of living areas. Encourage the patient's cousin to visit the physical therapy department to observe use of the adaptive equipment and observe correct performance of alternative approaches to functional activities. Work with the patient to generalize functional skills to as many different environmental contexts as available within the extended care facility.**

CLINICAL PROBLEM 10

Guiding Questions For First Position/Activity (Addressing Apprehension about Initiating Movement)

1. • Position/Activity: **Hooklying; lower trunk rotation (LTR).**
   • Technique: **Rhythmic rotation (RRo).**
   • Manual Contacts: **Both hands are placed on top of the patient's knees; the knees are slowly rocked back and forth; range of motion (ROM) in LTR is gradually increased as relaxation is achieved.**
   • Outcome (Goal) of Selected Intervention: **Promote relaxation; gain ROM.**

2. *Verbal commands (instructions):* **"Relax, relax, and let me move your legs."** *Patient actively involved:* **No, the patient is not involved; rhythmic rotation is a passive technique.**

3. *Positioning of upper extremities:* **Multiple options are available and represent a continuum of influence on the overall base of support; for example, the UEs can be gradually moved closer to the body on the mat; the UEs can be folded across the upper trunk; or the shoulders can be flexed above the head with the hands held in a prayer position.** *Positioning for this patient:* **Begin with a large base of support (shoulders extended and abducted, with the elbows in extension and hands supported on mat surface); as the patient's anxiety about movement is diminished, BOS provided by the UEs can be gradually reduced.** *Therapist position:* **The therapist is heel-sitting, positioned at the base of the patient's feet. The patient is in hooklying with both feet placed on the therapist's knees.**

Guiding Questions for Second Position/Activity
(Addressing Apprehension about Initiating Movement)

1. • Position/Activity: **Hooklying; lower trunk rotation (LTR).**
   • Technique: **Lower trunk guided movement (active-assistive movement), rhythmic initiation (RI).**
   • Manual Contacts: *Guided movement:* **Both hands are placed on top of the patient's knees; the knees are moved slowly away from and back toward the midline in both directions.** *Rhythmic Initiation (RI):* **Hands are fixed on top of the patient's knees during the first two phases; during the final resistive phase they slide to the side (medial side of one knee, lateral side of the opposite knee) to resist both knees as they pull away and then slide to the opposite sides of the knees to resist the return movement. Manual contacts must "pivot" in order to resist the complete return movement of the knees down to the mat.**
   • Outcome (Goal) of Selected Intervention: **Reduce anxiety; promote relaxation, initiation of movement.**

2. *Quality of verbal commands:* **To reduce anxiety and promote relaxation, cues (verbal input) should be calm, soothing, slow, rhythmic, and well timed with movements.**

3. *Quality of movement:* **Movements should be smooth, slow, and rhythmic. Abrupt or quick movements will heighten anxiety and may increase pain and diminish movement responses. Movements should require low effort to maximize performance.** *Type of movement:* **Several phases of movements are sought: the progression includes movements that are first passive, then active-assistive, and then lightly resisted (tracking resistance).** *Progression:* **Progression to a more challenging phase is determined by the patient's ability to participate in an earlier phase.**

Guiding Questions for Third Position/Activity
(First Intervention Addressing Weakness and Instability)

1. • Position/Activity: **Hooklying; lower trunk rotation (LTR).**
   • Technique: **Hold-relax active movement (HRAM).**
   • Manual Contacts: **On top of the knees.**
   • Outcome (Goal of Selected Intervention: **Facilitate movement; strengthen weak muscles.**

2. *Type of movement:* **Isometric hold, active relaxation, resisted isotonic contraction.** *Sequence:* **An isometric contraction is performed first in the middle to shortened range, followed by active relaxation, followed by a resisted isotonic contraction from the lengthened to the shortened range.**

3. *Therapist positioning:* **Half-kneeling at the side of the patient; hands are positioned on top of the knees.** *Sequence:* **from a hooklying position, the patient's knees are moved to the side (away from midline) a quarter range; the patient is asked to hold in this position with a gradual build up of the isometric contraction; the patient is then asked to actively relax**—*completely, before progressing to next phase.* **The therapist then returns the knees quickly back past midline and asks the patient to actively contract (isotonic) through the range back to the original starting position. Light (tracking) resistance is used with the isotonic movement.**

4. *Sensory input:* **A quick stretch to contracting muscle applied with manual contacts at the knees.** *Threshold response:* **Low threshold, which achieves a relatively short-lived response; facilitates isotonic contraction via reciprocal innervation effects.** *Applied during isotonic movement:* **A quick stretch is applied in the lengthened range (muscle fibers on stretch) to facilitate return movement.** *Sensory input eliminated:* **The quick stretch is phased out as soon as desired response is achieved.**

5. *Type of verbal commands:* **Vigorous, dynamic, challenging verbal input is used.** *Goal of verbal commands:* **To maintain patient involvement and focus on desired holding pattern or movement response; enhance isotonic contraction.**

Guiding Questions for Fourth Position/Activty (Second Intervention Addressing Weakness and Instability)

1. • Position/Activity: **Hooklying; lower trunk rotation (LTR).**
   • Technique: **Alternating isometrics (AI).**
   • Manual Contacts: **At the knees; hand placement will change as resistance is moved from one side of the joint to the other (resistance is alternated between opposing muscles).**
   • Goal of Selected Intervention: **Promote stability control (holding).**

2. *Application of resistance:* **Resistance is built up gradually, starting with light resistance and progressing to a maximal response; the isometric contraction is held for several counts.** *Direction of resistance:* **Resistance is applied either side to side or diagonally.**

3. *Transitional verbal command:* **"Now, don't let me pull (or push) you the other way."** *Verbal commands critical to achieving goals:* **Transitional commands prepare the patient for the next phase of the technique; they allow the patient an opportunity to make appropriate postural adjustments in anticipation of the changed direction of resistance.**

CLINICAL PROBLEM 11

Guiding Questions

1. • Position/Activity: **Sidelying, holding in extension. The supporting LE in contact with the mat is flexed slightly; the head is slightly extended. The upper arm is extended with the elbow flexed; the trunk and uppermost LE are in midline.**
   • Technique: **Shortened held resisted contraction (SHRC).**
   • Manual Contacts: **Head, UE, pelvis, LE. One hand supports the head and applies resistance to the neck extensors using the base of the hand; the opposite hand is placed on the upper trunk, or alternately, on the patient's elbow, resisting shoulder extension and scapular adduction.**
   • Outcome (Goal) of Selected Intervention: **Stability control; strengthen postural extensors. Improved functional sitting—reduce kyphosis; reduce forward head position.**

2. *Patient position:* **Sidelying, with head, arm, and trunk extended (non-weight-bearing position reduces patient effort to control against gravity).** *Benefits and treatment implications:* **This is a unilateral activity. Focus of control is placed on the uppermost trunk segments; attention can be directed toward weak, upper postural extensors.**

3. *Next area addressed:* **As control is achieved in one segment of the trunk, progression would be made to the next (lower) segment. Each segment is resisted and progressively added to the overall extension activity.**

4. *More challenging:* **Increase the number of segments involved in the holding; increase level of antigravity control (i.e., progress to modified pivot prone in supported sitting).** *Less challenging:* **Reduce the number of segments involved in the holding.**

5. *Pattern of Movement:* **Pivot prone pattern.** *Benefit:* **Incorporates a strong, total extension pattern.** *Contraindications:* **Influence of the tonic labyrinthine reflex in prone position (increased tone); cardiovascular disease or respiratory insufficiency.**

CLINICAL PROBLEM 12

Guiding Questions

1. • Position/Activity: **Prone-on-elbows (PoE); holding. Patient may require assist-to-position; may require modified positioning by placing a wedge underneath the upper trunk.**
   • Technique: **Alternating isometrics; rhythmic stabilization, active movement (active holding).**

- Manual Contacts: **Medial/lateral alternating isometrics: one hand is on contralateral side of trunk, pushing on vertebral border of scapula or pulling on the axillary border of scapula; opposite hand on the near side of the upper trunk, pushing on the axillary border of scapula, or cupped and pulling on the vertebral border of the scapula. Anterior/posterior alternating isometrics: both hands are positioned on inferior border of scapula, pushing forward and upward and upward or over top of shoulders or onto the anterior trunk (hands cupped over clavicle), pulling backward. Rhythmic Stabilization: both hands are positioned on upper trunk; one hand on lateral border of scapula (posterior trunk), the opposite hand is on the contralateral anterior trunk. Resistance is applied in a twisting motion, trying to rotate the upper trunk as the patient resists the movement.**
- Outcome (Goal) of Selected Intervention: **Stability control (active holding) of head, upper trunk, shoulders; development of static balance control in prone-on-elbows position.**

2. *Indications for use:* **Difficulty initiating or sustaining movement; absent or diminished motor control.** *Influences on effectiveness of response:* **Level of intactness of the central nervous system, tone, arousal levels, type and amount of stimulation, specific activity of motoneurons.** *Determination to phase out:* **Sensory stimulation techniques should be used during the early phase of treatment to facilitate initiation of a contraction response; they should be phased out as soon as active movement can be supported without them.**

3. *Quick stretch:* **Quick stretch would be applied to muscle as muscle attempts to hold, or by tapping directly over muscle belly; this facilitates agonist contractions.** *Joint approximation:* **Inherent in prone-on-elbows position; it can be enhanced with manual compression at the shoulder and head. Approximation facilitates postural extensors and enhances joint awareness.**

CLINICAL PROBLEM 13

Guiding Questions

1.
   - Position/Activity: **Bridging.**
   - Technique: **Active holding.**
   - Manual Contacts: **The patient and spouse are instructed in placement and use of Theraband tubing; the Theraband is placed bilaterally around the distal thighs.**
   - Outcome (Goal) of Selected Intervention: **Promote contraction of the lateral hip muscles (gluteus medius). Within the bridging position, simultaneous contraction of the gluteal muscles (gluteus medius and gluteus maximus) is achieved.**

2. *Sensory stimulation:* **Theraband tubing placed around distal thighs will increase proprioceptive loading.**

3. *Precautions:* **Avoid hip flexion beyond 90 degrees for both LEs. Be careful to avoid breath holding during this and all isometric work. Contractions should be carefully balanced with rest intervals.** *Information:* **Specific numeric values for both the "hold" and "rest interval" should be provided to the patient in writing; indicate that on subsequent outpatient visits you will determine the need for Theraband capable of imposing greater resistance.**

CLINICAL PROBLEM 14

Guiding Questions

1.
   - Position/Activity: **Sitting; PNF D1F, flexion-adduction-external rotation (elbow flexing).**
   - Technique: **Repeated contractions (RCs).**
   - Manual Contacts: **On forearm and arm.**
   - Outcome (Goal) of Selected Intervention: **Promote balanced contraction through the range; improve strength, promote coordinated movement.**

2. *Description of technique:* **Repeated isotonic contractions (RCs), induced by quick stretches, and enhanced by resistance performed through the range or part of range**

at point of weakness. RCs are used as a unidirectional technique. *Neuromuscular response:* **Application of a quick stretch will facilitate agonist and inhibit antagonist response via reciprocal innervation effects (low-threshold response; relatively short-lived; resistance assists in maintaining response).**

3. *Addition to technique:* **An isometric hold can be added at point of weakness.** *Advantages(s):* **The hold uses reciprocal innervation effects, which promote stretch sensitivity of spindle and improved kinesthetic awareness.**

CLINICAL PROBLEM 15

Guiding Questions

1. • Position/Activity: **Transitions from supine to sidelying to sitting.**
   • Technique: **Guided movements (active-assistive movement).**
   • Movement transition: **From the supine position the patient rolls onto the side. The hips and knees are flexed, and the legs are moved off the bed or mat. The legs act as counterweights as they lower down to rotate the patient up into sitting. The patient simultaneously uses both UEs to push up into sitting.**
   • Manual Contacts: **Hand placement at the upper trunk and pelvis can be used to assist the initial roll into the sidelying position. Hand placement on the legs assists movement of the legs in lowering off the mat or bed, or the lifting of the upper trunk can be guided with manual contacts at either side of trunk.**
   • Outcome (Goal) of Selected Intervention: **Independent movement transition; supine-to-sit.**

2. *Types of feedback:* **Both major types of feedback will be useful here.** *Intrinsic feedback* **is inherent information derived from an individual's own sensory and perceptual systems, such as visual, auditory, proprioceptive, and tactile feedback.** *Augmented feedback* **is supplemental or added information derived from external sources, such as verbal cues, or viewing a videotaped performance. Augmented feedback is subdivided into knowledge of results and knowledge of performance.** *Knowledge of results* **is information related to the nature of the result (outcome produced) in terms of the environmental goal.** *Knowledge of performance* **is information about the nature and quality of the movement characteristics produced.**

3. *Strategies to optimize effectiveness of feedback:*
   A. **Feedback should be precise and accurate. Initially, feedback given after every trial improves performance; this is followed by feedback given after several trials, which improves learning and retention.**
   B. **Early training should focus on visual feedback (cognitive phase of learning); later training should emphasize proprioceptive feedback or the "feel of the movement" (associative phase of learning).**
   C. **Augmented feedback should be provided about both knowledge of results and knowledge of performance. During early learning, focus should be on correct aspects of performance; during later learning the focus shifts to errors as they become consistent.**
   D. **Use of feedback should be monitored carefully. Feedback dependency should be avoided by reducing augmented feedback as soon as possible and allowing the learner active introspection and decision making, which improves learning and retention.**

CLINICAL PROBLEM 16

Guiding Questions

1. Equilibrium Board

• Position/Activity: **Sitting on an equilibrium board; balance training.**

• Technique: **Guided movement (assisted maintenance of a balanced posture), progressing to active holding and independent practice.**

- Manual Contacts: **Initially, manual contacts can be placed on the pelvis and/or trunk to assist balance training. As control develops, independent practice (a hands-off approach) is optimal; as control continues to progress, hand placement on equilibrium board allows therapist-initiated manual tilting.**

- Outcome (Goal) of Selected Intervention: **Dynamic balance control.**

2. *Movements allowed:* **The amount of motion is determined by the design of the board. A curved-bottom board allows motion in two directions; a dome-bottom board allows motion in all directions.** *Patient information:* **Selection is based largely on the patient's dynamic balance control and the type and range of movements permitted.**

3. *Patient-initiated challenges:* **Active weight shifts on equilibrium board, tilting the board in varying directions to stimulate balance reactions. These challenges stimulate both** *feed-forward (preparatory) and feedback-driven* **adjustments to balance.** *Therapist-initiated challenges:* **Manually tilting the board to stimulate balance responses stimulates** *feedback-driven* **responses.** *Types included in treatment:* **Both should be included in treatment; the therapist will vary speed and range of displacement as the child gradually exhibits more control.**

Swiss Ball

1. - Position/Activity: **Sitting, on Swiss ball; holding.**
   - Technique: **Guided movement (assisted hold), progressing to active holding and independent practice.**
   - Manual Contacts: **Initially, manual contacts can be placed on the pelvis and/or trunk to assist holding; as control develops, independent practice (a hands-off approach) is optimal.**
   - Outcome (Goal) of Selected Intervention: **Dynamic balance control.**

5. *Initial directions:* **The patient is instructed to hold a steady position and not to allow the ball to roll in any direction.**

6. *Prerequisite to ball activities:* **Static balance control must be achieved on a stationary surface first (the patient must be able to hold steady while sitting on a mat).**

7. *Upright posture:* **Correct sitting height is important to ensure optimal responses (hips and knees should be flexed to 90 degrees). Approximation can be used effectively by having the patient sit and gently bounce up and down. A fairly immediate and automatic improvement in posture (that is, the patient sits up straight) can be anticipated.** *Sensory input:* **Approximation is facilitatory to postural extensors (stabilizers) and enhances joint awareness.**

CLINICAL PROBLEM 17

Guiding Questions

1. - Position/Activity: **Sitting on a Swiss ball; pelvic shifts.**
   - Technique: **Guided movement (active-assistive movement), progressing to active movement and independent practice.**
   - Manual Contacts: **Initially, manual contacts can be placed on the pelvis to assist the patient in the correct movements; as control develops, independent practice (a hands-off approach) is desired.**
   - Outcome (Goal) of Selected Intervention: **Dynamic balance control, controlled mobility; static-dynamic control.**

2. *Initial activities on the Swiss ball:* **The patient is sitting on a Swiss ball and shifts the hips forward and backward (anterior and posterior pelvic tilts), or side to side (lateral shifts). The patient is instructed to "roll the ball using the hips" in the desired direction.**

3. *Additional activities:*
   - **Sitting, upper extremity lifts, circles**
   - **Sitting, upper extremity lifts, marching in place**

- Sitting, alternate knee extension, side-steps
- Sitting, writing letters of the alphabet in space with one foot
- Sitting, alternate crossing of the lower extremities
- Sitting, jumping jacks (bouncing with upper extremity raises overhead)
- Sitting, Mexican hat dance (bouncing with alternate upper and lower limb flexion and extension)
- Sitting, head and trunk rotation with upper limb swinging side to side
- Sitting, balancing on ball with feet on a roller or small ball

CLINICAL PROBLEM 18

Guiding Questions

1. • *PNF unilateral upper extremity patterns (any two of the following could be used to promote dynamic postural control):*
   A. **D1F, flexion-adduction-external-rotation: The hand of the dynamic limb is positioned near the side of the ipsilateral hip with hand open and thumb facing down. The patient is instructed to close the hand, turn, and pull the arm up and across the face.**
   B. **D1E, extension-abduction-internal rotation: The patient opens the hand, turns, and pushes the arm down and out to the side.**
   C. **D2F, flexion-abduction-external-rotation: The hand of the dynamic limb is positioned across the body on the opposite hip with hand closed and thumb facing down. The patient is instructed to open the hand, turn, and lift the arm up and out.**
   D. **D2E, extension-adduction-internal rotation: The patient closes the hand, turns, pulls the arm down and across the body.**

2. *Selection of patterns:* **The therapist chooses pattern(s) based on the patient's level of control. Unilateral patterns are typically used initially when the patient is unfamiliar (any two of the following could be used to promote dynamic postural control) with the PNF patterns, or when one extremity is needed for weight-bearing and support. As control develops, the therapist can progress to the more difficult bilateral patterns.** *Precaution:* **Although not the case with the patient described in Clinical Problem 18, recall that upper extremity D2 patterns are contraindicated for patients recovering from stroke who are firmly locked in abnormal synergies.**

3. *Application of resistance:* **Resistance can be manual, or the patient can use free weights, Theraband tubing, or pulleys that are appropriately positioned.** *Advantage of use of resistance:* **Effective use of resistance enhances or facilitates the responses of weak muscles owing to the increased proprioceptive loading.**

4. *Focus on motor learning:* **Eeffective motor learning is emphasized through use of repetition and practice. Varying practice through pattern variations and combinations fosters continued learning and generalizability. Verbal commands (both preparatory and action commands) and manual contacts assist in learning.**

CLINICAL PROBLEM 19

Guiding Questions

1. • Position/Activity: **Prone-on-elbows (PoE); holding.**
   • Technique: **Alternating isometrics (medial/lateral and anterior/posterior); rhythmic stabilization.**
   • Manual Contacts:
   • Medial/lateral alternating isometrics: **One hand on contralateral side of trunk, pushing on vertebral border of scapula or pulling on the axillary border of scapula; opposite hand on the near side of the upper trunk, pushing on the axillary border of scapula, or cupped and pulling on the vertebral border of the scapula.**
   • Anterior/posterior alternating isometrics: **Both hands positioned on inferior border of scapula, pushing forward and upward and upward or over top of shoulders or onto the anterior trunk (hands cupped over clavicle), pulling backward.**

- Rhythmic stabilization: **Both hands are positioned on upper trunk; one hand on lateral border of scapula (posterior trunk), the opposite hand on the contralateral anterior trunk. Resistance is applied in a twisting motion, trying to rotate or twist the upper trunk as the patient resists the movement.**
- Outcome (Goal) of Selected Intervention: **Stability control (active holding) of upper trunk, shoulders; development of static balance control in prone-on-elbows position.**

2. *Increase proprioceptive loading:* **Use Theraband tubing tied around forearms. The patient is instructed to maintain the forearms apart, holding against the resistance of the rubber tubing.**

3. *Weakness of which muscle?:* **Serratus anterior.** *Would this alter Position/Activity?:* **Yes.** *Rationale for response:* **Weakness of the serratus anterior, as demonstrated by winging of the scapula, is a contraindication to use of the prone-on-elbows position; this weakness would limit the ability to assume or hold this posture.** *Change in Position/Activity:* **A wedge cushion could be used to reduce loading in prone-on-elbows. The patient could be positioned in supported sitting with elbow(s) weight bearing on a table top (in modified PoE), or in supported sitting with arm at side—unilateral weight bearing occurs through the elbow on a stool positioned at side.**

4. *Tonic holding:* **A term used to describe stability control achieved during holding in the shortened range; generally applied to the postural trunk extensors.** *Co-contraction:* **A term used to describe control achieved during holding in midrange during weight-bearing activities.**

5. *Medial/lateral alternating isometrics:* **"Hold this position; don't let me push you away; hold, hold. Now don't let me pull you toward me; hold, hold."** *For anterior/posterior alternating isometrics:* **"Hold; don't let me push you up and away; hold, hold. Now don't let me pull you back; hold, hold . . ."** *For rhythmic stabilization:* **"Hold—don't let me twist you; hold, hold. Now don't let me twist you the other way; hold, hold."**

CLINICAL PROBLEM 20

Guiding Questions

1. • *PNF trunk patterns:*
    A. *Sitting, with PNF chop:* **This is an upper trunk flexion and rotation pattern that involves both UEs moving together. The lead limb (UE) moves in D1E; the hand of the assist limb (UE) holds on from on top of the wrist and moves down and across the body with the lead UE. In the reverse chop pattern, the lead limb moves in D1F; the assist limb moves up and across the face.**
    B. *Sitting, with PNF lift:* **This is an upper trunk extension and rotation pattern that involves both UEs moving together. The lead upper extremity moves in D2F; the hand of the assist upper extremity holds on from underneath the wrist and moves up and out with the lead UE. In the reverse lift pattern, the lead limb moves in D2E; the assist limb moves down and across the body.**

2. *The benefits of PNF patterns are:*
    A. **They promote muscle activity in naturally occurring synergistic combinations.**
    B. **They encourage diagonal and rotational movements, and represent advanced control work for many patients.**
    C. **They promote crossing the midline.**

3. *Attention to arm movements:* **The patient's full attention is focused on the correct UE movements and not on movement of the trunk. The patient is instructed to follow the movements of the UE looking at the hand. This encourages head and neck rotation and assists in promoting automatic postural control of the head and trunk.**

4. *Selection of patterns:* **The therapist chooses pattern(s) based on the patient's level of control.** *Chop* and *lift* **are asymmetrical patterns that focus on the trunk and proximal joint control. The patterns are performed with the extremities in contact, creating a closed kinetic chain. An advantage of these patterns is the ability to promote trunk rotation in combination with trunk flexion or extension.**

5. *Level of resistance:* **Level of resistance is determined by the ability of the trunk to stabilize and maintain upright sitting.** *Therapist position:* **In order to resist the PNF** *chop,* **the therapist is positioned slightly in front and to the side of the patient in the direction of the chop; to resist the** *lift* **pattern, the therapist is positioned slightly behind and to the side of the patient in the direction of the lift.**

6. *Modification for lack of stability:* **If stabilization is deficient, resistance may be contraindicated and active movements should be promoted.**

CLINICAL PROBLEM 21

Guiding Questions for Mat Activity
(To Address Limitations Imposed by the Soleus)

1. • Position/Activity: **Half-kneeling, weight shifting.**
   • Technique: **Guided movement (active-assistive movement, progressing to active movement).**
   • Manual Contacts: **One hand on the pelvis on the side of the support limb; one hand on the knee of the forward support limb.** *Alternate Manual Contacts:* **If the foot of the forward (support) limb is not maintained in neutral alignment on the mat surface, one hand will assist foot positioning with the opposite hand on the patient's knee of the same limb or on the pelvis of the opposite limb (depending on patient stability).**
   • Outcome (Goal) of Selected Intervention: **Reduce errors and promote early learning (guided movements); active weight shifts forward over the support foot and then backward over the support limb; increase ROM of the forward support ankle; promote early eccentric control of the soleus.**

2. *Patient positioning:* **The patient is half-kneeling with weight borne equally on the posterior support knee and anterior support foot placed flat on the mat. The head and trunk are in an upright position.** *Therapist position:* **The therapist is also in half-kneeling in front of the patient in a reversed (mirror-image) position.**

3. *Less challenging:* **Provide UE support on a chair or stool placed in front of the patient on the mat.**

4. *Verbal commands:* **"Shift forward and toward me; now shift back away from me."**

5. *Facilitation technique:* **A prolonged stretch of the soleus muscle could be achieved in this position.** *Receptors influenced:* **Activitates muscle receptors; sensitive to length changes.** *Response:* **Inhibits or dampens muscle contraction and tone (soleus), largely through peripheral reflex effects.** *Response enhanced:* **Firm pressure, using manual contacts on the forward (support) knee (inhibitory pressure to further dampen response).**

CLINICAL PROBLEM 22

Guiding Questions for Upright Activity in Modified Plantigrade
(To Address Limitations Imposed by Both the Soleus
and Gastrocnemius)

1. • Position/Activity: **Modified plantigrade, weight shifting.**
   • Technique: **Guided movement (active-assistive movement); progressing to active movement.**
   • Manual Contacts: **Both hands are placed on the pelvis.**
   • Outcome (Goal) of Selected Intervention: **Reduce errors and promote early learning (guided movements); reduce anxiety about ROM exercises. Active weight shifts, first forward (ROM in ankle dorsiflexion can be promoted by weight shifts forward), then backward. Promote eccentric plantarflexion control.**

2. *Patient position:* **The patient is standing with both elbows extended, hands open and weight bearing on a treatment table or treatment plinth. The head and trunk are**

maintained forward with weight over extended UEs; the shoulders are flexed. The hips are flexed with the knees extended; the ankles are dorsiflexed.

3. *Progression of dorsiflexion range of motion:* **Work toward** *increments* **in ROM. Positioning the feet farther away from the treatment table will increase the ankle dorsiflexion range obtained.**

4. *Verbal Commands:* **"Shift forward and away from me; now shift back toward me."**

5. *Facilitation Technique:* **A prolonged stretch of the plantarflexors (inhibitory response).** *Response enhanced:* **Firm pressure can be applied using body weight. Alternate UE positions can be used, including placing both hands on a wall with the shoulders flexed and the elbows extended; this increases the weight (pressure) borne on the LEs.** *Greater focus on single lower extremity:* **The LEs can be placed in an asymmetrical** *step position* **to impose greater inhibitory pressure (from body weight) on posterior stance LE.**

CLINICAL PROBLEM 23

Guiding Questions for Standing Activity To Address the Hip Abductor Weakness

1. • Position/Activity: **Standing, side-stepping.**
   • Technique: **Guided movement (active-assistive movement), progressing to active movement and independent practice.**
   • Manual Contacts: **Initially, manual contacts (tapping) can be used on the pelvis to assist the patient in the correct movements; as control develops, independent practice using a hands-off approach is optimal.**
   • Outcome (Goal) of Selected Intervention: **Recruits abductors. Promotes standing without the use of the cane; controlled mobility, static-dynamic control; lead-up activity to bipedal gait.**

2. *Patient performance:* **The patient is in standing; weight is shifted laterally over the support limb and a side-step is taken with the dynamic limb (static-dynamic control). The activity begins with side-stepping, using the affected limb as the dynamic limb and the sound limb as the static limb; a progression is made to the opposite sequence.** *More challenging:* **The challenge can be increased by incorporating lateral step-ups. This involves having the patient place the dynamic limb up onto a low step positioned at the side.**

3. *Facilitation technique:* **Joint approximation (can be applied over the top of pelvis as the support limb assumes weight bearing).** *Stimulus:* **Compression of joint surfaces.** *Response:* **Facilitates postural extensors and stabilizers.** *Technique:* **Manual joint compression.**

4. *Facilitation technique:* **Quick stretch or light (tracking) resistance (applied to dynamic limb).** *Stimulus:* **Quick stretch—a quick stretch applied to a muscle. Light (tracking) resistance—an external force exerted on a muscle.** *Response:* **Quick stretch facilitates or enhances a muscle contraction. Light (tracking) resistance facilitates a very weak muscle.** *Technique:* **Quick stretch: tapping over muscle belly or tendon. Light (tracking) resistance: very light manual resistance.**

CLINICAL PROBLEM 24

Guiding Questions for Advanced Stabilization Activity in Standing (To Address the Hip Abductor Weakness)

1. • Position/Activity: **Standing, single-limb support with abduction.**
   • Technique: **Guided movement (active-assistive movement), progressing to active movement and independent practice.**
   • Manual Contacts: **Initially, manual contacts can be placed on the pelvis to assist the**

patient in maintaining the pelvis level; as control develops, independent practice using a hands-off approach is optimal.
- Outcome (Goal) of Selected Intervention: **Recruits abductors; controlled mobility, static-dynamic control.**

2. *Patient performance:* **The patient stands sideways next to a wall but does not lean on the wall. The LE closest to the wall becomes the dynamic limb while the opposite LE becomes the support limb. The patient flexes the knee and abducts the dynamic limb, pushing the knee against the wall. The static limb maintains the upright posture during unilateral stance with the knee flexed slightly.** *Less challenging:* **The challenge can be decreased by postponing** *standing, single limb support with abduction* **and beginning with** *standing, single limb support* **(the patient lifts one lower limb off the ground and maintains the standing position using single-limb support).**

3. *Directions to patient:* **Initially the weaker limb is the dynamic limb. As control develops the weaker limb becomes the static or support limb. The abductors on both sides work strongly to push into the wall and to maintain the unilateral stance position. Overflow from one side to the other is strong (reciprocal innervation effects).**

CLINICAL PROBLEM 25

Guiding Questions

1. • Position/Activity: **Standing, partial squats.**
   • Technique: **Guided movement (active-assistive movement), progressing to active movement and independent practice.**
   • Manual Contacts: **Initially, manual contacts can be placed on the pelvis to assist the patient in the correct movements; as control develops, independent practice using a hands-off approach is optimal.**
   • Outcome (Goal) of Selected Intervention: **Recruits quadriceps; promotes controlled mobility. Partial wall squats are an important lead-up activity for independent sit-to-stand transitions and stair climbing.**

2. *Patient performance:* **The patient stands with the back next to a wall, feet about 4 inches (10 cm) from the wall. The patient is instructed to bend both knees while sliding the back down the wall. Movement is restricted to partial range; the patient is instructed to stop when no longer able to see the tips of the toes. The hip is maintained in neutral rotation to ensure proper patellar tracking. The pelvis is also maintained in neutral.** *Modification secondary to low back discomfort:* **The patient performs a posterior pelvic tilt and maintains this position during the squat.**

3. *Facilitate sliding against wall:* **The patient can also stand with the back supported by a medium-size Swiss ball placed in the lumbar region; the feet are positioned directly underneath the body. The ball is resting on the wall. As the patient moves down into the partial squat position, the movement is facilitated by the ball rolling upward.**

4. *Recruit the vastus medialis oblique:* **A small towel roll can be placed between the knees. The patient is instructed to hold the towel roll in position by squeezing both knees together. This activity increases the activity of the vastus medialis oblique and improves knee stability and patellar tracking.**

5. *Increase challenge:* **The activity can progress to unilateral (single-limb) squats to practice descending stairs (starting with a 4-inch—10 cm—rise and progressing to an 8-inch—20-cm—rise).**

CLINICAL PROBLEM 26

Guiding Questions

1. *First strategy to promote motor learning:* **Before beginning the actual instruction, describe to the patient activities that will be included in treatment; emphasize the importance and desirability of learning the activities. Focus on the functional relevance of physi-**

cal therapy, perhaps in terms of promoting return to volleyball or other activities important to the patient. Involve the patient in setting goals for the session (for example, ask how far the patient needs to learn to walk to get to a favorite shopping mall, movie theater, to visit a friend or relative?).

2. *Practice schedule:* **Distributed practice.** *Features:* **Practice in which the rest time is relatively large (practice time is less than rest time).** *Appropriateness for patient:* **Distributed practice is used when the task is complex, long, or energy costly for the patient. This type of practice is also indicated when a relatively high level of performance is desired, when motivation is low, the learner has a short attention span or poor concentration, or fatigues easily.**

3. *Feedback:* **Visual, augmented, and supportive feedback.** *Approach to using feedback:* **Early training should focus on** *visual feedback* **(cognitive phase of learning); later training should emphasize** *proprioceptive feedback,* **or the "feel" of the movement (associative phase of learning).** *Augmented feedback* **should be provided about knowledge of results and knowledge of performance. Emphasis should be placed on correct aspects of performance (important for early learning); and on errors only as they become consistent (important for middle and later stages of learning). Use of feedback should be carefully monitored; feedback dependency should be avoided with attention focused on reducing augmented feedback as soon as possible.** *Supportive feedback* **can be used to motivate the patient and shape (reinforce) behavior.** *Environmental influences:* **Extraneous environmental stimuli must be reduced early in learning—practice in a closed environment. During later learning focus can shift to adapting performance to varying environmental demands—practice in an open environment.**

4. *Optimize influence of treatment session:* **Involve the parents in the treatment session. Focus on the parents' understanding of the treatment activities, their applications, and the rationale for their use, together with safety precautions. Have the parents observe each aspect of the treatment. Explain the importance of practice and feedback. Provide detailed written instructions (diagrams, if possible) on each component of the intervention. Allow time for the parents to practice with their child and provide them with feedback, as well.**

CLINICAL PROBLEM 27

Guiding Questions

Handling Intervention #1

Stimulus: **Maintained touch, contact, or pressure.** *Receptors activated:* **Tactile receptors, autonomic nervous system, parasympathetic division.** *Response:* **Calming effect, generalized inhibition, desensitizes skin.** *Techniques:* **Firm manual contacts; firm pressure applied to midline of abdomen, back, lips, palms, soles of feet, and firm rubbing.**

Handling Intervention #2

Stimulus: **Slow stroking applied to paravertebral spinal region (over posterior primary rami).** *Receptors activated:* **Tactile receptors, autonomic nervous system, parasympathetic division.** *Response:* **Calming effect, generalized inhibition.** *Techniques:* **Position the child in a supported position such as prone on lap. A flat hand is used to apply firm, alternate strokes to the paravertebral region for approximately 3 to 5 minutes; gentle rocking can also be used (providing slow, vestibular stimulation) to increase generalized inhibition effects.**

CLINICAL PROBLEM 28

Guiding Questions

1. *Patient movement sequence:* **The patient is in quadruped and pushes the hips back over the heels while extending and lifting the trunk into the upright position. Patients can**

also be instructed to use a chair or other support to "climb up" into kneeling using the UEs. *Therapist participation:* The therapist can assist the transition into kneeling by standing slightly behind and to the side of the patient and placing both hands on the trunk under the axillae. First one shoulder, then the other, is lifted. Assistance to hip extension is generally needed and can be provided by the therapist placing one foot between the patient's knees and using the side of the knee to gently push the patient's hips into extension. *Motor control goals:* Controlled mobility (active-assistive movements progressing to active movements); promotes functional independence in movement transitions from one posture to another.

2. *Quadruped (prone kneeling):*
   • Base of support (BOS) is large.
   • Center of mass (COM) is higher than in PoE but still remains low.
   • Quadruped is a stable, four-limb posture.
   • Shoulders are flexed to 90 degrees, elbows extended, with hands positioned directly under shoulders; hips are flexed to 90 degrees with knees positioned directly under hips; the back is straight (flat).
   • Requires head, neck, upper trunk, UE (shoulder and elbow), and lower trunk and hip control.
   • Normal righting reactions (ORR, LRR, BOH) contribute to the maintenance of head position.
   • Increased demands for balance, especially with dynamic shifting activities.

   Kneeling (kneel-standing):
   • Base of support (BOS) is decreased; limited to the length of the lower leg and foot.
   • Center of mass (COM) is intermediate; elevated over supine or prone positions, decreased from standing.
   • Posture is more stable to the posterior than to the anterior.
   • Kneeling involves head, trunk, and hip muscles for upright postural control.
   • The head and trunk are maintained vertical in midline orientation, with normal spinal lumbar and thoracic curves.
   • The pelvis is maintained in midline orientation with hips fully extended, knees flexed (similar to bridging but vertical).
   • Normal righting reactions contribute to upright head position (face vertical, mouth horizontal); equilibrium reactions contribute to maintenance of upright posture in response to displacement (fixation) or changes in the support surface (tilting reaction).

CLINICAL PROBLEM 29

Guiding Questions for First Intevention (To Promote Stability)

1. • Position/Activity: **Kneeling, holding.**
   • Technique: **Alternating isometrics (AI).**
   • Manual Contacts: **The patient is asked to hold the kneeling position while the therapist applies resistance to the pelvis, first on one side pushing the pelvis away from the therapist, then pulling the pelvis toward the therapist (medial/lateral resistance).**
   • Outcome (Goal) of Selected Intervention: **Stability.**

2. *Application of resistance:* The resistance is built up gradually, starting from very light resistance progressing to the patient's maximum. The isometric contraction is maintained for several counts. Resistance can also be applied in anterior/posterior directions. Because of the limited BOS in front, the patient will be able to take very little resistance anteriorly, and more resistance posteriorly.

3. *Alter position:* During initial training in kneeling, the patient with instability may benefit from using UE support on a chair or stool placed in front. Alternate positions include UEs moved forward (shoulders flexed and elbows extended) with the hands placed on the therapist's shoulders, a wall, or placed on a ball (the moveable surface presents a more difficult challenge). These positions are modified plantigrade positions, because weight bearing occurs on both hands and knees. As control develops, the patient can be progressed from bilateral to single UE support to free kneeling.

Guiding Questions for Second Intervention (To Promote Stability)

1. • *Position / Activity:* **Kneeling, holding.**
   • Technique: **Rhythmic stabilization (RS).**
   • Manual Contacts: **The patient is asked to hold the kneeling position while the therapist applies rotational resistance to the trunk. One hand is placed on the posterior pelvis on one side pushing forward while the other hand is on the anterior upper trunk, opposite side, pulling backward.**
   • Outcome (Goal) of Selected Intervention: **Stability.**

2. *Verbal commands / (input):* **"Don't let me twist you; now don't let me twist you the other way."**

3. *Proprioceptive loading and contraction:* **Theraband tubing placed around the distal thighs increases the proprioceptive loading and contraction of the lateral hip muscles (gluteus medius). Thus, simultaneous contraction of the gluteal muscles (maximus and medius) is achieved.**

CLINICAL PROBLEM 30

Guiding Questions for First Intervention (To Promote Controlled Mobility)

1. • Position/Activity: **Kneeling, weight shifting.**
   • Technique: **Slow reversals (SRs), medial/lateral shifts.**
   • Manual Contacts: **The therapist alternates hand placement, first on one side of the pelvis resisting the pelvis as it pulls away, then on the opposite side as the pelvis pushes back.**
   • Outcome (Goal) of Selected Intervention: **Controlled mobility; smooth reversal of antagonists.**

2. *Patient positioning:* **The patient is in kneeling positioned in a symmetrical stance. The head and trunk are maintained vertical in midline orientation, with normal spinal lumbar and thoracic curves. Initially, movement of the hips is assisted for several repetitions to ensure the patient knows expected movements. Active side-to-side movements are then lightly resisted.** *Therapist positioning:* **The therapist is positioned in kneeling or half-kneeling at the side of the patient.**

3. *Verbal commands:* **Smooth reversal of antagonists is facilitated by well-timed verbal commands ("Pull away" or "Push back.").**

Guiding Questions for Second Intervention (To Promote Controlled Mobility)

1. • Position/Activity: **Kneeling in step position, weight shifting.**
   • Technique: **Slow reversals (SRs), diagonal shifts.**
   • Manual Contacts: **Hand placements are at the pelvis.**
   • Outcome (Goal) of Selected Intervention: **Controlled mobility.**

2. *Application of resistance:* **Resistance is applied to the pelvis as the patient weight-shifts diagonally forward over the more advanced knee, then diagonally backward over the other knee.** *Verbal commands:* **"Shift forward and toward me; now shift back and away from me."**

3. *Patient positioning:* **The patient is positioned in kneeling with the knees in step position (one knee is advanced in front of the other, simulating normal step length).** *Therapist positioning:* **The therapist is positioned in half-kneeling diagonally in front of the patient.**

APPENDIX B

Suggested Answers to the Case Studies

Please note that the answers provided in Appendix B represent only one solution to a given problem. Owing to the variety of treatment options available, the selection of an alternative *position, activity,* or *technique* may be equally effective in accomplishing a desired outcome (goal). These situations warrant feedback from colleagues or instructors.

CASE STUDY 1: SPINAL CORD INJURY

1. *Key muscles:* **Top half of intercostals; long muscles of back (sacrospinalis and semi-spinalis).**

2. *Selected functional capabilities and expected outcomes of physical therapy (long-term goals):*
   A. *Activities of daily living:* **Independent in all areas.**
   B. *Standing:* **Physiologic standing only (not realistic for functional ambulation); requires use of knee-ankle-foot orthoses with spinal attachment; may be able to ambulate for short distances with assistance.**
   C. *Locomotion:* **Independent with manual wheelchair with standard handrims.**
   D. *Housekeeping:* **Independent with routine activities.**
   E. *Curb climbing in wheelchair:* **Able to negotiate curbs using a "wheelie" technique.**
   F. *Wheelchair sports:* **Full participation.**

3. YES: *Indicate approach, including data or information needed and test or measures required;*
   NO: *Indicate rationale for ruling out the assessment:*
   A. *Respiratory Assessment:*
      1. *Function of Respiratory Muscles:* Yes **X**   No __.
         Approach or Rationale: **Muscle strength and tone; function of the diaphragm, abdominals, and intercostals should be assessed; respiratory rate should be documented.**

      2. *Chest Expansion:* Yes **X**   No __.
         Approach or Rationale: **Circumferential measurements should be taken at the level of the axillae and xiphoid process using a cloth tape measure (remove plastic body jacket from patients in recumbent positions). Chest expansion is recorded as the difference in measurement between maximum exhalation and maximum inhalation. Normal chest expansion is approximately 2 1/2 to 3 inches (6.25 to 7.5 cm) at the xiphoid process.**

      3. *Breathing Pattern:* Yes **X**   No __.
         Approach or Rationale: **A determination should be made of muscles that are functioning and their contributions to respiration. This may be accomplished by manual palpation over the chest and abdominal region or by observation. Particular attention should be directed toward use of accessory muscles and alteration in breathing pattern when the patient is talking or moving.**

      4. *Cough:* Yes **X**   No __.
         Approach or Rationale: **Coughing allows the patient to remove secretions. Ineffective cough function will necessitate suctioning to avoid pulmonary complications. Cough classifications typically include: (a)** *functional*—**strong enough to clear secretions, (b)** *weak functional*—**adequate force to clear upper-tract secretions in small quantities but assistance required to clear mucus secondary to infection, and (c)** *nonfunctional*—**unable to produce any cough force.**

      5. *Vital Capacity:* Yes **X**   No __.
         Approach or Rationale: **Initial measures can be taken with a hand-held spirometer. Vital capacity measures also can be used as a baseline for defining respiratory muscle involvement.**

B. *Skin Assessment:* Yes **X** No __.
   Approach or Rationale: **The nursing admission note indicated the skin on both heels and elbows was dry and reddened. This would suggest that other areas of the patient's body may be at risk, as well. Skin inspection combines both** *observation* **and** *palpation.* **The patient's entire body should be observed regularly with particular attention to areas most susceptible to pressure (occiput, scapulae, vertebrae, elbows, sacrum, coccyx, and heels). Palpation is useful for identifying skin temperature changes that may be indicative of a hyperemic reaction. Skin reactions to excess pressure include redness, local warmth, local edema, and small open, cracked areas. Careful attention should be directed toward accidental skin abrasions or bruises, which increase the potential for skin breakdown. As the patient is wearing an orthotic device, contact points between the body and the plastic jacket must also be inspected.**

C. *Manual Muscle Test (MMT) and Range of Motion (ROM) Assessment:* Yes **X** No __.
   Approach or Rationale: **Standard techniques should be used for MMT and ROM. Inasmuch as mobility will be limited, deviations from standard positioning will be necessary and should be carefully documented. Discretion should be used in applying resistance around the trunk and hips with this patient. The contraindications for ROM are to avoid straight-leg raises of more than 60 degrees and avoid hip flexion beyond 90 degrees.**

D. *Cardiovascular Endurance:* Yes __ No **X**.
   Approach or Rationale: **This assessment would be premature and is not indicated. Once the patient achieves some wheelchair mobility skills, cardiovascular endurance can be assessed. This can be accomplished by upper extremity (UE) stress testing or telemetry monitoring during wheelchair propulsion. However, the patient's age and cardiac history should be taken into account in considering such an assessment. Recall that the patient's previous medical history has been unremarkable. There is no evidence of impaired cardiovascular adaptation to exercise.**

E. *Functional Assessment:* Yes **X** No __.
   Approach or Rationale: **The functional assessment provides baseline information for setting function-oriented outcomes (goals). It is also an indicator of the patient's initial abilities, which can then be used for comparison to assess later progress. In addition, data from this assessment provide guidelines for determining safety in performing a particular task. One might logically consider not including a functional assessment initially, since limited information will be available this early. This is the result of movement restrictions imposed by the plastic body jacket, together with the patient's recovery from surgery and relative inactivity during the past 2 weeks. However, if not included in the initial assessment, functional skills should be among the first priorities during the initial components of physical therapy intervention.**

F. *Sensory Assessment:* Yes **X** No __.
   Approach or Rationale: **A detailed assessment of superficial, deep, and combined sensations should be completed. A comparison should be made between the sensory level of injury and the motor level of injury (i.e., complete versus incomplete lesion).**

G. *Assessment of Tone and Deep Tendon Reflexes:* Yes **X** No __.
   Approach or Rationale: **Muscle tone should be assessed with reference to quality, muscle groups involved, and factors that appear to increase or decrease tone. An assessment of deep tendon reflexes is indicated. The specific tendons selected for testing will be influenced by the lesion level. The lower extremity deep tendon reflexes most commonly assessed are the quadriceps (L-3, L-4), and the gastrocnemius (S-1).**

H. *Sacral Sparing:* Yes **X** No __.
   Approach or Rationale: **Periodic checks should be made for the presence of sacral sparing, which may not have been evident on admission (check for perianal sensation, rectal sphincter tone, or active toe flexion).**

4. *Identify the four assessments you would place as highest priorities for this patient. Identify the rationale for placing each assessment among your choices:*

- **Priority 1: Respiratory Assessment.**
  Rationale: **Respiratory function varies considerably, depending on the level of lesion. However, all patients with high-level paraplegia demonstrate some compromise in respiratory function. The level of respiratory impairment is directly related to the lesion level and residual respiratory muscle function, additional trauma sustained at time of injury, as well as premorbid respiratory status. Respiratory assessment is a high priority since involvement can represent a serious and limiting feature of spinal cord injury (SCI). Pulmonary complications—especially bronchopneumonia and pulmonary embolism—are potentially life-threatening complications of SCI during the early stages of recovery.**

- **Priority 2: Skin Assessment.**
  Rationale: **Several factors make skin assessment a high priority for this patient. The development of skin breakdown (pressure sores) is related to impaired sensory function and the inability to make appropriate positional changes. Pressure sores are among the most frequent medical complications following SCI and a major contributor to increasing duration and subsequently cost of hospital stay. Pressure sores will develop over any bony prominence subjected to excessive pressure. Among the more common sites of involvement are the sacrum, heels, trochanters, and ischium. In addition, the patient already has reddened areas over the heels and elbows, suggesting potential for development of additional areas of skin irritation.**

- **Priority 3: Sensory Assessment.**
  Rationale: **Sensory assessment is a high priority because it adds to the data base of patient information. Following spinal cord injury, disruption of the ascending sensory fibers results in impaired or absent sensation below the level of the lesion. A sensory assessment can assist in identifying specific features of the injury. These include the neurologic level, the completeness of the lesion, the symmetry of the lesion (transverse or oblique), and the presence or absence of sacral sparing.**

- **Priority 4: Functional Assessment.**
  Rationale: **Analysis of function also adds to the data base of patient information. A functional assessment will provide an accurate and specific determination of the patient's ability to accomplish specific tasks. Data will assist in setting function-oriented outcomes, provide a baseline level for measuring progress, and assist with establishing guidelines for determining safety in performing a particular task.**

5. *For each of the problems identified, indicate your projected outcome of treatment (short-term goal), together with the treatment procedure(s) you would use to accomplish the outcome (goal):*

- **Clinical Problem:** Decreased chest expansion (3/4 inch—1.8 cm—measured at the xiphoid process).
  Outcome of Treatment (Short-Term Goal): **Increase chest expansion to 2 inches (5 cm) as measured from xiphoid process.**
  Treatment: **Deep breathing exercises (diaphragmatic breathing) should be encouraged. To facilitate diaphragmatic movement and to increase vital capacity, the therapist applies light pressure during both inspiration and expiration. Manual contacts can be made just below the sternum. This will assist the patient to concentrate on deep breathing patterns even in the absence of thoracic and abdominal sensation. To facilitate expiration, the therapist should make manual contacts over the thorax with the hands spread wide. This creates a compressive force on the thorax, resulting in a more forceful expiration followed by a more efficient inspiration. Inflation hold and incentive spirometry are also useful adjuncts to deep breathing exercises.** *Note:* **Respiratory management will vary according to the level of injury and the individual patient's respiratory status. However, general outcomes (goals) of respiratory management for patients with SCI typically include improved ventilation, increased effectiveness of cough *and* prevention of chest tightness and ineffective substitute breathing patterns.**

- **Clinical Problem:** Dependent in skin inspection: FIM level* = 2; patient unaware of importance of skin inspection.

---

*The FIM level is measured from 1 to 7 using the Functional Independence Measure Scale (FIM^SM instrument). FIM^SM is a service mark of the Uniform Data System for Medical Rehabilitation, a division of UB Foundation Activities, Inc.

Outcome of Treatment (Short-Term Goal): **Independent in skin inspection (FIM level = 7);** patient will be knowledgeable about skin reactions to excess pressure, implications of impaired sensation, prevention techniques, and rationale for positioning program.
Treatment: Initially, regular skin inspection is a shared responsibility of the patient and the entire rehabilitation team. As management progresses, the patient will gradually assume greater responsibility for this activity. Patient education related to skin care is crucial and should be initiated early. This should include detailed information about the cause and prevention of skin breakdown, the areas of greatest susceptibility, use of pressure relief techniques, and how to respond to the appearance of an abnormal skin reaction. Long-handled or adapted mirrors will allow the patient to inspect areas that are not easily visible. Inexpensive wall mirrors adjacent to the bed may assist in achieving independence with this activity. In addition, it is important that the patient be instructed in how to direct others to complete this assessment. Continued emphasis by the therapist should be placed on the importance of skin inspection and the rationale for pressure relief throughout the course of rehabilitation. Skin inspection must become a regular and life-long component of the patient's daily routine.

- **Clinical Problem:** Tightness in heel cords (0–10 degrees).
  Outcome of Treatment (Short-Term Goal): **Increase ROM in dorsiflexion (0–20 degrees).**
  Treatment: **Plastic ankle boots or splints are indicated to maintain alignment and to prevent heel-cord tightness. The ankles should be positioned at a 90-degree angle. ROM exercises are indicated for the ankles with emphasis on dorsiflexion. In addition, a full program of ROM exercises should be initiated for both lower extremities (LEs), except for those areas which are contraindicated or require selective stretching. Some motions of the hip are contraindicated for this patient. Straight-leg raises greater than 60 degrees and hip flexion beyond 90 degrees (during combined hip and knee flexion) should be avoided. This will prevent strain on the lower thoracic and lumbar spine. Range of motion (ROM) exercises should be completed in both the prone and supine positions. In the prone position, attention should be directed toward shoulder and hip extension and knee flexion. Full ROM exercises should be included for both lower extremities (LEs). Patients with SCI do not require full ROM in all joints. In some instances, allowing tightness to develop in certain muscles will enhance function. For example, with this patient, slight tightness of the lower trunk musculature will improve sitting posture by increasing trunk stability. Conversely, some muscles require a fully lengthened range. The hamstrings will require stretching to achieve a straight-leg raise of approximately 100 degrees. This ROM is required for many functional activities such as sitting, transfers, LE dressing, and self-directed ROM exercises.**

- **Clinical Problem:** Dependent in bed mobility (positional changes): FIM level = 2.
  Outcome of Treatment (Short-Term Goal): **Independent in bed mobility and positional changes: FIM level = 7.**
  Treatment: **Mat program—rolling. The functional significance of rolling is related to improved bed mobility, preparation for independent positional changes in bed (for pressure relief), and for LE dressing. Rolling will be among the initial mat activities for this patient and provides an early lesson in developing functional patterns of movement. It will require the patient to learn to use the head, neck, and UEs as well as momentum to move the trunk and/or LEs. It is usually easiest to begin rolling activities in sidelying using small ranges, progressing to large ranges and finally to full range of motion, such as movement from supine to prone position. UE movements and momentum can assist rolling. The shoulders can be flexed with the elbows extended and brought up and across the body to facilitate rolling from supine to sidelying. The addition of weights (wrist cuffs) can assist in momentum and functional training. A variety of UE PNF patterns can be used to promote rolling from supine to sidelying, including D1F, reverse chop pattern, and lift pattern. Although rolling is initially taught on a mat, this activity must also be mastered on the surface of a bed similar to the one that the patient will use at home.**

- **Clinical Problem:** Proximal UE muscles all graded as good using MMT with modified positions.
  Outcome of Treatment (Short-Term Goal): **Normal UE muscle strength (normal grade using MMT).**
  Treatment: **Upper extremity (UE) strengthening can be initiated immediately. All muscles with active movement remaining should be strengthened maximally. During the first few weeks of treatment intervention, application of resistance to musculature of the upper trunk must be strengthened very cautiously to avoid stress at**

the fracture site. An important consideration in planning initial exercise programs is to emphasize bilateral UE activities, because these will avoid asymmetric, rotational stresses on the spine. Several forms of UE strengthening exercises are appropriate during this early phase: bilateral manually resisted motions in straight planes; bilateral UE PNF patterns (i.e., bilateral symmetrical D2F with elbow extending); and progressive resistive exercises using cuff weights or dumbbells. All UE musculature should be strengthened, with emphasis on shoulder depressors, triceps, and latissimus dorsi, which are required for movement transitions and transfers (i.e., PNF bilateral symmetrical D1E). Early involvement in functional activities should be stressed. In addition to their intrinsic value, many activities afford the important benefit of progressive strengthening. For example, bed mobility activities, dressing, movement transitions, and involvement in personal care activities will assist with strengthening the shoulder and elbow flexors. Another example of a functional activity with important benefits is wheelchair propulsion, which strengthens deltoids, biceps, and shoulder rotators.

- **Clinical Problem:** Postural hypotension (tolerance: 4 to 6 minutes with head of bed elevated to 30 degrees).
  Outcome of Treatment (Short-Term Goal): **Acclimation to upright posture/orientation to the vertical sitting position (tolerance: 2 to 3 hours using a manual wheelchair).**
  Treatment: **Radiographic findings have established stability of the fracture site, clearing the patient for upright sitting activities. A very gradual acclimation to upright postures is most effective. Use of the plastic body jacket (abdominal support) and elastic stockings will retard venous pooling. During early upright positioning, elastic wraps (placed on top of the stockings) may be used in combination with the elastic stockings. Upright activities are typically initiated by elevating the head of the bed and progressing to a reclining wheelchair with elevating leg rests. Use of the tilt table provides another option for orienting the patient to a vertical position. Vital signs should be monitored carefully and documented during this acclimation period.**

6. *Describe how you would respond to the couple's request for advice.* (Feedback on your response is provided in the answers to question 7.)

7. **Decision 1:** Is the response compatible with your own decision making? Yes ___ No **X** ("No" is the best choice).
   Justification for your decision about response: **Therapist response represents *faulty clinical decision making.***
   A. Concealing compassion and empathy are contradictory to the important notion of therapeutic use of self. Feeling compassion for our patients, which is quite different from pity or feeling sorry for someone in unfortunate circumstances, helps the practitioner to envision what is possible from the patient's perspective. Empathy also assists this process by putting one's self in the place of another.
   B. Use of humor here would be *inappropriate*. It would likely detract from the overall healing process and make the couple feel as if their interactions with you have been depersonalized. This may cause the patient to feel you have little concern for his individuality or unique circumstances.
   C. Not being knowledgeable about the specific rules and regulations of every managed-care company may be a reality of the situation. However, this information is not relevant to assisting the couple with the problems presented. There is no indication the wife is not a good source of information. In addition, such a response indicates an unwillingness to act on provided information or a refusal to obtain information available to you directly from the managed-care company.
   D. Suggesting that this information should not alter the plan for rehabilitation intervention is irresponsible. The health care insurance providers are clearly focused on cost containment. Prior authorization, limited hospital stays, and maximum number of visits are realities of the current system. It is the therapist's responsibility to assist the patient and family to work within the system to achieve desired outcomes (goals).

   Decision 2: Is the response compatible with your own decision making? Yes ___ No **X** ("No" is the best choice).
   Justification for your decision about response: **Therapist response represents *faulty clinical decision making.***
   A. The therapist may have been very well intentioned. Perhaps writing the letter is a reasonable idea. However, using this approach did not address the couple's immediate dilemma. In fact, the therapist inadvertently showed some indifference to their problem. The therapist's re-

sponse showed lack of interest and detachment from the immediate problem by deciding to address the issue on a more global scale.

B. It is apparent that the therapist is unhappy and wants the treatment time allocation for patient's with spinal cord injury to be increased. Perhaps the therapist did not know how to address the couple's immediate concerns. The therapist's automatic, emotion-based response was an opportunity to "let off steam" about the topic at hand; however, such a spontaneous outburst was inappropriate. The impact of the therapist's response did not address the problem. In addition, it is difficult to determine the impact on the patient of such open, aggressive expressions.

C. If the therapist truly did not know how to help, assistance from a colleague should have been sought. An important component of the role of the physical therapist is recognizing the limits of one's own knowledge, acknowledging the need for advice from someone else, and asking for help in a timely fashion.

Decision 3: Is the response compatible with your own decision making? Yes **X** No __
("Yes" is the best choice).
Justification for your decision about response: **Therapist response represents *sound clinical decision making.***

A. Expressions of concern and understanding are foundation to the healing process. Putting oneself in the described circumstances, helps with understanding the concerns and fears of the couple.

B. The therapist did not offer an "on-the-spot" solution to the complex problem at hand. However, logical choices were made based on sound decision making. The therapist was not only open and honest about the need for more information but offered solutions for how it could be obtained.

Now consider the therapist's response from the perspective of the steps that comprise the clinical decision-making process. Examine the information provided below under each of the interrelated steps of the process. Compare this information to your own response provided earlier for question 6. This will provide preliminary feedback on your own responses. Recall, however, that these represent only one appropriate response to the situation. Although not listed here, your responses may be appropriate. To confirm acceptability, feedback from colleagues or instructor is warranted.

- **Step 1—Collect Data:** Data gathered by the therapist indicated:
  1. Insufficient information was available to completely define the couple's problem.
  2. The couple is faced with limited allocation of insurance funds.
  3. Their home and business are potentially threatened.
  4. The husband requires extensive rehabilitation intervention, which potentially could exceed the time allocated by the HMO.
  5. The couple is in a new hospital environment and they appear to be facing a harsh, apathetic health care environment.
  6. Identification of resources to address the problem: case manager for the HMO, and rehabilitation team members.
- **Step 2—Analyze Data and Identify Problems:** The therapist identified two immediate problems:
  1. More information is needed from the HMO regarding specific details of coverage. Once additional data are obtained, the decision-making process may need to begin again in light of new findings.
  2. The therapist also identified a second problem: The couple was feeling helpless, cut off, and fragmented by an unfamiliar health care system. By communicating trust, respect, and interest, the therapist facilitated the couple's belief that an advocate was available. The therapist also focused on addressing the inherent strength of the situation by indicating that the rehabilitation team would have many creative suggestions for maximizing use of available time.
- **Step 3—Set Outcomes (Goals) and Priorities:** The therapist set two outcomes (goals):
  1. First priority: Establish overall plan of care designed to make best use of the time and achieve optimal outcomes (goals).
  2. Second priority: Function as an advocate for the patient with the managed-care company.

- **Step 4—Formulate Plan:** The interventions required to meet the outcomes (goals) include:
  1. Meeting of the entire rehabilitation team together with the patient and his wife.
  2. Contact the managed-care company directly to obtain details of coverage; establish line of communication with case manager; function as an advocate for the patient during the course of rehabilitation.
- **Step 5—Implement Plan:** How the plan will be carried out will be determined:
  (1) At the rehabilitation team meeting. (2) The plan may also be influenced by information obtained from case manager.
  8. *General strategies for optimizing use of treatment time allocated:*
     - *General Strategy 1:* **Education.** The patient and his family should have the benefit of full knowledge of all aspects of the injury. A major feature of the rehabilitation program will include a focus on assisted management with progression to self-management. This might also include development of patient teaching materials to initially be used as an in-patient and then taken home, participation in peer support groups, and when and how to obtain follow-up care. A coordinated plan must be developed for long-term periodic rehabilitation, including follow-up visits.
     - *General Strategy 2:* **Incorporate family support system.** Family members can effectively address issues of community reintegration. Consideration must be given to multiple issues, including housing (and any modifications needed), transportation, maintaining functional skills and level of physical fitness, employment or further education, and methods for involvement in desired social or recreational activities. Each of these issues must be addressed early in the course of rehabilitation in consultation with the physical therapist and appropriate team members. The patient and family also should be encouraged to contact and to explore the resources available through the local chapter of the National Spinal Cord Injury Association. Family members may also assist by setting up *trial use periods* with equipment vendors.
     - *General Strategy 3:* **Delegate appropriate segments of treatment to the physical therapist assistant.** Utilize group class activities (for example, UE strengthening, wheelchair mobility skills, range of motion exercises, and so on).

CASE STUDY 2: STROKE

1. *Significance of the patient's past medical history:* **The history of angina suggests the presence of coronary artery disease. Although the stress test was negative, it does not rule out the development of atherosclerotic involvement. The importance of family history is difficult to judge. The father's death at age 59 from a "heart attack" suggests early coronary disease. The mother's stroke, at a more advanced age, suggests atherosclerotic disease.**
   - *Atherosclerosis* **is a major contributing factor in occlusive vascular disease and is characterized by plaque formation and progressive narrowing of the vessel. The principle sequelae of this process are stenosis, ulceration of the atherosclerotic lesion, and thrombosis.**
   - *Cerebral thrombosis* **refers to the formation or development of a blood clot or thrombus within the cerebral arteries or their branches. Thrombi result from platelet adhesion and aggregation, coagulation of fibrin, and decreased fibrinolysis.**
   - *Cerebral emboli* **are traveling bits of matter such as thrombi, tissue, fat, air, bacteria, or other foreign bodies that are released into the bloodstream and travel to the cerebral arteries, where they produce occlusion and infarction. They are commonly associated with cardiovascular disease.**
   - *Hypertension* **is also a precipitating factor, as the affected vessel is often weakened by atherosclerosis.**

2. *Sites of predilection for atherosclerotic plaques:* **These sites generally include bifurcations, constrictions, dilation, or angulation of arteries. The most common sites for lesions to occur are at the origin of the common carotid artery, in the internal carotid artery at the level of the carotid sinus or at its transition into the middle cerebral artery, at the main bifurcation of the middle cerebral artery, and at the junction of the vertebral arteries with the basilar artery.**

3. *Structures supplied by middle cerebral artery:* **The middle cerebral artery (MCA) is the second of the two main branches of the internal carotid artery and supplies the lateral aspect of the cerebral hemisphere (frontal, temporal, and parietal lobes) and subcorti-**

cal structures, including the internal capsule (posterior portion), corona radiata, globus pallidus (outer part), most of the caudate nucleus, and the putamen.

4. *Focal signs:* **Differentiation between** *superficial occlusions* **and** *deep syndromes.* **The middle cerebral artery is the most common site of stroke. A superficial MCA occlusion results in contralateral hemiparesis or hemiplegia and sensory deficits, with the face and upper extremity more involved than the lower extremity. Homonymous hemianopsia (visual field defect) and loss of conjugate gaze to the opposite side also results. A deep MCA syndrome results in a pure motor hemiplegia without sensory or visual deficits.**

5. *General behavior patterns:*
   - **General Affect: Frequently described as being negative, anxious, and depressed; likely to be slower, more cautious, uncertain, and insecure. Tendency to be more hesitant when performing tasks; typically realistic in appraisal of existing problems. Teaching strategies require increased and more frequent use of feedback and support.**
   - **Cognitive Style: Difficulties demonstrated in processing information in a sequential, linear manner; and in observing and analyzing details.**
   - **Perception and Cognition: Deficits in processing and producing language.**
   - **Academic Skills: Impaired ability to read (sound-symbol relationships, word recognition, reading comprehension); impaired performance of mathematical operations.**
   - **Motor Responses: Difficulties in sequencing movements and performing movements and gestures to command.**
   - **Emotional Responses: Difficulties with expressions of positive or optimistic emotions.**

6. *List of six most important assessments (not prioritized yet):*
   1. **Perception**
   2. **Functional assessment**
   3. **Mental status**
   4. **Skin condition and edema**
   5. **Sensation**
   6. **Communication ability**

7. *Prioritized list of six most important assessments:*
   1. **Mental status**
   2. **Communication ability**
   3. **Sensation**
   4. **Perception**
   5. **Skin condition and edema**
   6. **Functional assessment**

8. *Prioritized list of assessments, rationale for high priority, needed information, and need for collaborative input:*
   - **Priority 1: Mental Status.** *Rationale:* **It is important to assess cognitive status first, because it may affect the results of other assessments.** *Information Needed:* **Level of consciousness, memory (immediate recall, short- and long-term), orientation (to person, place, time), ability to follow instructions (one-, two-, and three-level commands), higher cortical functions (calculation ability, abstract reasoning), and attention span should be included, as well as investigation of behavioral and emotional responses. Learning deficits, including retention and generalization deficits, can significantly impede rehabilitation efforts and should be identified early.** *Collaborative Input:* **Not needed immediately.**
   - **Priority 2: Communication ability.** *Rationale:* **Because communication deficits may severely limit the validity of other assessments, patient comprehension must be assessed early.** *Information Needed:* **Impairments in receptive language (word recognition, auditory comprehension, reading comprehension) and/or expressive language function (word finding, fluency, writing, spelling) should be noted. The functional deficits of dysarthria (disordered motor production of speech) should be carefully examined. Alternate forms of communication (gestures, movements, pantomime) should be documented.** *Collaborative Input:* **Close collaboration with the speech language pathologist will be important in making an accurate determination of the patient's communication deficits.**
   - **Priority 3: Sensation.** *Rationale:* **Because of the close relationship between sensory input and motor output, sensory deficits will influence assessments of motor perfor-**

mance. *Information Needed:* **Data on superficial, proprioceptive, and combined sensations. The visual system should be carefully investigated, including tests for acuity, peripheral vision, depth perception, and hemianopsia. Hearing status should be determined.** *Collaborative Input:* **Not needed.**

- **Priority 4: Perception.** *Rationale:* **Deficits can present as impaired ability to detect relevant cues from the environment or to discriminate between relevant and irrelevant stimuli. Assessment of movement disorders will therefore be affected by perceptual limitations.** *Information Needed:* **Data on body scheme, body image, spatial relations, agnosia, and apraxia.** *Collaborative Input:* **Close collaboration with occupational therapist. Note: Perceptual impairments are most often associated with right hemisphere lesions. However, all patients with stroke should be asssessed for: (a) how information is processed and (b) the behavioral style adopted in performance of functional tasks.**

- **Priority 5: Skin condition and edema.** *Rationale:* **Swelling has been documented in the patient's hand; this may be a precursor to development of reflex sympathetic dystrophy (shoulder-hand syndrome). Early diagnosis and treatment are critical to preventing or minimizing its progression.** *Information Needed:* **Evidence of sympathetic vasomotor changes such as warm, red, and glossy skin; trophic changes of the fingernails (nails may appear white, opaque). Presence of pain at rest or with movement; location of any skin areas that appear red, dry, or cracked.** *Collaborative Input:* **Collaboration with entire rehabilitation team to monitor skin condition and potential development of hand or shoulder pain.**

- **Priority 6: Functional assessment.** *Rationale:* **Provides baseline information for setting functional outcomes, serves as indicator of patient's initial abilities (which can be compared to level of progression later in treatment), contributes to establishing guidelines for safety and potential risk of injury for an individual patient, and provides evidence of the effectiveness of specific treatment interventions; later in treatment, data from assessment can also be used as criteria for discharge or transition to another level of care (i.e., home, extended care facility, rehabilitation facility, and so on).** *Information Needed:* **Level of functional skill in bed mobility and transfers, in basic activities of daily living (BADLs), assistance required, and adaptive equipment used or needed.** *Collaborative Input:* **Not needed immediately; during treatment intervention collaboration with entire rehabilitation team to ensure consistency in approach.**

9. *Selection of treatment:* **Feedback on the features (type of contraction, application, and motor goals) and indications of techniques appropriate to address decreased trunk stability in sitting is provided in answers to questions 10 and 11 below.**

10. *Needed features of and indications for techniques appropriate to address decreased trunk stability in sitting:* ***The features of techniques are:* Isometric contractions in the shortened range (postural extensors), progressing to midrange control (co-contraction). Description of application should promote weight bearing and holding in antigravity postures; the motor control goal is stability.** *Indications are:* **Instability in sitting.**

11. *Features of and indications for each technique, compatibility with needs,* include or rule out:
    A. **Alternating Isometrics (AI).** *Application:* **Isometric holding is facilitated first on one side of the joint, followed by alternate holding of the antagonist muscle groups. May be applied in any direction (anterior/posterior, medial/lateral, diagonal).** *Indications:* **Instability in weight bearing and holding, poor antigravity control.** *Contraction:* **Isometric.** *Compatible with needs:* **Yes.** *Include/Rule Out:* **Include.**
    B. **Rhythmic Initiation (RI).** *Application:* **Voluntary relaxation followed by passive movements through increments in range, then by active-assistive movements progressing to resisted movements using tracking resistance. Movements may be unidirectional or in both directions.** *Indications:* **Inability to relax, hypertonicity, inability to initiate movement.** *Contraction:* **Isotonic.** *Compatible with needs:* **No.** *Include/Rule Out:* **Rule out.**
    C. **Hold-Relax (HR).** *Application:* **A relaxation technique usually performed at the point of limited ROM in the agonist pattern. An isometric contraction of the range-limiting antagonist pattern is performed against slowly increasing resistance, followed by voluntary relaxation and passive movement into the newly gained range of the agonist pattern.** *Indications:* **Limitations caused by muscle tightness, muscle spasm, and pain.** *Contraction:* **Isometric.** *Compatible with needs:* **No.** *Include/Rule Out:* **Rule out.**
    D. **Rhythmic Stabilization (RS).** *Application:* **Simultaneous isometric contractions of both agonist and antagonist patterns, performed without relaxation but using**

careful grading of resistance; results in co-contraction of opposing muscle groups. *Indications:* **Instability in weight bearing and holding, poor antigravity control.** *Contraction:* **Isometric.** *Compatible with needs:* **Yes.** *Include/Rule Out:* **Include.**

  E. **Slow Reversals (SRs).** *Application:* **Slow isotonic contractions of first agonist, then antagonist patterns, using careful grading of resistance and optimal facilitation; reversal of antagonists; progression through increments of range.** *Indications:* **Inability to reverse directions, muscle imbalances, weakness.** *Contraction:* **Isotonic.** *Compatible with needs:* **No.** *Include/Rule Out:* **Rule Out.**

  F. **Placing and Holding.** *Application:* **Stability control is developed in weight-bearing postures. A patient with stability control deficits may be unable to hold a posture. Early stability outcomes (goals) may be achieved by assisting to position (placing) and holding (manual contacts) after positioning.** *Indications:* **Tonal imbalance; impaired voluntary control.** *Contraction:* **Isometric.** *Compatible with needs:* **Yes.** *Include/Rule Out:* **Include.**

  G. **Agonist Reversals (ARs).** *Application:* **A slow isotonic, shortening contraction through the range followed by an eccentric, lengthening contraction using the same muscle groups; performed through increments of range (typically used in bridging, sit-to-stand transitions, and stepping).** *Indications:* **Inability to eccentrically control body weight during movement transitions; weak postural muscles.** *Contraction:* **Isotonic; eccentric.** *Compatible with needs:* **No.** *Include/Rule Out:* **Rule Out.**

CASE STUDY 3: RHEUMATOID ARTHRITIS

1. *Response to patient who has difficulty with early morning activity:* **Explain that morning stiffness is very common. Difficulty moving after awakening and generalized stiffness are classic symptoms of rheumatoid arthritis. It results from changes in cellular content and volume of the fluid surrounding the joint. This increased content within the joint space impairs free movement of the joint, causing it to feel stiff even after early morning activity.**

2. *Steps in clinical decision-making process:* **Feedback on mental review of interrelated steps in the decision-making process is provided in question 3 below.**

3. *Key steps in decision-making process omitted:*

> ■ Collect Data   ■ **Analyze Data/Identify Problems**
> ■ **Set Outcomes (Goals)/Priorities**   ■ **Formulate a Plan**   ■ Implement the Plan
> ■ **Evaluate the Outcome**

- **Step 1: Collect Data:** *Question(s) to ask yourself:* Do I have sufficient information to define the clinical problems(s)? Can I identify resources available to address the problem(s)? Do I have adequate subjective and objective data?
- **Step 2: Analyze Data/Identify Problems:** *Question(s) to ask yourself:* Have I mentally organized and analyzed the available data? do I have a thorough understanding of the problem(s) identified, the needs of the patient, and the resources available? Can I generate an asset list (to optimize inherent strengths in the situation)?
- **Step 3: Set Functional Outcomes (Goals)/Priorities.** *Question(s) to ask yourself:* Have I determined the appropriate outcome (goal) for the clinical problems(s)? What are my greatest concerns about the problem(s) identified? What do I want to see happen? How will I measure progress? How will I involve the patient in the decision-making process? Do I need to set more than one outcome (goal) to address the problem? Have I established priorities?
- **Step 4: Formulate a Plan.** *Question(s) to ask yourself:* What interventions or activities will be required to meet the outcome (goal)?
- **Step 5: Implement the Plan.** *Question(s) to ask yourself:* How will I carry out the plan? How will I optimize its effectiveness? How will I explain the plan to the patient? How will the plan influence the clinical problem(s) identified?

- **Step 6: Evaluate Outcome.** *Question(s) to ask yourself:* How will I determine the effectiveness of the plan?

4. *Formulation of clinical problem list:* **Right (R) knee pain (PS* = 6); (R) knee instability; (L) knee swelling; ill-fitting/worn cane; decreased LE ROM; worn shoes; decreased LE strength; morning stiffness. Increased hip adduction (0–20 degrees); genu valgum (20 degrees); subtalar pronation (0–15 degrees); stair climbing (FIM level* = 4). Gait: decreased (R) stance; IADL†(FIM level = 4); uneven step length. Shoulder pain (PS = 7); shoulder tightness at end of range; decreased ROM at elbow; slight inflammation at elbow. Fingers: minimal swelling, MCP‡ ulnar drift; wrist: bilateral volar subluxation (10 degrees).**

5. *List of Clinical Problems, Outcome of Treatment (OT) or Short-Term Goal (STG), and Treatment (TR) to achieve the outcome:*

Problem 1: (R) knee pain (PS = 6).	**OT/STG:** Reduce (R) knee pain to manageable levels (PS = 3).	**TR:** Patient education; moist hot pack; dry heating pad (home use).
Problem 2: Shoulder pain (PS = 7).	**OT/STG:** Reduce shoulder pain to manageable levels (PS = 3).	**TR:** Patient education; moist hot pack; dry heating pad (home use).
Problem 3: Genu valgum (25 degrees)/ (R) knee instability.	**OT/STG:** Genu valgum (10 degrees) maintained in stance.	**TR:** Stabilize with rigid knee orthosis (Miami Knee Orthosis); consult with orthotist.
Problem 4: Subtalar pronation (0–15 degrees).	**OT/STG:** Subtalar neutral (0–0 degrees).	**TR:** Strengthen posterior tibialis; recommend foot orthoses (to be worn inside shoe); consult with orthotist.
Problem 5: Ill-fitting/worn cane.	**OT/STG:** Correct use of well-fitted cane.	**TR:** Recommend/order new cane; patient education; gait training.
Problem 6: Worn shoes contributing to subtalar malalignment.	**OT/STG:** Subtalar neutral via positioning.	**TR:** Recommend shoe components; assist with order; consult with orthotist.
Problem 7: Increased hip adduction (0–20 degrees) in weight bearing.	**OT/STG:** Neutral hip adduction alignment (0–0 degrees) in weight bearing.	**TR:** Subtalar (0–0 degrees) and knee positioning (10 degrees genu valgum) through orthotic intervention.
Problem 8: Decreased LE strength.	**OT/STG:** Increase or maintain strength sufficient for function.	**TR:** Patient education; home exercise program (isotonic); outpatient clinic exercise (isotonic and isokinetic); isometric exercise during acute flare-ups.
Problem 9: Decreases in UE and LE ROM.	**OT/STG:** Increase/maintain ROM sufficient for function.	**TR:** Patient education; proper positioning when resting; self-performed ROM exercises.
Problem 10: Gait deviations: decreased (R) stance; uneven step length.	**OT/STG:** Safe, efficient gait pattern; even stance time and step length.	**TR:** Gait training.

---

*Reminder: A summary of grading scales for balance, pain, the Functional Independence Measure (FIMˢᴹ scale), and sensation is located on pp. 240–241.
†IADL = Instrumental activities of daily living.
‡MCP = Metacarpophalangeal.

- **Problem 11:**
Stair climbing
(FIM level = 4).

  OT/STG:
Stair climbing
(FIM level = 6).

  TR:
Stair climbing training using
standard cane; appropriate
LE sequence.

- **Problem 12:**
IADLs (FIM level = 4);
decreased endurance for
ambulation.

  OT/STG:
IADLs (FIM level = 6);
increase endurance to within
functional limits.

  TR:
Assess cardiovascular status;
gradual increase in
functional activity level;
home exercise program; outdoor and community gait
training and travel.

- **Problem 13:**
Joint swelling
(multiple areas); MCP ulnar
drift; volar subluxation.

  OT/STG:
Decrease biochemical stress
on all affected joints.

  TR:
Patient education; joint
conservation techniques.

6. *Prioritized list of clinical problems:*
   1. **(R) knee pain** (PS = 6)
   2. **Stair climbing** (FIM level 4)
   3. **Genu valgum** (20 degrees)
   4. **Subtalar pronation** (0–15 degrees)
   5. **Worn shoes**
   6. **Ill-fitting/worn cane**

7. *General treatment or strategy:* **A logical treatment approach for this patient is to incorporate elements of patient education and therapeutic exercise with components of compensatory training. This treatment approach should be developed with integration of
   appropriate practice and feedback. Patient and family member education will also
   constitute a substantial segment of the overall plan.** *Rationale for priorities:* **In establishing the order of priority, putting the patient's most pressing needs first is critical to
   the decision-making process:**
   - **Priority 1:** *Pain.* **One factor that demands immediate attention is responding to the
     patient's pain. Responding first to pain or severe discomfort is typically very high in
     establishing priorities.**
   - **Priority 2:** *Sequence of stair climbing.* **Pain and additional potential damage to the
     joint place this item high on the list.**
   - **Priorities 3, 4, 5, and 6:** *Genu valgum, subtalar pronation, worn shoes, and ill-fit-
     ting/worn cane.* **These items actually constitute a second-level "group priority." They
     are all contributing factors to the cause of the malalignment and one might logically
     argue a somewhat different order. Recall that although the arthritic involvement is
     long standing, the history of the chief complaint goes back only 2 months, when the
     bicycle fall occurred. In addition, during non-weight-bearing assessment, relative
     neutral alignment was achieved at the hip and ankle; genu valgum was reduced to
     10 degrees. This would indicate the alignment problems are amenable to interven-
     tion. Resolution of problems 3, 4, 5, and 6, collectively, will assist in maintaining
     more normal alignment and move the patient toward her stated outcome (goal) of
     early resumption of functional independence.**

8. *Clinical problem and projected number of visits (PNV) for each problem; rationale for decisions:*
   - **Problem:** Joint swelling (multiple areas); morning stiffness; MCP ulnar drift volar subluxa-
     tion; **PNV: 1.**
   - **Problem:** Gait deviations; decreased (R) stance; uneven step length; **PNV: 2.**
   - **Problem:** Ill-fitting/worn cane; **PNV: 1.**
   - **Problem:** Stair climbing (FIM level = 4); **PNV: 1.**
   - *Rationale for Projected Number of Visits:* **This case has a number of unique aspects that
     influence required number of visits. The patient asset list includes: intact cognitive
     function, high motivation level, high patient compliance, medically stable, no com-
     plicating factors to achieving outcomes (goals), and supportive family member will-
     ing to assist with care.**

9. *Time allocation for treatment:*
   A. **Yes, 8 visits are sufficient.**

B. **No, additional treatments at private expense would not be necessary.**
C. **Frequency of treatment and distribution over the month: Considering that several items need to be ordered for the patient (shoes, orthosis, cane, and so forth), it would be logical to have slightly more visits toward the latter portion of the month, after all items have arrived.**
D. **There is clearly no set formula for such decisions. A reasonable suggestion might be: week 1, 2 visits; week 2, 1 visit; week 3, 2 visits; and week 4, 3 visits.**

CASE STUDY 4: CONSTRUCTION ACCIDENT (TRAUMA)

1. *Prioritized Physical Therapy Problem List:*
    1. **Pain:** Left (L) hip—PS = 5; (L) ankle—PS = 7; (L) shoulder—PS = 8; (L) elbow—PS = 7.
    2. **Tightness and swelling of left (L) hand and fingers.** Finger flexion (mass grasp): end ranges unavailable.
    3. **Sensory deficits:** Left hand—Sharp/Dull: 2, Light Touch: 2, Temperature: 2. Proprioceptive sensations: 2. Cortical sensations: 2.
    4. **Decreased chest expansion:** Circumferential chest measurement = 1 inch (2.5 cm difference between maximum exhalation and inhalation).
    5. **Decreased lower trunk rotation, weakness of the low back extensor muscles.**
    6. **Decreased ROM in left (L) upper and lower extremities, especially hamstring tightness; tightness in right (R) lower extremity (extremes of range).**
    7. **Decreased strength in (L) upper and lower extremities** (MMT: F− to G− range; dorsiflexion strength is P).
    8. **Functional mobility skills:** (a) Bed mobility: Supine-to-sit transfer; FIM level = 4; Bridging: FIM level = 3. (b) Transfers: Sit-to-stand: FIM level = 3; non-weight-bearing on (L) lower extremity. Stand-to-sit: FIM level = 3; non-weight-bearing on (L) lower extremity. Stand pivot to wheelchair on right (R) lower extremity: FIM level = 4. (c) Basic activities of daily living (BADLs*): Bathing: FIM = 4. Dressing: FIM = 4.
    9. **Low sitting tolerance (approx 20 minutes).**
    10. **Non-weight-bearing (L) lower extremity.**

2. *Patient Asset List:* **(1) Medical history essentially unremarkable; (2) medically stable; (3) intact cognitive function; (4) cooperative; (5) anxious to regain complete independence; high patient compliance anticipated; (6) no apparent complicating factors limiting achievement of desired outcomes; and outpatient care is not restricted by the patient's medical benefits; (7) bed mobility—supine-to-sit: FIM level = 4; (8) transfers—stand pivot to wheelchair on right lower extremity: FIM level = 4; (9) basic activities of daily living (BADLs*)—bathing: FIM =4 , dressing: FIM = 4.**

3. *Outcomes of Physical Therapy (Long-Term Goals) and Outcomes of Treatment (Short-Term Goals).*
    * **Outcome(s) of Physical Therapy:**
        1. **The patient will be independent in ambulation on all surfaces for unlimited distances (FIM level = 7).**
        2. **The patient will be independent in all IADLs† (FIM level = 7).**
    * **Outcomes of Treatment:**
        1. **Reduction of pain in left hip, ankle, shoulder, elbow from PS = 5–8 to PS 2–3.**
        2. **Elimination of swelling in left hand and increased ROM in mass grasp from three-quarters range to full range.**
        3. **Independence (FIM = 7) in use of protective and compensatory strategies to substitute for sensory deficits of left hand.**
        4. **Increased chest expansion from 1 inch to 2 inches (2.5 cm to 5 cm) using circumferential chest measurement.**
        5. **Increased lower trunk rotation toward right from 0–30 degrees to 0–40 degrees, and toward left from 0–25 degrees to 0–40 degrees.**
        6. **Increased ROM of left upper and lower extremities (UEs and LEs) to within functional limits.**
        7. **Increased strength of trunk extensors from MMT = F+ to MMT = G+.**

---

*BADLS = Basic activities of daily living
†IADLs = Instrumental activities of daily living

8. **Increased left LE strength: hip and knee from MMT = G−/F− to MMT = G+; ankle musculature from MMT = F−/P to G−.**
9. **Increased left UE strength: shoulder and elbow from MMT = G−/F− to MMT = G+; forearm, wrist, and hand musculature from MMT = G−/F− to G−.**
10. **Independence in supine-to-sit transfers: from FIM level = 4 to FIM level = 7.**
11. **Independence in bridging: from FIM level = 3 to FIM level = 7.**
12. **Independence in transfer activities (sit-to-stand: from FIM level = 3 to FIM level = 7; stand-to-sit: from FIM level = 3 to FIM level = 7).**
13. **Independence in performance of basic activities of daily living (BADLs)—bathing: from FIM level = 4 to FIM = 7; dressing: from FIM level = 4 to FIM level = 7.**
14. **Increased sitting tolerance from approx 20 minutes to 90 minutes, with appropriate positional changes.**
15. **Tightness eliminated in the extremes of range for the right LE.**
16. **Gradual acclimation to upright standing posture with assistance (FIM level = 3).**

4. *Physical Therapy Plan of Care:* **Problem and Outcome of Treatment (OT), or short-term goal; sequential order of the three advanced therapeutic exercise interventions or procedures (A, B, or C). For each intervention, describe Position/Activity (P/A) or Movement Transitions and Technique:**
   - **Problem 1:** Decreased lower trunk rotation (toward right 0–30 degrees; toward left 0–25 degrees). **OT: The patient gains increased rotation of lower trunk (0–40 degrees bilaterally).**
     A. *First Intervention:* **P/A: Hooklying, lower trunk rotation. Technique: Rhythmic initiation (RI):** The lower trunk is rotated as the knees are moved slowly from side to side. As the patient relaxes, range is gradually increased until the knees move laterally down to the mat on each side. The movements are first passive (identical to rhythmic rotation), then active-assistive, then lightly resisted (tracking resistance). Progression to next phase is dependent upon patient's ability to relax and participate in the active and resistive phases.
     B. *Second Intervention:* **P/A: Hooklying, holding. Technique: Alternating isometrics (AI):** The patient is asked to hold the position while the therapist applies resistance to the knees. Side-to-side resistance is applied with one hand on the medial side of the knee and the opposite hand on the lateral side of the other knee; hand placements are then reversed to resist holding in the other direction. The resistance is built up gradually, starting from very light resistance and progressing to the patient's maximum. The isometric contraction is maintained for several counts. The therapist must give a **transitional verbal command** ("now don't let me pull you the other way") before sliding his or her hands to resist the opposite muscles; this allows the patient the opportunity to make appropriate preparatory postural adjustments. Resistance can be applied side to side, or diagonally. The position of the therapist will vary according to the line of force that needs to be applied. Resistance applied to both hip abductors may be used to gain overflow from strong to weak muscles. In this situation, resistance to abductors is typically maximized while resistance to adductors is minimal.
     C. *Third Intervention:* **P/A: Hooklying, lower trunk rotation. Technique: Slow reversals (SRs):** In hooklying, the patient moves both knees together in side-to-side movements. Depending upon available range of motion (ROM), the knees can move all the way down to the mat on one side, then the other. The knees are moved passively from side to side for a few repetitions to ensure that the patient knows the movements expected. The movements are then resisted. The therapist alternates hand placement, first on one side to resist the knees pulling away from midline, then on the other side to resist the return movement. Smooth reversals of antagonists are facilitated by well-timed **verbal commands** ("Pull away" or "Push back") and by a quick stretch to initiate the reverse movement. Progression is from partial-range to full-range control.
   - **Problem 2: Weakness of low back extensors and gluteal muscles: bridging—FIM level = 3. OT: Bridging—FIM level = 7; the patient performs sit-to-stand and stand-to-sit transfers (FIM = 7).**
     A. *First Intervention:* **P/A: Bridging, pelvic elevation. Technique: Slow reversals (SRs):** The therapist is positioned in half-kneeling at the side of the patient. The hips are assisted up and down for a few repetitions to ensure that the patient knows the movements expected. The movements are then lightly resisted. The therapist alternates hand placement, first on the top of the pelvis, resisting the hips as they rise up, then on the buttocks, giving a directional cue for the return to the mat. Resistance is minimal in the return motion. **Verbal commands:** Smooth motions of opposing muscle groups (reversals of antagonists) are facilitated by well-timed verbal commands ("Push up" or "Pull down"). **Slow reversal-hold (SRH):** A hold may be added in the direction of pelvic elevation if difficulty is experi-

enced in maintaining the contraction in the shortened range. The hold is a momentary pause (held to one count); the antagonist contraction is then facilitated. **Note:** if this P/A is too challenging for the patient it can be preceded by a less challenging intervention— **P/A: Bridging, pelvic elevation. Technique: Active or guided movement (active-assistive).** The patient is positioned in supine with the knees flexed and feet flat on the mat (hooklying). The patient is instructed to raise the hips from the mat until the hips are fully extended and the pelvis is elevated and level. The patient then lowers the pelvis down to the mat slowly, rather than "plopping" or collapsing down. Pelvic elevation can be facilitated by the therapist placing both hands on the patient's lower thighs and pushing down on the knees, pulling the distal thighs toward the feet. Tapping over the gluteus maximus can also be used to stimulate muscle contraction.

   B. *Second Intervention:* **P/A: Bridging, pelvic elevation. Technique: Agonist reversals (ARs):** This technique provides resistance to low back and hip extensors during both the concentric (shortening) contractions and eccentric (lengthening) contractions. The therapist is in half-kneeling at the patient's side, with both hands positioned on the anterior pelvis during the elevation and lowering phases of bridging. **Verbal commands** include "Push up" and "Now go down slowly."

   C. *Third Intervention:* **P/A: Bridging, holding. Technique: Alternating isometrics (AI):** The patient is asked to hold the bridge position while resistance is applied to the pelvis, first on one side pushing the pelvis away from the therapist, then pulling the pelvis toward the therapist (medial/lateral resistance). The resistance is built up gradually, starting from very light resistance and progressing to the patient's maximum. The isometric contraction is maintained for several counts. The therapist must give a transitional command ("Now don't let me pull you the other way") before sliding his or her hands to resist the opposite muscles; this allows the patient to make appropriate preparatory postural adjustments.

- **Problem 3:** Weakness of left foot and ankle musculature (MMT = F−/P). **OT: The patient achieves improved medial/lateral foot/ankle control in preparation for gait (MMT = G−).**
  - A. *First Intervention:* **P/A: Bridging, holding. Technique: Alternating isometrics (AI):** Resistance applied at the knees increases the length of the lever arm and recruits more lower limb muscles, especially foot and ankle muscles. The position of the therapist will vary according to the line of force required.
  - B. *Second Intervention:* **P/A: Bridging, weight shifts. Technique: slow reversals (SRs):** The therapist is positioned in kneeling at the side of the patient. Manual contacts at the knees increase the length of the lever arm and recruit medial and lateral ankle and foot muscles to shift the body from side to side.
  - C. *Third Intervention:* **P/A: Bridging, advanced stabilization. Technique: Bridging, leg lifts:** The patient is asked to lift one leg up while maintaining the bridge position using single-limb support. Lifts can include knee extension or marching in place (hip and knee flexion). The patient is asked to alternate limbs, lifting first one LE, then the other. Movements can be assisted with tactile or verbal cueing. UE stabilization (abducted and extended on mat) is essential during initial training; as control progresses, difficulty can be increased by reducing the UE support (increasing shoulder adduction by crossing the arms over chest or by holidng the hands in a prayer position). Speed and range of movements can be varied to increase the difficulty of the activities. Patients can work up to marching, then running in place, or running side to side.
- **Problem 4: Supine-to-sit transfer (FIM level = 4). OT: Patient independently performs movement transitions from supine to sitting (FIM level = 7). Technique: Movement transitions:** teaching strategy and method of assistance—two options could be considered:

   P/A: Transitions from supine to sidelying to sitting: From the supine position, the patient rolls onto the right side. The hips and knees are flexed, and the legs are moved off the bed or mat. The pelvis acts as a fulcrum with the legs as counterweights as they lower down to rotate the patient up into sitting. The patient simultaneously uses both UEs to push up into sitting (this may be difficult at first, owing to left UE involvement). The therapist can assist the initial rolling sequence into the sidelying position, the movement of the legs lowering off the mat or bed, or the lifting of the upper trunk.

   P/A: Transitions from supine to sidelying-on-elbow to sitting: From the supine position the patient rotates the head and upper trunk up and rolls onto the flexed elbow placed nearest the edge. Once in the sidelying-on-elbow position, the knees are flexed and the legs moved off the mat or bed. Individuals with increased control can move from lying to sitting in one smooth motion without using the UEs to assist. The therapist can assist movement into the sidelyng-on-elbow position by holding onto the sides of the trunk and rotating and lifting the upper trunk. Movement into the sitting position can also be assisted by pulling down on the iliac crest, providing an anchoring point for the trunk side flexors. If the patient requires additional assistance, the therapist's opposite hand can be placed around the shoulder on the weight-bearing side to lift the patient into sitting.

- **Problem 5:** Decreased strength of left shoulder/proximal upper extremity (MMT = F−); **OT:** The patient is able to stabilize the shoulder in all positions needed for UE function (MMT = G+).

    A. *First Intervention:* **P/A: Shoulder stabilization, active holding. Technique: Guided movement (active assistive) to active movement (holding):** The patient is positioned in supine. The elbow is extended and the UE is passively positioned at 90 degrees of shoulder flexion. The patient is asked to actively hold this position. This is a good initial position for stabilization training of the shoulder because of the minimized influence of gravity. The patient can then be asked to maintain the position of the shoulder while flexing and extending the elbow. These simultaneous movements increase the difficulty of the task and promote independent or isolated joint activity. The position can be modified for the patient to promote active holding in alternate positions such as sidelying or sitting, or standing, when full weight bearing is permitted. Upright positioning with the shoulder holding at 90 degrees of flexion with the elbow extended imposes a greater challenge due to maximum effects of gravity acting on the shoulder and the increased demands for upright trunk stability. The therapist can provide initial support (assistance) and remove support as soon as the patient is able to assume voluntary control.

    B. *Second Intervention:* **P/A: Shoulder stabilization, active holding. Technique: Hold-relax active motion (HRAM):** The patient is positioned in supine with the limb positioned in D1 extension; the shoulder is holding at approximately 30 degrees of shoulder flexion. (The position is analogous to the UE position needed during ambulation with an assistive device or in the parallel bars.) The patient is asked to hold while the therapist applies gradually increasing isometric resistance to shoulder extensors, abductors, and internal rotators. The patient is then asked to actively relax. The therapist moves the UE quickly in the opposite D1F pattern and provides a quick stretch and a **verbal command** to "push the arm down and out" back to the original start position. The patient actively contracts and pushes the arm down. The sequence is then repeated. This is an effective procedure to improve shoulder stabilization within a functional position needed for weight bearing. Muscles needed for assisted ambulation or for push-up transfers (that is, latissimus dorsi, teres minor, triceps) are strengthened.

    C. *Third Intervention:* **P/A: Shoulder stabilization, active holding. Technique: Rhythmic stabilization (RS):** The patient is positioned in supine and instructed to move in the PNF D1 flexion pattern (the UE moves up into flexion, adduction, and external rotation with the elbow straight). As the UE moves up and across into D1F, the patient is asked to hold at approximately 90 degrees of flexion. The therapist applies isometric resistance to shoulder flexors, adductors, and external rotators. The therapist then switches hands to the opposite side of the limb to resist the D1E pattern (resistance is now applied to shoulder extensors, abductors, and internal rotators). A **verbal command** ("Now hold here—don't let me move you up and across") is given before resistance is applied. Resistance is gradually built up; the patient is expected to hold the UE steady. The technique is continued for several repetitions. The patient is then asked to complete the D1E pattern and push the arm down and out to the side. Isometric training is specific to the range of joint motion where it is applied. The therapist, therefore, must vary the shoulder joint angle and apply resistance using RS to the UE at various points in the range in order to ensure shoulder stability throughout the entire range of motion. Rhythmic stabilization (RS) can also be applied in sitting and standing positions (when weight bearing allows) to increase the difficulty of the task. Upright positioning requires stabilization control of shoulder as well as trunk and LE muscles. Alternating isometrics (AI) is a technique that can also be used to promote shoulder stabilization. The difference between the two techniques is the absence of isometric resistance to rotators in AI.

5. *Justification for Treatment—Outcome of Treatment (OT) 1 through 5: Therapeutic Exercise or Movement Transition (T/MT), and Rationale for Selection of the intervention, including Techniques with Motor Control Goal and/or Indications—(GI).*

    - **OT 1: The patient gains increased rotation of lower trunk. T/MT: Hooklying, lower trunk rotation. Rhythmic initiation (RI), Alternating isometrics (AI), Slow reversals (SRs). The patient is positioned in supine with both hips and knees flexed and feet flat on the mat.** Rationale for Selection: Base of support (BOS) is large; center of mass (COM) is low. Posture is very stable. The activity primarily involves lower trunk, hip and knee control: activation of lower trunk rotators and hip abductors/adductors allows the patient to actively move the knees from side to side away from midline; activation of hamstrings allow the patient to maintain the knees flexed in the hooklying position. Hooklying activities are important lead-up activities for controlled bridging, kneeling, and bipedal gait. Patients with gluteus medius weakness benefit from hooklying activities to activate abductors in a less stressful, non-weight-bearing position. **Techniques and GI: Rhythmic initiation (RI):** Mobility; decreased lower trunk rotation. **Alternating isometrics (AI):** Stability; weak lower trunk rotators. **Slow reversals (SRs):** Controlled mobility; diminished control of lower trunk/pelvic movements.

- **OT 2: Patient independently performs sit-to-stand and stand-to-sit transfers. T/MT: Bridging, pelvic elevation. Active or guided movement; Agonist reversals (ARs); Alternating isometrics (AI). Rationale for Selection: Base of support (BOS) is large; center of mass (COM) is low. Posture is very stable.** Activity is similar to hooklying in that it primarily involves the lower trunk, hip, and knee muscles; the lower trunk muscles and hip abductors and adductors stabilize the pelvis and lower trunk. The low back and hip extensors elevate the pelvis, and the hamstrings keep the knees flexed, with the feet under the knees. Bridging activities are important lead-up activities for later functional activities such as moving in bed, scooting to the edge of the bed, sit-to-stand transitions, and stair climbing. Bridging allows for early weight bearing through the foot and ankle without the body weight constraints of a fully upright posture. It is an appropriate early posture for patients who are recovering from ankle injury. **Techniques and GI: Active or guided movement:** Active movement control is overall goal; effective problem solving; inability to complete full range of movement (weakness). **Agonist reversals (ARs):** Controlled mobility; weakness of the low back extensors and gluteals; important for patient with poor eccentric control who has difficulty sitting slowly. **Alternating isometrics (AI):** Stability; weakness of low back extensors and gluteals.

- **OT 3: The patient is able to ambulate with normal medial/lateral foot/ankle control. T/MT: Bridging, holding; Bridging, weight shifts; Bridging, advanced stabilization. Alternating isometrics (AI); Slow reversals (SRs); Bridging, leg lifts. Rationale for Selection: Base of support (BOS) is large; center of mass (COM) is low. Posture is very stable.** Similar to hooklying in that it primarily involves the lower trunk, hip, and knee muscles; lower trunk muscles and hip abductors and adductors stabilize the pelvis and lower trunk. Low back and hip extensors elevate the pelvis; hamstrings maintain the knees flexed, feet under knees. Bridging activities are important lead-up activities for later functional activities such as moving in bed, scooting to the edge of the bed, sit-to-stand transitions, and stair climbing. Bridging allows for early weight bearing through the foot and ankle without the body weight constraints of a fully upright posture. It is an appropriate early posture for patients who are recovering from ankle injury. **Techniques and GI: Alternating isometrics (AI):** Stability; resistance applied at the knees increases the length of the lever arm and recruits more lower limb muscles, especially foot and ankle muscles. **Slow reversals (SRs):** Controlled mobility; manual contacts at the knees increase the length of the lever arm and recruit medial and lateral ankle and foot muscles to shift the body from side to side. **Bridging, leg lifts:** Controlled mobility (static-dynamic work); places greater demands on weight-bearing ankle.

- **OT 4: Patient independently performs movement transitions from supine to sitting. T/MT: Supine-to-sit.**
  1. **Supine to sidelying to sitting: transitions from the supine position. Rationale for Selection: This method is frequently used for patients with low back pain when trunk rotation is contraindicated due to pain.**
  2. **Supine to sidelying-on-elbow to sitting: transitions from the supine position. Rationale for Selection: Requires patient to use head and upper trunk rotation; weight bearing on the affected elbow provides joint compression and proprioceptive stimulation and is useful for problems of shoulder weakness and instability.**

- **OT 5: The patient is able to stabilize the shoulder in all positions needed for UE function. T/MT: Shoulder stabilization, active holding. Guided movement (active-assistive) to active movement (holding); Hold-relax active motion (HRAM); Rhythmic stabilization (RS). Rationale for Selection: Promotes postural stability and proximal UE control before focusing on grasp. Techniques and GI: Guided movement (active-assistive) to active movement (holding):** Active movement control is overall goal; effective problem solving; inability to complete full range of movement (weakness). **Hold-relax active motion (HRAM):** Promotes shoulder stabilization (isometric holding) within a functional position needed for weight bearing; strengthens weak shoulder extensor muscles moving from the lengthened to shortened range. **Rhythmic stabilization (RS):** Stability; promotes shoulder stabilization.

CASE STUDY 5: STROKE

1. *Prioritized Physical Therapy Problem List and Terminology:*
   1. **Cognitive impairments:** *direct impairment.*
   2. **Pain—Right (R) Upper Extremity:** PS = 7: *indirect impairment.*
   3. **Sensory deficits—Right (R) Upper Extremity:** Sharp/Dull: 2, Light Touch 2, Temperature: 4, Proprioceptive sensations: 5, Cortical sensations: 5. **(R) Lower Extremity:** Sharp/Dull: 2, Light Touch: 4, Temperature: 4; Proprioceptive sensations: 5; Cortical sensations: 5; *direct impairment.*
   4. **Functional mobility skills: bed mobility—rolling:** FIM level = 3. **Supine to sit:** FIM level = 2. **Transfers—sit-to-stand:** FIM level = 2; **stand-to-sit:** FIM level = 2, **stand pivot to wheelchair:** FIM level = 2. **Wheelchair mobility:** In unobstructed, open areas: FIM level = 3 (verbal cueing required). **Basic activities of daily living (BADLs):** Eating: FIM = 4 (once set up), bathing: FIM = 3, dressing: upper extremity/trunk: FIM level = 3, dressing: lower extremity/feet: FIM level = 2: *functional disability.*
   5. **Balance—sitting: Static:** Poor (FIM level = 2); *dynamic:* Poor−(FIM level = 2): *composite impairment.*
   6. **Posture—sitting:** Asymmetrical positioning, lateral flexion of right side of trunk; fair head control: *composite impairment.*
   7. **Muscle Tone:** Moderate to severe increase in muscle tone in both right upper and lower extremities (LEs): *direct impairment.*
   8. **Motor control:** No volitional movement outside of synergy in right UE and LE, right UE neglect, extension synergy present with effort; right LE, extensor pattern dominant: *direct impairment.*
   9. **Range of motion (ROM):** Tightness in extremes of range for (R) shoulder flexion; right dorsiflexion: 0–5 degrees: *indirect impairment.*

2. *Patient Asset List:* **(1) Language skills are functional; (2) early transfer to a rehabilitation facility; (3) lives with wife (level of support not determined); (4) recently gave up smoking; (5) hypertension controlled; (6) young age (generally, better prognosis); (7) uncomplicated medical history; (8) eating: FIM = 4 (once set up).**

3. *Outcomes of Physical Therapy (Long-Term Goals):* **The patient will be independent in ambulation using an ankle-foot orthosis and a quadruped cane on level surfaces for unlimited distances (FIM level = 7).**
   - *Outcomes of Treatment (Short-Term Goals):*
     1. **Reduced pain in right (R) UE and LE from PS 7 to 3.**
     2. **Minimal assistance (FIM = 4) required in use of protective and compensatory strategies to substitute for sensory deficits.**
     3. **Able to roll supine to prone (from FIM level 3 to 7).**
     4. **Able to stabilize trunk in postural extension (static sitting balance from FIM level 2 to 7).**
     5. **Able to perform segmental trunk patterns (from FIM level 1 to 7).**
     6. **Able to perform reciprocal trunk patterns (from FIM level 1 to 7).**
     7. **Able to maintain sitting with weight bearing on extended right arm (from FIM level 2 to 5).**
     8. **Able to stabilize in the quadruped posture (from FIM level 1 to 4).**
     9. **Tolerance for treatment increased from 30 to 45 minutes.**

4. *Physical Therapy Plan of Care:* Problem; Outcome of Treatment (OT), or short-term goal; sequential order of the three advanced therapeutic exercise procedures (A, B, or C). For each procedure, describe Position/Activity (P/A) and Movement Transitions; for movement transitions, describe the method of assistance and teaching strategy; describe Techniques. **Note:** The order of treatment interventions suggested here begin functional mobility training with early focus on supine and sidelying activities with progression to sitting activities. However, many therapists intersperse supported sitting activities within the supine and sidelying progression to promote early weight bearing through the upper extremity.
   - **Problem 1: Rolling—supine to prone: FIM level = 3 (greater difficulty rolling toward sound side; difficulty initiating movement). OT: The patient is able to roll from supine to prone.**
     A. *First Intervention—***P/A: Rolling, supine to sidelying (onto the sound side). Technique: Guided movement (active-assistive movement, AAM); Note:** Practicing the pattern first with the sound left lower extremity (LE) will reinforce motor learning of the desired patterns of movement. Patient is positioned in supine. Therapist is standing next to

treatment table or half-kneeling next to platform mat. The therapist assists the motion of the trunk and/or limbs. The patient is assisted to lift the right LE off the mat and swing it up and across the body in a D1F pattern (an out-of-synergy pattern); the trunk and remaining extremity follow. Maximum assistance is given in the beginning of the range (maximum effects of gravity) and reduced from midrange on as patient can move more easily. The patient's affected UE can be supported using a prayer position to keep the shoulder forward and elbow extended. The patient is given only as much assistance as necessary to accomplish the motion; active-assistive movements should progress toward active movements (voluntary control) as soon as possible. The therapist's position and movements should not restrict or limit ease of movement.

B. *Second Intervention*—**Technique: Rolling onto sidelying-on-elbow position:** The patient turns and lifts up into the sidelying-on-elbow position. The therapist assists the rotation of the upper trunk and lifts the trunk with both hands on patient's sides under the axillae. The patient's lowermost UE is pre-positioned with the elbow in 90 degrees of flexion. The patient's uppermost UE is pre-positioned with the elbow extended and hand placed on the therapist's shoulder (this minimizes the effect of gravity dragging the shoulder back). The patient is gently placed into the sidelying-on-elbow position; the elbow should not be "slammed" into support surface. One leg can be crossed over the other to facilitate the roll or can be flexed with foot flat. *Teaching Strategy:* The patient has difficulty with new learning. Consideration should be given to use of both visual feedback and available proprioceptive feedback. Augmented feedback should be provided about knowledge of results and knowledge of performance. Emphasis should be placed on correct aspects of performance (important during early phases of learning). Errors should be addressed only as they become consistent. Feedback should be carefully monitored in order to avoid dependency. Supportive feedback can be used to motivate the patient and shape behavior. The patient will benefit from reduction of extraneous environmental variables early in learning. During late learning, focus can be shifted to adapting to performance with varying environmental demands.

C. *Third Intervention*—**P/A: Sidelying (on sound side), logrolling. Technique: Rhythmic initiation (RI):** Patient is positioned in sidelying LEs extended in midposition or in slight flexion. UEs are positioned with the lowermost limb flexed overhead; the patient's uppermost limb can be positioned overhead or with the arm at the side, hand resting on pelvis. The therapist heel-sits or kneels in front or behind patient. One hand is placed on the side of trunk under the axilla or over the top of the shoulder; one hand on the pelvis. The upper trunk/shoulder moves together as one unit with the lower trunk/pelvis. Movements are first passive, then active-assistive, then lightly resisted (tracking resistance). Progression to next phase of movement is dependent upon patient's ability to relax and participate in each phase of the movements. The therapist's manual contacts are fixed during the first two phases; during the final resistive phase the hands slide forward or backward on trunk to resist the movement. **Verbal commands:** "Relax; let me move you back and forth" (passive movements). "Now move with me, back and forth" (active movements). "Now pull forward; and push backward" (resisted movements).

• **Problem 2: Poor upright sitting (antigravity) control; weak trunk extensors; inability to hold posture. OT: Patient is able to stabilize trunk in postural extension.**

A. *First Intervention*—**P/A: Sidelying (on sound side), holding in extension. Technique: Shortened held resisted contraction (SHRC). Note:** Several important precautions are indicated for this patient in using (a) the sidelying position; and (b) in application of resistance.

(a) **Positioning:** When using sidelying on the sound side, the trunk should be straight; the affected shoulder protracted with the UE well forward on a supporting pillow, with the elbow extended and the forearm in neutral or supinated. The pelvis should be protracted and the affected LE flexed at the knee with the hip extended, in neutral rotation and supported on a pillow. This positioning will place the patient out of the tone-dependent extensor posture.

(b) **Application of Resistance:** Use of resistance must be carefully monitored. Inappropriate levels of resistance leading to excess patient effort can result in unwanted movement and increase spasticity. Generally, when dealing with hypertonicity, resistance should initially be minimal to ensure correct muscular responses. As control develops, greater challenges can be used. The patient is positioned in sidelying, head is extended slightly with the trunk and lower extremity in midline; the uppermost shoulder is extended with the elbow flexed (a modified pivot prone position). The lowermost LE can be flexed slightly and the lowermost UE flexed, supporting the head. Therapist heel-sits behind patient. Manual contacts for trunk extensor weakness: one hand can be on the upper trunk or arm; one hand on the pelvis/lower trunk or thigh. Resistance to extension is applied at multiple points (head, upper trunk, arm, pelvis); an isometric hold is built up gradually to achieve a contraction and maintained; overflow to other extensor muscles throughout the trunk is expected. **Verbal commands:** "Hold—don't let me push you forward; hold . . . hold."

B. *Second Intervention*—**Position/Activity: Sidelying (on sound side), holding. Technique: Alternating isometrics (AI):** Patient is positioned in sidelying, with trunk in midrange, lowermost extremities are flexed slightly to increase BOS; uppermost LE is in extension, uppermost UE is flexed overhead. Therapist heel-sits behind or in front of patient. Manual contacts are on the upper trunk, either under axilla or over top of shoulder; hands are slid over top of trunk from anterior to posterior surfaces. Flat open hands are used to apply resistance, not tightly grasped fingers. The patient is asked to hold the position while therapist applies resistance alternately, first to trunk extensors, then to flexors. The resistance is built up gradually, starting from very light resistance progressing to the patient's maximum. The isometric contraction is maintained for several counts. **Verbal commands:** "Hold—don't let me push you forward; hold, hold. Now don't let me pull you backward—hold, hold." The therapist must give the transitional command ("Now don't let me pull you the other way") before sliding the hands to the opposite surface (this allows the patient to make preparatory postural adjustments). *Note:* Precautions must be taken with this treatment choice by positioning the patient in out-of-tone-dependent postures and careful use of resistance to avoid unwanted movement or spasticity.

C. *Third Intervention*—**P/A: Sidelying (on sound side), holding. Technique: Rhythmic stabilization (RS):** The patient is asked to hold the position while the therapist applies resistance: one hand resists upper trunk flexors while the other hand resists lower trunk extensors. Resistance is then reversed: one hand resists upper trunk extensors while the other hand resists lower trunk flexors. **Verbal commands:** "Hold—don't let me twist you; hold, hold. Now don't let me twist you the other way—hold, hold." **Note:** Precautions must be taken with this treatment choice by positioning the patient in out-of-tone-dependent postures and careful use of resistance to avoid unwanted movement or spasticity.

- **Problem 3: Impaired segmental trunk patterns; unable to isolate upper and lower trunk rotation. OT: (1) Patient is able to perform segmental trunk patterns. (2) Patient is able to perform reciprocal trunk patterns.**
    A. *First Intervention:* **P/A: Sidelying (on sound side), upper trunk rotation (UTR); lower trunk rotation (LTR). Technique: Rhythmic initiation (RI):** The patient is instructed to relax while the therapist passively moves each trunk segment in opposite directions (the lower trunk/pelvis moves forward while the upper trunk/shoulder moves backward). The movements are reversed and continued until the patient moves easily. The patient is then asked to participate actively in the movements. **Verbal commands** are "Relax—let me move you, let me twist you; now let me twist you the other way. Now move with me; twist the other way. . ." Therapist heel-sits behind or in front. Manual contacts are on the upper trunk and pelvis. Movements are assisted passively at first, slowly progressing to active-assistive.

    B. *Second Intervention:* **P/A: Sidelying, upper trunk rotation (UTR), lower trunk rotation (LTR). Technique:**
        1. **Slow reversals (SR):** The therapist keeps one hand on the stationery segment being stabilizing while the other hand resists the movement first on anterior trunk, then slides posterior to resist the opposite movement. Verbal commands: "Keep your pelvis still and pull your shoulder forward. Now push back—pull forward; now push back." **Note:** Application of resistance in a posterior direction must be carefully monitored to avoid increased pelvic retraction.
        2. **Slow reversal-hold (SRH):** A hold may be added if the patient demonstrates difficulty in completing the movement into the shortened range (the isometric hold adds additional muscle spindle support). The hold is a momentary pause, held to one count; the antagonist movement is then facilitated. The hold can be added in one direction only or in both directions.

    C. *Third Intervention:* **P/A: Sidelying, trunk counterrotation. Technique: Rhythmic initiation (RI):** Patient is positioned in sidelying. The upper trunk/shoulder moves forward while the lower trunk/pelvis move backward in the opposite direction. The movements are then reversed. Therapist heel-sits behind or in front. Manual contacts are on the upper trunk under axilla and on pelvis. The patient is instructed to relax while the therapist passively moves each trunk segment in opposite directions (lower trunk/pelvis moves forward while upper trunk/shoulder moves backward). The movements are reversed and continued until patient moves easily. The patient is then asked to actively participate in the movements. **Verbal commands:** "Relax—let me move you, let me twist you; now let me twist you the other way. Now move with me, twist; now twist the other way." This is a particularly difficult movement to achieve—some patients will be unable to accomplish this activity.

- **Problem 4: Strong UE flexor spasticity and trunk weakness. OT: The patient is able to maintain sitting with weight bearing on extended right arm (FIM level = 2 to 5).**

A. *First Intervention*—**P/A: Sitting, holding with weight bearing on extended right arm:** The patient is positioned in sitting with head and trunk vertical, both hips and knees flexed to 90 degrees, and feet flat on the floor. Posture is symmetrical with weight bearing equal over both lower extremities. Feet are flat on the floor. The right UE is positioned in shoulder and elbow extension, external rotation with the hand open and flat on the support surface. This is a useful position to counteract UE flexor spasticity evident with this patient. Rhythmic rotation (RRo) may be required to initially move the UE into the extended position. Additional stimulation (tapping or stroking) over the triceps and deltoid can be used to assist the patient in maintaining the extended position. The dorsum of the hand can also be stroked to maintain the hand open with extended fingers. This patient presents with excess right UE flexor tone and will likely benefit from initial weight shifting forward and back with the elbow extended and hand weight bearing. The rocking provides slow vestibular stimulation and additional inhibition to the spastic muscles (rhythmic rotation, inhibitory positioning, and stroking to antagonist muscles also provide inhibitory influences). This patient also demonstrates a drooping down and forward of the right shoulder as well as right UE neglect; the patient will benefit from weight bearing and compression through an extended UE (promote stability in extension and proprioceptive input). The proprioceptive loading that occurs increases the action of stabilizing muscles around the shoulder. The therapist can add additional stimulation by lightly compressing the top of the shoulder downward while stabilizing the elbow as needed. **Technique: Alternating isometrics (AI):** The patient is asked to hold the sitting position while therapist applies medial/lateral resistance to the upper trunk, first on one side pushing the upper trunk away from the therapist, then pulling the upper trunk toward the therapist. Manual contacts are on the lateral aspect of one side of the trunk and the medial portion (vertebral border of the scapula) of the other side; the hands are then reversed. The resistance is built up gradually, starting from very light resistance and progressing to the patient's maximum. The isometric contraction is maintained for several counts. The therapist must give a **transitional command** ("Now don't let me pull you the other way") before sliding the hands to resist the opposite muscles; this allows the patient the opportunity to make appropriate preparatory postural adjustments. Resistance can also be applied in anterior/posterior directions, or diagonally. The position of the therapist will vary according to the line of force that needs to be applied.

B. *Second Intervention*—**P/A:** Sitting, holding with weight bearing on extended right arm. Technique: Rhythmic stabilization (RS): The patient is asked to hold the sitting position while the therapist applies rotational resistance to the upper trunk. One hand is placed on the posterior trunk of one side (on the axillary border of the scapula), pushing forward, while the other hand is on the opposite side, anterior upper trunk, pulling back. Hands are then reversed for the opposite movement (each hand remains positioned on the same side of the trunk). **Verbal commands** include "Don't let me twist you—now don't let me twist you the other way."

C. *Third Intervention*—**P/A: Sitting, weight shifting:** The patient is encouraged to shift weight from side to side, forward and backward and diagonally. Re-education of limits of stability (LOS) is one of the first activities in a balance training sequence. The patient is encouraged to shift as far as possible without losing balance and then to return to the midline position. Initially, weight shifts may begin with bilateral or unilateral UE support and progress to no arm support (arms crossed or cradled). **Technique: Active reaching, cone stacking, PNF UE D1F pattern:** To promote dynamic balance control, the patient continues to support himself with weight bearing on the extended right arm. The sound UE (dynamic limb) is used for a variety of activities such as active reaching, cone stacking, and use of UE PNF patterns. This places further challenges on the affected support limb. Active reaching activities can be used to promote weight shifting in the direction of the patient's instability. The therapist provides a target ("Reach out and touch my hand"), or a functional task like cone stacking can be used to promote reaching in any direction. The patient can also be instructed to reach down and touch the floor or pick up objects from the floor. The PNF D1F pattern was selected here (flexion-adduction-external-rotation). However, many other patterns would also provide the ability to gradually (progressively) challenge postural control. As the patient progresses and gains more control, crossing one lower limb over the other can be used to promote an initial weight shift to unload and free up the dynamic limb for movement. The therapist can facilitate the action of crossing one limb over the other by appropriate verbal cues (ensuring the initial weight shift) and by manual cues or guided movement of the dynamic limb. This is a useful activity for the patient, because crossing the affected LE over the sound limb represents out-of-synergy, isolated control.

- **Problem 5: Strong UE and LE spasticity. OT: The patient is able to stabilize in the quadruped posture (from FIM level = 1 to 4).**
  A. *First Intervention*—**Movement transition to quadruped from sidesitting:** The patient is positioned in sidesitting, with upper trunk rotated and both hands weight bearing with

extended elbows (the hands should be shoulder-width apart); the hips and knees are pre-positioned to 90 degrees. The patient twists (rotates) the lower trunk from the sidesit into quadruped. The therapist is half-kneeling near the patient's hips or squatting over both legs. Manual contacts are on both hips. The therapist assists the movement of the hips (lower trunk rotation) into quadruped. **Verbal commands:** "On the count of three, I want you to twist your hips around, coming up onto your hands and knees. One, two, three." Maximum assistance is required at the beginning of the movement; as the hips move closer to the final position, less assistance is given; pre-positioning of the limbs is important to achieving the correct final position. *Teaching Strategy:* Use of visual and proprioceptive feedback. Augmented feedback (knowledge of results; knowledge of performance). Emphasis on correct aspects of performance. Errors addressed as they become consistent. Feedback carefully monitored. Supportive feed back to motivate; shape behavior. Reduction of environmental variables (early). Performance with varying environmental demands (late).

B. *Second Intervention—***P/A: Quadruped, holding:** Patient is positioned in quadruped, with the head in midposition and the back flat. The patient actively holds in the all-fours posture. **Techniques:**

1. **Alternating isometrics (AI): Medial/lateral:** The therapist is half-kneeling at patient's side. Resistance is given in M/L directions. One hand is positioned on contralateral side of upper trunk, and resists either on the vertebral or axillary borders of scapula; the other hand is positioned on the ipsilateral lower trunk, and resists either on the lateral border of pelvis or is cupped and pulls on the midpelvic region. Alternately, both hands can resist on the sides of the trunk, switching from ipsilateral to contralateral. **Verbal commands:** "Hold this position—don't let me push you away; hold, hold. Now don't let me pull you toward me; hold, hold."

2. **Alternating isometrics (AI): Anterior/posterior:** The therapist is positioned in kneeling directly behind the patient. Resistance is given in A/P directions. Both hands are positioned on pelvis pushing forward (hands slide down over lower pelvis/ischium) or pulling backward (hands slide up over top of iliac crest). Alternately, one hand can be on upper trunk and one hand on pelvis. **Verbal commands:** "Hold—don't let me push you up and away; hold, hold. Now don't let me pull you back; hold, hold. . ."

3. **Alternating isometrics (AI): Diagonal:** The therapist is half-kneeling next to the patient, positioned on the diagonal. Resistance is given in diagonal directions. **Verbal commands:** "Hold—don't let me push you up and over your right arm; hold, hold. Now don't let me pull back and over your left hip—hold, hold."

C. *Third Intervention:* **P/A: Quadruped, holding. T/MT: Rhythmic stabilization (RS):** The therapist is standing (knees flexed) or half-kneels next to patient. One hand is positioned on upper trunk: either on lateral border of scapula (posterior trunk), or on the anterior trunk/shoulder. The other hand is positioned either on the posterior or anterior pelvis. The therapist applies resistance to trunk rotation; the therapist pushes forward and downward on the upper trunk while pulling upward and backward on the pelvis (twisting the trunk). The hands are then reversed maintaining their respective positions on the pelvis and upper trunk. The patient resists the movement, holding steady. **Verbal commands:** "Hold—don't let me twist you; hold, hold. Now don't let me twist you the other way—hold, hold . . ."

5. *Justification for Treatment Procedure or Movement Transition—Outcome of Treatment (OT) 1 through 5: Therapeutic Exercise or Movement Transition (T/MT) selected and Rationale for Selection of the intervention, including Techniques (with Motor Control Goal and Indications—(GI).*

- **OT 1: The patient is able to roll from supine to prone position. T/MT: Rolling from supine to prone; guided movement (active-assistive movement, AAM). Movement Transition: Rolling into sidelying-on-elbows. Sidelying, log rolling; rhythmic initiation. Rationale for Selection: Rolling is a lead-up skill to independent transition from supine to sitting and dressing in bed. Base of support (BOS) in supine is large. Center of mass (COM) is low. Posture is very stable; does not require upright postural control. Weight bearing occurs through large segments of body. Minimal antigravity postural control is required.** Supine to sidelying movements are resisted by gravity acting on trunk and extremities. Sidelying to prone movements are assisted by gravity. Head/neck motions are combined with upper trunk rotation (UTR) as normal components of movement—head/neck flexion and rotation with UTR assist in supine to sidelying movement. Head/neck extension and rotation with UTR assist in prone to sidelying movement. Rolling can also be used to promote perceptaul awareness of the environment. This patient recovering from a stroke needs to practice rolling both over onto the affected side and over onto the sound side (a more difficult activity). **T/MT: Rolling into sidelying-on-elbows position.** For this patient recovering from stroke, this is an important exercise to initiate early weight bearing on the affected shoulder (important for promoting facilitation of shoulder stabilizers); and elongation of the trunk on the affected side (important for inhibition of spastic trunk side muscles). **Techniques and GI: Guided movement (active-assistive movement, AAM):** Active movement control is the overall goal; effective problem solving is promoted as the key to independent function; promotes early learning during the acquisition phase of motor learning. Indications: inability to move, impaired tactile and kinesthetic inputs that normally guide movement. **Motor Control Goal: Mobility (active-assistive movement, AAM), progressing to controlled mobility (active movement, AM).** Indications: Dependent function due to disordered motor control. **Rhythmic initiation (RI):** Mobility. **Indications:** Dependent function due to spasticity; impaired ability to initiate rolling (dyspraxia), impaired cognition and motor learning (as is evident in this case).

- **OT 2: Patient is able to stabilize trunk in postural extension. T/MT: Sidelying, holding in extension. Shortened held resisted contraction (SHRC); alternating isometrics (AI); rhythmic stabilization. Rationale for Selection: Base of support (BOS) is large. Center of mass (COM) in sidelying is low. Posture is very stable; it does not require upright postural control. Tonic reflex activity is reduced in sidelying.** The posture can be used to work on trunk extension and trunk rotation patterns in patients who lack upright (antigravity) control. The focus is on developing initial extensor control. Sidelying, modified pivot prone (SHRC) is a lead-up activity to sitting stability control. **Techniques and GI: Shortened held resisted contraction (SHRC):** Stability; static control. **Indications:** Weak postural extensors, inability to sustain a contraction, poor sitting control and posture. **Alternating isometrics (AI):** Stability, static control. Steady holding of the posture is the goal. Isometric holding is facilitated. **Indications:** Instability in weight bearing and holding; poor antigravity control. **Rhythmic stabilization (RS):** Stability, static control; stabilize trunk in postural extension. Indications: weakness of trunk muscles; rhythmic stabilization increases emphasis on stabilizing action of trunk rotators.

- **OT 3: Patient is able to perform segmental trunk patterns. T/MT: Sidelying, upper trunk rotation (UTR); lower trunk rotation (LTR); rhythmic initiation (RI); slow reversal (SRs); slow reversal-hold (SRH); sidelying, trunk counterrotation; rhythmic initiation (RI). Rationale for Selection: Lower trunk rotation:** For this patient, the selection of procedures allows movements to begin with small-range control and progress to larger ranges. Light, tracking resistance can be used to promote smooth reversal of antagonists. A facilitatory quick stretch can be used to initiate the movement and should be timed to coincide with verbal commands. This patient may find it easier to move one segment more than the other (lower trunk rotation is usually more problematic). Upper trunk rotation can be combined with PNF scapular patterns to promote scapula/shoulder movements. **Sidelying, upper trunk rotation (UTR); lower trunk rotation (LTR) and trunk counterrotation. Techniques and GI: Rhythmic initiation:** RI is the technique of choice to assist in motor learning of difficult tasks such as isolated UTR and LTR and trunk counterrotation, which is a particularly difficult movement to achieve. Movements are assisted passively at first, slowly progressing to active-assistive movements. The resisted movement is usually very difficult and may not be attempted during early practice attempts. If the resistive phase is used, the hands must slide forward and backward on the trunk to resist the movements. Once learning occurs, rhythmic initiation (RI) can progress to slow reversals (SRs). Active reciprocal extremity movements simulating arm swing and stepping movements in gait can be asked for. (This allows the complete motor program to be called up.) Smooth reversals of antagonists is the goal—the movements should look coordinated, the movement sequence continuous; the therapist and patient must be in rhythm together. **GI: Rhythmic initiation (RI):** Skill-level control for trunk. **Indications:** Impaired reciprocal trunk movements during gait (trunk counterrotation). **Slow reversals (SRs); slow reversal-hold (SRH):** Controlled mobility, static-dynamic control of trunk. **Indications:** Impairment of segmental trunk patterns; an important lead-up skill for independent rolling, supine-to-sit transfers, and trunk counterrotation and reciprocal arm and trunk movements in gait.

- **OT 4: The patient is able to maintain sitting with weight bearing on extended right arm (FIM level = 2 to 5). P/A and T/MT: Sitting, holding with weight bearing on extended right arm: alternating isometrics (AI), rhythmic stabilization (RS); sitting, weight shifting: active reaching, cone stacking, PNF UE D1F pattern. Rationale for Selection: Sitting is an important lead-up skill for many activities of daily living (dressing, grooming, toileting, feeding) as well as later transfer training. Active reaching (controlled mobility) in sitting is an important lead-up skill to performing weight shifts (pressure relief) and transfers. Base of support (BOS) is moderate. Center of mass (COM) is elevated over supine or prone positions. Posture is relatively stable.** The head and trunk are maintained vertical in midline orientation (upright sitting); this patient has several deficits in postural alignment which can be worked on in sitting: diminished head control and an asymmetric sitting posture. The pelvis is maintained in midline orientation. Righting reactions contribute to upright head position (face vertical, mouth horizontal). Dynamic balance reactions contribute to maintenance of upright posture in response to displacement. BOS can be varied to alter postural stabilization requirements and difficulty. The type of seating surface used in supported sitting can influence postural alignment. Therapist position and level of support for sitting can vary with the patient's level of control and anxiety. **Techniques and GI: Sitting, holding with weight bearing on extended right arm: alternating isometrics (AI), rhythmic stabilization (RS). Motor Control Goal:** Stability. **Indications:** Impaired static balance control. **Sitting, weight shifting: active reaching, cone stacking, PNF UE D1F pattern:** Promote weight shifting in all directions. **Motor Control Goal:** Controlled mobility. **Indications:** Impaired dynamic balance control.

- **OT 5: The patient is able to stabilize in the quadruped posture (from FIM level 1 to 4). P/A and T/MT: Movement transition into quadruped; quadruped, holding; alternating isometrics (AI): medial/lateral; alternating isometrics (AI): Anterior/posterior; alternating isometrics (AI): diagonal; rhythmic stabilization (RS). Rationale for Selection: Base of support (BOS) is large. Center of mass (COM) in quadruped is higher than in prone-on-elbows position (PoE) but still low.** The patient presents with increased LE extensor tone and finger flexor hypertonicity. He may benefit from the effects of inhibitory pressure inherent in this posture; quadruped can be a useful lead-up activity to relax tone before standing and walking, or prior to hand (reaching and grasping) activities. The patient also demonstrates UE spasticity (retracted scapula with shoulder internal rotation and adduction, elbow flexion) and may benefit from rounding the back, then hollowing it (requires active scapular protraction movements). The UE should be positioned in elbow extension, forearm supination, and shoulder external rotation. **Techniques and GI: Guided movement (active-assistive movement, AAM):** Mobility (active-assistive movements), progressing to controlled mobility (active movements). **Indications:** Dependent function due to weakness; disordered motor control. **Alternating isometrics (AI):** Stability, static control. Steady holding of the posture is the goal. **Rhythmic stabilization (RS):** Stability, static control of head, upper and lower trunk, shoulders. Isometric control is the goal—resistance should build up gradually; the hold should be steady. **Indications:** Dependent function due to weakness, disordered motor control.

CASE STUDY 6: PARKINSON'S DISEASE

1. *Prioritized Physical Therapy Problem List and Terminology:*
   1. **Bed mobility—rolling, supine to sitting (FIM level = 4):** *functional disability.*
   2. **Transfers—sit-to-stand and stand-to-sit (FIM level = 4):** *functional disability.*
   3. **Inability to weight-shift in sitting:** *functional disability.*
   4. **Seating surfaces impair sit-to-stand transfers:** *functional disability.*
   5. **Gait and stair climbing lack timing and sequencing:** *functional disability.*
   6. **Impaired dynamic balance control (sitting = fair; standing = fair):** *composite impairment.*
   7. **Diminished postural responses:** *composite impairment.*
   8. **Generalized rigidity:** *direct impairment.*
   9. **Akinesia:** *direct impairment.*
   10. **Diminished coordination:** *direct impairment.*
   11. **Faulty posture:** *indirect impairment.*
   12. **ROM: tightness in extremes of range for all extremities and trunk:** *indirect impairment.*
   13. **Weakness of trunk extensors and rotators; gluteal muscles, hamstrings:** *indirect impairment.*

2. *Patient Asset List:* **(1) Independent in gait (FIM level = 7); (2) motivated to improve function; (3) knowledgeable about disease; (3) able to identify specific functional goals; (4) independent in activities of daily living (requires adaptive equipment); (5) good tolerance for treatment activities (40 minutes with rest intervals); (6) supportive family; (7) without other medical problems.**

3. *Functional Outcomes of Physical Therapy (Long-Term Goals):*
   1. **The patient ambulates with functional sequencing and timing on level surfaces and stairs using a small-based quad cane for functional distances.**
   2. **The patient is independent in functional mobility skills, including rolling and transfers (FIM level = 7).**

- *Outcomes of Treatment (short-term goals):*
  1. **Perform bed mobility activities (FIM level = 4 to 6).**
  2. **Perform sit-to-stand and stand-to-sit transfers (FIM level = 4 to 6).**
  3. **Perform seated weight shifts.**
  4. **Perform sit-to-stand transfers from a variety of surfaces (FIM level = 4 to 6).**
  5. **To ambulate using appropriate functional timing and sequencing.**

4. *Physical Therapy Plan of Care:* Problem; Outcome of Treatment (OT), or short-term goal; sequential order of the three advanced therapeutic exercise procedures (A, B, or C). For each procedure, describe: Position/Activity (P/A) and Movement Transitions for movement transitions, describe the method of assistance and teaching strategy; describe Techniques.

   - **Problem 1: Bed mobility—rolling, supine to sitting: FIM level = 4. OT: The patient is able to perform bed mobility activities: FIM level = 6.**
     A. *First Intervention*—**P/A: Hooklying, lower trunk rotation. Technique: Rhythmic rotation (RRO):** Rhythmic rotation is a passive technique designed to promote relaxation in the patient with lower extremity hypertonicity. The patient is positioned in hooklying, with both feet placed flat on the mat or on the therapist's knees; the therapist is heel-sitting at the base of the patient's feet. The patient is instructed to relax and let the therapist move the lower extremities (LEs). The therapist places both hands on top of the patient's knees and slowly rocks the knees side to side. Range in lower trunk rotation is gradually increased as tone decreases. An alternate approach involves positioning the patient's legs on a Swiss ball (hips and knees are flexed to approximately 90 degrees). The therapist is in half-kneeling, holding onto the patient's legs just below the knees. The ball is slowly rocked from side to side. The ball also allows for easy side-to-side movement and may be more effective for patients with high levels of rigidity. Rhythmic rotation is repeated until relaxation occurs, generally up to several minutes.

     B. *Second Intervention*—**P/A: Hooklying, lower trunk rotation. Technique: Rhythmic initiation (RI):** The lower trunk is rotated as the knees are moved slowly from side-to-side; as the patient relaxes, range is gradually increased until the knees move laterally down to the mat on each side. The movements are first passive (identical to rhythmic rotation), then active-assistive, then lightly resisted (tracking resistance). Progression to next phase is dependent upon patient's ability to relax and participate in the active and resistive phases. The therapist is positioned at the patient's side in a half-kneeling position. Manual contacts are fixed on top of the knees during the first two phases; during the final resistive phase they slide to the side (medial side of one knee; lateral side of the opposite knee) to resist both knees as they pull away and then slide to the opposite sides of the knees to resist the return movement. The therapist's hands will need to pivot in order to resist the complete return movement of the knees down to the mat.

     C. *Third Intervention*—**P/A: Hooklying, lower trunk rotation. Technique: Slow reversals (SRs).** In hooklying, the patient moves both knees together in side-to-side movements. Depending upon available range of motion, the knees can move all the way down to the mat on one side, then the other. The knees are moved passively from side to side for a few repetitions to ensure the patient knows the movements expected. The movements are then resisted. The therapist alternates hand placement—first on one side to resist the knees pulling away from midline, then on the other side to resist the return movement. Smooth reversals of antagonists are facilitated by well-timed **verbal commands** ("Pull away" or "Push back") and a quick stretch to initiate the reverse movement. Progression is from partial-range to full-range control. As the patient's control progresses, she can be taught to use this procedure with active movement for self-relaxation.

   - **Problem 2: Transfers—sit-to-stand and stand-to-sit: FIM level = 4. OT: The patient independently performs sit-to-stand and stand-to-sit transfers: FIM level = 7.**
     A. *First Intervention*—**P/A: Bridging, pelvic elevation. Techniques:**
        1. **Slow reversals (SRs):** The therapist is half-kneeling at the side of the patient. The patient's hips are assisted up and down for a few repetitions to ensure the patient knows the movements expected. The movements are then lightly resisted. The therapist alternates hand placement, first on the top of the pelvis resisting the hips as they rise up, then on the buttocks giving a directional cue for the return to the mat. Resistance is minimal in the return motion. **Verbal commands:** Smooth motions of opposing muscle groups (reversals of antagonists) are facilitated by well-timed verbal commands ("Push up" or "Pull down").
        2. **Slow reversal-hold (SRH):** A hold may be added in the direction of pelvic elevation if difficulty is experienced in maintaining the contraction in the shortened range. The hold is a momentary pause (held to one count); the antagonist contraction is then facilitated. **Note:** If the above activity is too challenging for the patient, it can be started with using active or guided movement as described below.

3. **P/A: Bridging, pelvic elevation. Technique: Active or guided movement (active-assistive):** The patient is positioned in supine with knees flexed and feet flat on the mat (hooklying). The patient is instructed to raise the hips from the mat until the hips are fully extended, and the pelvis is elevated and level. The patient then lowers the pelvis slowly down to the mat, rather than "plopping" or collapsing down. Pelvic elevation can be facilitated by the therapist placing both hands on the patient's lower thighs and pushing down on the knees, pulling the distal thighs toward the feet. Tapping over the gluteus maximus can also be used to stimulate muscle contraction.

B. *Second Intervention*—**P/A: Bridging, pelvic elevation. Technique: Agonist reversals (ARs):** This technique provides resistance to low back and hip extensors during both the concentric (shortening) contractions and eccentric (lengthening) contractions. The therapist is half-kneeling at the patient's side, with both hands positioned on the anterior pelvis during the elevation and lowering phases of bridging. **Verbal commands** include "Push up" and "Now go down slowly."

C. *Third Intervention*—**P/A: Bridge and place. Technique: Active or guided movement (active-assistive) with verbal/tactile cueing:** The patient is instructed to move up into the bridge position, shift the pelvis laterally to one side, and lower the pelvis down to the new side position. The therapist manually assists the lateral motion for the first few repetitions; tactile cueing (tapping on the side of the pelvis) and verbal cueing are used to assist the patient.

- **Problem 3: Inability to weight-shift in sitting. OT: The patient is able to perform seated weight shifts.**
  A. *First Intervention*—**P/A: Sitting, weight shifts with a large ball. Technique: Active or guided movement (active-assistive) with verbal/tactile cueing:** The patient is sitting with both elbows extended forward, hands resting on a large ball. The patient is instructed to move the ball slowly forward and backward and side to side. Initially, the therapist can stand on the opposite side of the ball to assist in controlling the range and speed of movements. This activity has a number of benefits. The ball provides upper extremity support. It also reduces anxiety that may occur with weight shifting, because the patient does not feel threatened with falling forward to the floor. Movements can be easily assisted using the ball. Rocking activities can incorporate moving the ball forward and backward in sitting. The patient can also be instructed in active reaching activities, which will promote weight shifting in all directions. The therapist provides a target ("Reach out and touch my hand") to promote reaching in any direction. The patient can also be instructed to reach down and touch the floor or pick up objects from the floor. Altering target position of the target can be effectively used to promote upper trunk rotation (UTR).
  B. *Second Intervention:* **P/A: Sitting, weight shifts with upper trunk rotation (UTR). T/MT: Slow reversals (SRs):** The patient is moved passively from side to side (in medial/lateral shifts) for a few repetitions to ensure the patient knows the movements expected. The movements are then lightly resisted. The therapist alternates hand placement—first on one side to resist the upper body pulling away, then on the other side to resist the return movement. Manual contacts are on the trunk to effectively resist the trunk muscles, not on the lateral shoulders. Typically one hand is on the side of the trunk and the other hand is on the vertebral border of the scapula. The hands are then reversed to the opposite side of trunk and opposite scapula for the return movement. Smooth reversals of antagonists are facilitated by well-timed **verbal commands** ("Pull away" or "Push back") and a quick stretch to initiate the reverse movement. Progression is from partial-range to full-range control. Shifts may be resisted in all directions: medial/lateral, anterior/posterior, diagonal, and diagonal with rotation.
  C. *Third Intervention:* **P/A: Sitting. T/MT: Bilateral symmetrical PNF D2F:** The patient moves both UEs together into the D2F pattern: the hands open and the limbs turn, and lift up and out. As the UEs move up and out, trunk extension is promoted. The therapist is positioned behind the patient to resist the UEs as they move up and out. A hold (SRH) is typically performed in the D2F position to further emphasize trunk extension. **Note:** Rhythmic initiation (RI) can be used to facilitate the pattern (RI promotes relaxation and learning).

- **Problem 4: Seating surfaces impair sit-to-stand transfers. OT: Patient is able to perform sit-to-stand transfers from a variety of surfaces.**
  A. *First Intervention*—**Movement Transition: Sit-to-stand transfers, push-up assist:** The patient scoots to the front of the chair and positions the feet under the hips (positioning center of mass over the base of support). The patient is instructed to lean forward, and push up into standing, using both UEs for support. Adequate height of the armrest is necessary to assist the UEs as they push up into standing. The therapist can assist the transfer by counting ("On three, I want you to shift forward and stand up. One, two, three.") and initiating a rocking motion in time to the counts. This enables the patient to use momentum to

stand up. During initial training, the height of the armrests can be varied (for example, by using a wheelchair with adjustable height armrests) to increase or decrease the level of assistance. *Teaching Strategy:* For this patient, early activities would focus on visual feedback together with verbal and manual guidance (cognitive phase of learning). A shift could then be made to emphasis on proprioceptive feedback to reinforce the "feel" of the movement (associated phase of learning). Augmented feedback will provide input about knowledge of results and knowledge of performance. Emphasis should be placed on correct aspects of performance (important during early phases of learning). Errors should be addressed only as they become consistent (important for middle and late stages of learning). Feedback should be carefully monitored in order to avoid dependency. Supportive feedback will assist to motivate the patient and reinforce behaviors.

B. *Second Intervention*—**Movement Transition: Sit-to-stand transfers, without upper limb support:** The sit-to-stand transfer is similar to the above sequence, with the exception that the upper limbs are not used to push up. The therapist can facilitate the initial weight transfer forward by placing a stool or low table in front of the patient. The patient then practices partial stand-ups with the hands bearing weight (sit-to-plantigrade transfers). A rocking chair could also be used with this patient to facilitate forward weight transfer and momentum. It would assist her to overcome the effects of akinesia and rigidity. The height of the seat can be varied depending on patient performance. A higher seat decreases the total excursion and facilitates early independent standing. The seat can then be progressively lowered as the patient develops control. The support surface should be firm (such as a stool or mat), as opposed to a soft bed, to facilitate ease of transfer. The therapist can assist the transfer by counting ("On three, I want you to shift forward and stand up. One, two, three.") and initiating a rocking motion in time to the counts. This enables the patient to use momentum to stand up. *Teaching Strategy:* (1) Early activities: Visual feedback; verbal, manual guidance, as needed. (2) Later training: proprioceptive feedback. (3) Augmented feedback (knowledge of results and knowledge of performance). (4) Emphasis on correct aspects of performance (early). (5) Errors addressed when consistent. (6) Feedback carefully monitored. (7) Supportive feedback to motivate patient and shape behavior. (8) Environmental variables reduced (early). (9) Varying environmental demands (late).

C. *Third Intervention*—**P/A: Sit-to-stand, placing to one side. Technique: Active or guided movement (active-assistive) with verbal/tactile cueing:** During this activity the patient practices standing up, rotating the hips to one side, and sitting down adjacent to the original start position. The feet are then repositioned directly in front. The patient can move completely around the mat in one direction by repeating this sequence.

- **Problem 5: Impaired timing and sequencing during gait. OT: The patient ambulates using functional timing and sequencing.**
  A. *First Intervention*—**P/A: Standing, stepping. Technique: Slow reversals (SRs), stepping:** This activity is initiated with the lower extremities (LEs) in step position. The patient shifts weight diagonally forward over the anterior support limb (stance limb) and takes a step forward with the dynamic (swing) limb. The movements are then reversed: the patient shifts diagonally back and takes a step backward using the same dynamic limb. The therapist is in front of the patient, either sitting on a rolling stool or standing. Manual contacts are on the pelvis. The therapist applies light stretch and resistance to facilitate the forward pelvic rotation as the swing limb moves forward. Approximation can be given as needed over the top of the pelvis as the dynamic limb comes into extension and weight bearing. **Verbal commands** are "Shift forward and step; now shift back and step."
  B. *Second Intervention*—**P/A: Walking forward. Technique: Resisted progression (RP):** The therapist is in front of the patient, either in standing or sitting on a rolling stool. As the patient moves forward the therapist also moves in a reverse or mirror image of the patient's movements. The therapist provides maintained resistance to the forward progression by placing both hands on the pelvis. Resistance should be light (facilitatory) to encourage proper timing of the pelvic movements. Stretch to pelvic rotators can be used to facilitate the initiation of the pelvic motion. Resistance can also be applied with manual contacts on the pelvis and contralateral shoulder. The position and movements are reversed for backwards walking. The therapist's movements must be synchronized with the patient's. The pacing of the activity is dependent upon the timing of the therapist's verbal commands (a metronome can also be used to provide a steady rhythm to pace activity for this patient). Movements can become uncoordinated or out of synchronization if the manual resistance on the pelvis is too great. The patient will feel as if she is "walking uphill" and may respond with exaggerated movements of the trunk (for example, forward head and trunk flexion). This defeats the overall purposes of facilitated walking, that is, to improve timing and sequencing of gait and to decrease effort. Also useful for this patient are the use of wands to promote reciprocal arm swing and trunk counterrotation. The therapist walks

behind the patient. Both patient and therapist hold onto the wands. The therapist is then able to assist in sequencing the arm swings during forward progression.

C. *Third Intervention*—**P/A: Standing, stepping up. Technique: Active or guided movement (active-assistive) with verbal/tactile cueing:** From a symmetrical stance position, the patient weight-shifts laterally toward the support limb and places the dynamic limb up on a step positioned directly in front of her. The limb is then returned to the original stance position; the patient does not move up onto the step. Normal postural alignment is maintained during the activity. Excessive trunk flexion should be avoided. This patient would benefit from altering the height of the step to gradually increase difficulty. For example, activity could be initiated with a 4-inch (10-cm) aerobic step. The height can then be progressed to a standard 7-inch (17.5-cm) step. As control develops, the patient can be progressed to stepping up onto the step, then stepping up and over the step or walking through an "obstacle course" of items randomly placed on the floor.

5. *Justification for Treatment Procedure or Movement Transition—Outcome of Treatment (OT) 1 through 5: Therapeutic Exercise or Movement Transition (T/MT) selected and Rationale for Selection of the intervention, including Techniques (with Motor Control Goal and Indications—GI).*

- **OT 1: The patient is able to perform bed mobility activities at FIM level = 6. P/A and T/MT: Hooklying, lower trunk rotation: rhythmic rotation (RRO); hooklying, lower trunk rotation: rhythmic initiation (RI); hooklying, lower trunk rotation: slow reversals (SRs). Rationale for Selection of Hooklying (crooklying): Base of support (BOS) is large. Center of mass (COM) is low. Posture is very stable. Hooklying primarily involves lower trunk, hip, and knee control.** (1) Activation of lower trunk rotators and hip abductors and adductors allows the patient to actively move the knees from side to side away from midline. (2) Activation of hamstrings allows the patient to keep the knees flexed in the hooklying position. Hooklying activities are important lead-up activities for controlled bridging, kneeling, and bipedal gait. Patients with gluteus medius weakness (for example, this patient with Parkinson's disease) may benefit from hooklying activities to activate abductors in a less stressful, non-weight-bearing position. **Technique and GI—Motor Control Goals (for RRo and RI):** Mobility. **Indications:** Impaired function due to hypertonia (lower extremity rigidity) and decreased lower trunk rotation. **Motor Control Goals (for SRs):** Controlled mobility. **Indications:** Lead-up skill for functional trunk/pelvic movements during gait; as the patient's control improves, the technique can be used for self-relaxation.

- **OT 2: Patient independently performs sit-to-stand and stand-to-sit transfers: FIM level = 7. P/A and T/MT: Bridging, pelvic elevation: slow reversals (SRs), active or guided movement; Bridging, pelvic elevation: agonistic reversals (ARs); alternating isometrics (AI); bridge and place: active or guided movement (active-assistive) with verbal/tactile cueing. Rationale for Selection: Base of support (BOS) is large. Center of mass (COM) in bridging is low. Posture is very stable.** Bridging is similar to hooklying in that it involves primarily lower trunk, hip, and knee muscles. (1) Lower trunk muscles and hip abductors and adductors stabilize the pelvis and lower trunk. (2) Low back and hip extensors elevate the pelvis. (3) Hamstrings maintain the knees flexed, feet under knees. Bridging activities are important lead-up activities for later functional activities such as moving in bed, scooting to the edge of the bed, sit-to-stand transitions, and stair climbing. **Techniques and GI:**

  1. **Bridging, pelvic elevation: slow reversals (SRs), agonist reversals (ARs):** Controlled mobility. **Indications:** Weakness of the low back extensors and gluteals; important for the patient with poor eccentric control who has difficulty sitting slowly; important lead-up activities for upright stance and balance training.

  2. **Bridge and place, active or guided movement:** Active movement control is overall goal; lower trunk rotation is fostered. **Indications:** Effective problem solving; inability to complete full range of movement (weakness); controlled mobility. **Indications:** Diminished mobility in preparation for sit-to-stand transfers (for example, inability to scoot side to side, or scoot to the edge of the bed prior to sitting up); an important lead-up for sit-to-stand transfers.

- **OT 3: The patient is able to perform seated weight shifts. P/A and T/MT: Sitting, weight shifts with a large ball. Active or guided movement (active-assistive) with verbal/tactile cueing; sitting, weight shifts with upper trunk rotation (UTR); slow reversals (SRs); sitting: bilateral symmetrical PNF D2F. Rationale for Selection: Base of support (BOS) in sitting is moderate; center of mass (COM) is elevated over supine or prone positions. Posture is relatively stable.** Sitting involves head, trunk, and lower extremity muscles for upright postural control; extensor activity of the pelvis and lumbar spine are the primary muscles for antigravity control. The head and trunk are maintained on the vertical in midline orientation (upright sitting); the pelvis is maintained in midline orientation. Righting reactions contribute to upright head position (face vertical, mouth horizontal). Dynamic balance reactions contribute to maintenance of upright posture in response to displacement. BOS can be varied to alter postural stabilization requirements and difficulty. The type of chair used in supported sitting can influence postural alignment. Therapist position and level of support for unsupported sitting can vary with the patient's level of control and anxiety. **Techniques and GI:**

1. **Sitting, weight shifts with a large ball: active or guided movement (active-assistive) with verbal/tactile cueing:** Controlled mobility. **Indications:** Impaired dynamic control; impaired antigravity control of the upper trunk. **Active or guided movement:** Active movement control is overall goal. **Indications:** Effective problem solving; inability to complete full range of movement (weakness).

2. **Sitting, weight shifts with upper trunk rotation (SRs):** Controlled mobility. **Indications:** Impaired dynamic control; impaired antigravity control of the upper trunk; important lead-up for weight shifts (pressure relief).

3. **Sitting: bilateral symmetrical PNF D2F:** Controlled mobility. **Indications:** Impaired dynamic balance control; impaired antigravity control of the upper trunk. This pattern emphasizes trunk extension, which is particularly useful with this patient, who presents with kyphosis and rounded forward shoulders. Another advantage of using PNF patterns is that the patient's full attention is focused on the correct limb movements and not on the movements of the trunk; this assists in promoting automatic postural control of the head and trunk.

- **OT 4: Patient is able to perform sit-to-stand transfers from a variety of surfaces. T/MT: Movement transition: sit-to-stand transfers; sit-to-stand transfers without upper limb support; sit-to-stand, placing to one side transfers: active or guided movement (active-assistive) with verbal/tactile cueing. Rationale for Selection: Movement transitions: (1) Sit-to-stand transfers and (2) sit-to-stand transfers without upper limb support:** The goal of these activities is independent assumption of standing. They are also important lead-up activities to independent gait and stair climbing. **Techniques and GI:** Sit-to-stand, placing to one side transfers: active or guided movement (active-assistive) with verbal/tactile cueing: Controlled mobility, static-dynamic control. **Indications:** Weakness of the low back extensors and gluteals, hamstring muscles; promotes dynamic balance control.

- **OT 5: The patient ambulates using functional timing and sequencing. P/A and T/MT: Standing, stepping: slow reversals (SRs), stepping; standing, stepping-up; active or guided movement (active-assistive) with verbal/tactile cueing. Walking forward and backward: resisted progression (RP); Rationale for Selection:**
  1. **Standing, Stepping: (SR) Stepping; Standing, Stepping-up:** Stepping is an important functional goal for this patient; it is an important lead-up activity for the patient to be independent in community ambulation. **GI:** Walking forward: resisted progression (RP): Skill. **Indications:** To promote timing and sequencing of bipedal gait. **Standing, Stepping: (SR); Stepping Standing, Stepping-up (Active or Guided Movement):** Static-dynamic control. **Indications:** Stepping is an important lead-up activity for gait and stair climbing and independence in community ambulation; it promotes early learning during the acquisition phase of motor learning.
  2. **Resisted Progression (RP):** Manual contacts can be used to guide movements and facilitate missing elements of the patient's pelvic and trunk movement. The technique allows variable hand placement for application of facilitatory resistance at different points in the gait cycle. Resistance can also be used to encourage proper timing of the pelvic movements. Stretch to pelvic rotators can be used to facilitate the initiation of the pelvic motion.

CASE STUDY 7: MULTIPLE SCLEROSIS

1. *Prioritized Physical Therapy Problem List and Terminology:*
   1. **Diminished upright trunk control:** *direct impairment.*
   2. **Weakness of hip extensors; poor eccentric control:** *direct impairment.*
   3. **Diminished pelvis and lower trunk rotation:** *direct impairment.*
   4. **Diminished upright weight-shift control in half-kneeling:** *composite impairment.*
   5. **Diminished upright dynamic balance control:** *composite impairment.*
   6. **Floor-to-stand transfers (FIM level = 3):** *functional disability.*
   7. **Transient double vision:** *direct impairment.*
   8. **Diminished ankle dorsiflexion ROM:** *indirect impairment.*
   9. **Hypertonicity of quadriceps, adductors, and plantarflexors:** *direct impairment.*
   10. **Incoordination:** *direct impairment.*
   11. **Multiple gait deviations:** *functional disability.*
   12. **Diminished LE proprioception:** *direct impairment.*

13. **UE intention tremor; limb ataxia:** *direct impairment.*
14. **Fair−dynamic standing balance:** *composite impairment.*
15. **Diminished strength (LE: gluteals, hip rotators, hamstrings, and foot/ankle musculature):** *composite impairment* (since it is likely due to a combination of *direct* effects of the diagnosis and *indirect* effects of loss of mobility and disuse atrophy).

2. *Patient Asset List:* **(1) Cognitive function intact; (2) motivated, compliant; (3) maintains a regular home exercise program; (4) knowledgeable about disease; (5) good UE strength and function; (6) supportive family; (7) home environment is completely accessible; (8) patient integrated into community, holds a full-time job; (9) independent in all BADLs; (10) independent in approximately 85% of IADLs.**

3. *Functional Outcomes of Physical Therapy (Long-Term Goals):*
   1. **The patient will be independent in floor-to-stand transfers (FIM level = 7).**
   2. **The patient will be independent in ambulation with forearm crutches using functional balance reactions.**
      • *Outcomes of Treatment (short-term goals):*
      1. **Able to stabilize and weight-shift during upright kneeling.**
      2. **Able to assume upright kneeling.**
      3. **Able to move in upright kneeling using a reciprocal trunk and limb pattern.**
      4. **Able to assume and maintain the half-kneeling position.**
      5. **Able to assume and maintain upright standing.**

4. *Physical Therapy Plan of Care:* Problem; Outcome of Treatment (OT), or short-term goal; sequential order of the three advanced therapeutic exercise procedures (A, B, or C). For each procedure, describe the Position or Activity (P/A) and Movement Transition (T/MT); for movement transitions, describe method of assistance and teaching strategy; describe Techniques.
   • **Problem 1: Diminished upright trunk and hip control. OT: The patient is able to stabilize and weight-shift during upright kneeling.**
      A. *First Intervention*—**Movement transition into kneeling from quadruped:** The patient is in quadruped and pushes the hips back over the heels while extending and lifting the trunk into the upright position. The patient will require use of a chair or other support to climb up into kneeling using the arms. The therapist can assist the transition into kneeling by standing slightly behind and to the side of the patient and placing both hands on the trunk under the axillae. First one shoulder, then the other, is lifted back. The therapist can assist tip extension by placing one foot between the patient's knees and using the side of the knee to gently push the patient's hips into extension. *Teaching Strategy:* Early activities should focus on visual feedback (cognitive phase of learning) and manual or verbal guidance, as needed. Later training will emphasize proprioceptive feedback (associative phase of learning). Augmented feedback should be provided about knowledge of results and knowledge of performance. Emphasis should be placed on correct aspects of performance (important during early phases of learning). Errors should be addressed only as they become consistent. Feedback should be carefully monitored in order to avoid dependency. Supportive feedback can be used to motivate the patient and shape behavior. Environmental variables should be reduced early in learning. During late learning, focus can be shifted to adapting to performance with varying environmental demands.
      B. *Second Intervention*—**P/A: Kneeling, holding:** The patient is kneeling, weight bearing on both knees and legs with head and trunk upright and hips extended. The patient will require UE support on a chair placed in front (or UEs extending forward with the hands placed on the therapist's shoulders). **Techniques:**
      1. **Alternating isometrics (AI):** The patient is asked to hold the kneeling position while therapist applies resistance to the pelvis, first on one side, pushing the pelvis away from the therapist, then pulling the pelvis toward the therapist (medial/lateral resistance). The resistance is built up gradually, starting from very light resistance and progressing to the patient's maximum. The isometric contraction is maintained for several counts. The therapist must give a **transitional verbal command** ("Now don't let me pull you the other way") before sliding the hands to resist the opposite muscles; this allows the patient an opportunity to take appropriate preparatory postural adjustments Theraband tubing placed around the distal thighs increases the proprioceptive loading and contraction of the lateral hip muscles (gluteus medius). Thus, simultaneous contraction of gluteal muscles (maximus and medius) is achieved. Resistance can also be applied in anterior/posterior directions. Because of the limited BOS in front, the patient will be able to take very little resistance anteriorly, and more resistance posteriorly. The position of the therapist will vary according to the direction of the line of force applied.

2. **Rhythmic stabilization (RS):** The patient is asked to hold the kneeling position while the therapist applies rotational resistance to the trunk. One hand is placed on the posterior pelvis on one side, pushing forward, while the other hand is on the anterior upper trunk on the opposite side, pulling backward. **Verbal commands** are "Don't let me twist you; now don't let me twist you the other way."

C. *Third Intervention*—**P/A: Kneeling, weight shifting:** The patient actively shifts the pelvis side to side with the knees in a symmetrical-stance position or diagonally forward and backward with the knees in a step position. The patient's UEs remain forward with the hands placed on the therapist's shoulders. Small-range shifts are stressed and are important lead-up skills for normal gait. Active reaching activities are particularly important for this patient, to promote weight shifting in all directions. The therapist provides a target ("Reach out and touch my hand") or a functional task such as cone stacking can be used to promote reaching. **Techniques:**

1. **Slow reversals (SRs), medial/lateral shifts:** The therapist is positioned in kneeling or half-kneeling at the side of the patient. The movement of the hips is assisted for a few repetitions to ensure the patient knows the movements expected. Side-to-side movements are then lightly resisted. The therapist alternates hand placement, first on one side of the pelvis resisting the pelvis as it pulls away, then on the opposite side as the pelvis pushes back. Smooth reversals of antagonists is facilitated by well-timed **verbal commands** ("Pull away" or "Push back.")

2. **Slow reversals (SRs), diagonal shifts:** The patient is positioned in kneeling with the knees in step position (one knee is advanced in front of the other, simulating normal step length). The therapist half-kneels diagonally in front of the patient. Resistance is applied to the pelvis as the patient weight-shifts diagonally forward over the more advanced knee, then diagonally backward over the other knee. **Verbal commands** are "Shift forward and toward me; now shift back and away from me."

3. **Slow reversals (SRs), diagonal shifts with rotation:** Once control is achieved in diagonal shifts, the patient then is instructed to shift weight diagonally forward on the more advanced knee while rotating the pelvis forward on opposite side; then diagonally backward while rotating the pelvis backward. **Verbal commands** are "Shift forward and twist; now shift back and twist." **Note:** The upper trunk may move forward as the pelvis rotates forward, producing an ipsilateral trunk rotation pattern. This is not the desired pattern. The therapist can isolate the pelvic motion by having the patient put both hands forward on the therapist's shoulders or on a wall in front. The patient is instructed to keep both elbows straight and move only the pelvis forward and backward during the weight shifts. The forward supported positioning of the UEs effectively locks up the upper trunk and allows the patient to move the pelvis in isolation. This is an important lead-up activity for the weight transfers and pelvic rotation needed for normal gait.

- **Problem 2: Weakness of hip extensors; poor eccentric control. OT: The patient is able to assume kneeling.**
  A. *First Intervention*—**P/A and T/MT: Kneeling to heel-sitting:** The patient is kneeling, with the knees normal-stance width apart. The patient's UEs are forward, with the hands placed on the therapist's shoulders. The patient lowers the hips down to a sitting position on both heels. The patient then flexes the trunk forward and moves up into the kneeling position, extending both hips. As in sit-to-stand transitions, the forward trunk lean is important to ensure success in assuming the upright position and should be verbally cued. The patient is encouraged to lower the body slowly rather than "plopping" or collapsing down. **Verbal commands** are "Go down slowly into sitting. Now, come up into kneeling." As this patient has weak hip extensors, he may not be able to go down slowly or get up from the full heel-sitting position. A prayer seat (a small wooden seat) can be used to decrease the range. The patient's legs fit underneath the seat while he sits. Since the seat is only part way down, the range of excursion is decreased. The therapist can verbally cue the patient or tap over the gluteal muscles to facilitate muscle contraction. *Teaching Strategy:* Early activities: visual feedback; verbal, manual guidance, as needed. Later training: proprioceptive feedback. Augmented feedback (knowledge of results and knowledge of performance); emphasis on correct aspects of performance (early); errors addressed when consistent. Feedback carefully monitored—supportive feedback used to motivate patient and shape behavior. Environmental variables reduced (early); and varying environmental demands (late).
  B. *Second Intervention*—**PA and T/MT: Kneeling to side-sitting:** From kneeling, the patient lowers both hips down to a side-sitting position. The patient's UEs are forward, with the hands placed on the therapist's shoulders. The trunk elongates on one side and the patient rotates the head and upper trunk slightly to maintain the UEs in the forward weight-bearing position. The patient then flexes the trunk forward, extends both hips, and moves back up into the kneeling position. The upper extremities are maintained in front of the pa-

tient. The therapist can assist the movement by guiding the upper trunk rotation and providing verbal and tactile cues. The patient has weak hip extensors and initially may not be able go down into or up from the full side-sitting position. A side seat (sandbag or firm cushion) placed at the patient's side can be used to decrease the range of excursion and provide a platform for sitting. *Teaching Strategy:* Early activities: visual feedback; verbal, manual guidance, as needed. Later training: proprioceptive feedback. Augmented feedback (knowledge of results and knowledge of performance); emphasis on correct aspects of performance (early); errors addressed when consistent. Feedback carefully monitored—supportive feedback used to motivate patient and shape behavior. Environmental variables reduced (early); and varying environmental demands (late).

C. *Third Intervention*—**P/A: Kneeling to heel-sitting. Technique: Agonist reversals (ARs):** The therapist is in kneeling in front of the patient with both hands positioned on the anterior pelvis. The patient's UEs are forward, with the hands placed on the therapist's shoulders. The patient lowers both hips down into the heel-sitting position, then moves up into kneeling. Resistance is applied to the anterior pelvis during both the lowering and elevation phases. Thus both eccentric (lengthening) contraction and the concentric (shortening) contractions are resisted. Resistance is variable in different parts of the range—it is greatest initially as the patient starts to sit down, and minimal during middle and end ranges, where the maximum effects of gravity take hold. In the reverse heel-sitting to kneeling transition, resistance is minimal through the early and middle range and builds up by the end of the transition as the patient moves into the shortened range to emphasize hip extensors. **Verbal commands** are "Go down slowly into sitting on your heels; now push up into kneeling."

- **Problem 3: Diminished pelvic and lower trunk rotation. OT: The patient is able to move in kneeling using a reciprocal trunk and limb pattern.**
  A. *First Intervention*—**P/A: Kneeling, weight shifting:** For this activity, the patient will require UE support on a chair placed in front (or UEs extending forward with the hands placed on the therapist's shoulders). **Technique: Slow reversals (SRs), diagonal shifts:** The patient is positioned in kneeling with the knees in step position (one knee is advanced in front of the other, simulating normal step length). The therapist half-kneels diagonally in front of the patient. Resistance is applied to the pelvis as the patient shifts weight diagonally forward over the more advanced knee, then diagonally backward over the other knee. **Verbal commands** are "Shift forward and toward me; now shift back and away from me."
  B. *Second Intervention*—**P/A: Kneel-walking:** For this activity, the patient may require UE support either from a small stool or chair placed in front (and moved forward in a manner similar to use of a walker) or UEs can be brought forward with the hands placed on the therapist's shoulders. **Technique: Resisted progression (RP).** The therapist provides maintained resistance to the forward or backward progression by placing both hands on the pelvis. Resistance should be light (facilitatory) to encourage proper timing of the pelvic movements. Approximation can be applied down through the top of the pelvis to assist in stabilizing responses as weight is taken on the stance limb. Alternate hand placements can include pelvis and opposite shoulder, both shoulders, or shoulder/head.
  C. *Third Intervention*—**P/A: Kneeling, balance training activities:** For this activity, the patient will require UE support on a chair placed in front (or UEs extending forward with the hands placed on the therapist's shoulders). As balance control improves, UE support is eliminated. **T/MT:**
    1. **Weight shifts:** In the kneeling position, the patient initially practices weight shifts to the limits of stability (LOS) and returns to the centered position. Additional activities that challenge balance in the kneeling position include: look-arounds (head and trunk rotation) and UE reaching.
    2. **Kneeling, manual perturbations (disturbances of the patient's center of mass):** The patient is kneeling on a stationary surface (mat). The therapist provides a displacing force (manual perturbation) to the trunk. It is important to ensure appropriate compensatory responses with perturbations in varying directions. With backward displacements, hip and trunk flexor activity is required. With forward displacements, hip and trunk extensor activity is required. Lateral displacements require head and trunk inclination. Rotational displacements (twisting and displacing the trunk) require movement combinations of the trunk. Protective extension of the UEs can be initiated if the displacements move the center of mass near the limits of stability or outside of the base of support. If patient responses are lacking, the therapist may need to guide the initial attempts either verbally or manually. The patient can then progress to active movements. Perturbations should be appropriate for patient's range and speed of control. It is important to use gentle disturbances with varied, asymmetrical manual contacts (tapping out of position). The therapist can vary the base of support (for example, by moving the patient's knees apart or together) to increase or decrease difficulty.

- **Problem 4: Diminished upright weight-shift control in half-kneeling. OT: The patient is able to assume and maintain the half-kneeling position.**
  A. *First Intervention*—**P/A and T/MT: Half-kneeling from kneeling:** For this activity, the patient may require UE support either from a small stool or chair placed in front (and moved forward in a manner similar to use of a walker) or UEs can be brought forward with the hands placed on the therapist's shoulders. From kneeling, the patient brings one limb up into the foot-flat position with both the hip and knee flexed while keeping the other knee weight bearing. The therapist is half-kneeling to the side and slightly behind the patient. Manual contacts are on the pelvis. The therapist assists the patient's weight shift onto the static limb by rotating the pelvis laterally and backward onto the weight-bearing limb. This unloads and facilitates movement of the dynamic limb into the hip flexion, foot-flat position.
  B. *Second Intervention*—**P/A: Half-Kneeling, holding:** For this activity, the patient may require UE support either from a small stool or chair placed in front (and moved forward in a manner similar to use of a walker) or UEs can be brought forward with the hands placed on the therapist's shoulders. The patient is half-kneeling, bearing weight equally on the posterior (knee-down) and anterior (foot-flat) support limbs. The head and trunk are upright. The therapist is also in half-kneeling in front of the patient, in a reversed (mirror-image) position. During initial training, the patient with instability may benefit from support provided by forward placement of the UEs on the therapist's shoulders. Alternately, both hands can be positioned on the patient's elevated anterior knee for support. **Technique: Alternating isometrics (AI):** The patient is asked to hold the half-kneeling position while therapist applies resistance to the pelvis, first pushing the pelvis diagonally back toward the posterior (knee-down) limb, then pulling the pelvis forward toward the anterior (foot-flat) limb. The resistance is built up gradually, starting from very light resistance and progressing to the patient's maximum. The isometric contraction is maintained for several counts. Resistance is applied only diagonally, in the direction of the BOS. The therapist must give a **transitional verbal command** ("Now don't let me move you the other way") before sliding the hands to resist the opposite muscles. This allows the patient an opportunity to make appropriate preparatory postural adjustments.
  C. *Third Intervention*—**P/A: Half-kneeling, weight shifting:** For this activity, the patient may require UE support either from a small stool or chair placed in front (and moved forward in a manner similar to use of a walker) or UEs can be brought forward with the hands placed on the therapist's shoulders. The patient actively shifts weight diagonally forward over the foot-flat support limb; then diagonally backward over the knee-down support limb. **Technique: Slow reversals (SRs), diagonal shifts:** The patient is positioned in half-kneeling. The therapist is diagonally in front of the patient. Light resistance is applied to the pelvis as the patient shifts weight diagonally forward over the support foot, then diagonally backward over the support knee. **Verbal commands** are "Shift forward and toward me; now shift back and away from me."
- **Problem 5: Diminished upright dynamic balance control. OT: The patient is able to assume and maintain upright standing.**
  A. *First Intervention*—**P/A and T/MT: Half-kneeling to standing:** In the half-kneeling position, the patient flexes and rotates the trunk, transferring weight diagonally forward over the foot. The patient then comes up into the standing position by extending the hip and knee and placing the other foot parallel to the weight-bearing foot. This activity can be practiced with UE support. Both hands are placed on the patient's elevated knee and assist in the rise to standing by pushing off. The UEs can also be held in a forward prayer position, which helps get the weight forward over the anterior limb. The therapist stands behind the patient and assists the forward weight transfer by placing both hands on the upper trunk under the axillae. Alternately, in the half-kneeling position next to the patient, the therapist can place both hands on the pelvis and assist the forward weight shift. Since the upward movement is largely unassisted, this requires more independent control by the patient. **Note:** For independence at home, practicing this activity will require a chair or low table in front of the patient. The patient then comes up into standing with both UEs bearing weight in a modified plantigrade position.
  B. *Second Intervention*—**P/A: Modified plantigrade, holding:** The patient is in modified plantigrade, with weight borne equally on both UEs and LEs. The LEs can be positioned in a symmetrical-stance position or in step position. During initial training, the patient will benefit from bilateral upper limb support. As control develops the patient can be progressed from bilateral to single-limb support to free standing. **Techniques:**
    1. **Alternating isometrics (AI):** The patient is asked to hold the plantigrade position while therapist stands behind the patient and applies resistance to the trunk. Hands can be placed on the pelvis, pelvis/contralateral shoulder, or both shoulders. Resistance is applied first in one direction, then the other (anterior/posterior, medial/lateral, or diagonal

with the LEs in the step position). The position of the therapist will vary according to the direction of the line of force. Resistance is built up gradually, starting from very light resistance and progressing to the patient's maximum. The isometric contraction is maintained for several counts. The therapist must give a **transitional verbal command,** ("Now don't let me move you the other way") before sliding the hands to resist the opposite muscles; this allows the patient an opportunity to make appropriate preparatory postural adjustments. Theraband tubing can be placed around the thighs (LEs in symmetrical-stance position) to increase the proprioceptive loading and contraction of the lateral hip muscles (gluteus medius).

2. **Rhythmic stabilization (RS):** The patient is asked to hold the plantigrade position while the therapist stands behind the patient and applies rotational resistance to the trunk. One hand is placed on the posterior pelvis on one side pushing forward while the other hand is on the anterior upper trunk, contralateral side, pulling backward. **Verbal commands** are "Don't let me twist you—hold, hold. Now don't let me twist you the other way."

C. *Third Intervention—***P/A: Modified plantigrade, weight shifting:** The patient actively shifts weight first forward (increasing loading on the upper extremities), then backward (increasing loading on the lower extremities). Weight shifts can also be performed side to side (medial/lateral shifts) with the LEs in a symmetrical-stance position, or diagonally forward and backward with the LEs in a step position. Active reaching activities can be used to promote weight shifting in all directions. **Techniques:**

1. **Slow reversals (SRs):** The therapist is standing at the patient's side (for medial/lateral shifts), or behind (for anterior/posterior shifts). Manual contacts can be placed on the pelvis, the pelvis/contralateral upper trunk, or on upper trunk. The movement is assisted a few repetitions to ensure the patient knows the expected movements. Movements are then lightly resisted. The therapist alternates hand placement, resisting the movements first in one direction, then the other. Smooth reversal of antagonists is facilitated by well-timed **verbal commands** ("Pull away; now push back.")

2. **Slow reversals (SRs), diagonal shifts:** The patient is positioned in plantigrade with the LEs in step position. The therapist stands diagonally behind the patient. Resistance is applied to the pelvis as the patient weight shifts diagonally forward over the more advanced LE, then diagonally backward over the other LE. **Verbal commands** are "Shift forward and away from me, now shift back and toward me."

5. *Justification for Treatment Procedure or Movement Transition—Outcome of Treatment 1 through 5: Therapeutic Exercise or Movement Transition (T/MT) selected and Rationale for Selection of the intervention, including Techniques (with Motor Control Goal and Indications—(GI).*

   • **OT 1: The patient is able to stabilize and weight-shift in upright kneeling. P/A and T/MT: Movement transition into kneeling from quadruped; kneeling, holding (AI, RS); kneeling, weight shifting: slow reversals (SRs), medial/lateral shifts, diagonal shifts, diagonal shifts with rotation. Rationale for Selection: Base of support (BOS) in kneeling is decreased—it is limited to the length of the lower leg and foot. Center of mass (COM) is intermediate—elevated over supine or prone positions but decreased from standing; the posture is more stable posteriorly than anteriorly. Kneeling involves head, trunk, and hip muscles for upright postural control.** The head and trunk are maintained on the vertical in midline orientation, with normal spinal lumbar and thoracic curves. The pelvis is maintained in midline orientation with hips fully extended and knees flexed (as in to bridging but vertical). Balance reactions contribute to maintenance of upright posture. **The lower COM and wider BOS than in standing make this a safe posture for initial training of upright trunk and hip control;** if the patient loses control, the distance to the mat is small and likely would not result in injury. The degrees of freedom problem is reduced; the patient does not need to demonstrate control of the knee or foot/ankle to develop upright trunk and hip control. **Prolonged positioning in kneeling is particularly helpful for this patient because it provides strong inhibitory influences (inhibitory pressure) acting on the quadriceps;** it is a useful treatment activity to dampen extensor hypertonicity in patients with LE spasticity. Kneeling is an important lead-up activity to upright stance in plantigrade and standing. Kneeling (weight shifting) is an important lead-up activity to upright control in stepping and gait. Theraband tubing can be used to facilitate weak abductors and inhibit adductor tone. **Techniques and GI: Movement transition into kneeling from quadruped:** Controlled mobility (active-assistive movements, progressing to active movements). **Indications:** Useful as a lead-up activity to independent floor-to-standing transfers. **Kneeling, holding (AI, RS):** Stability. **Indications:** Weakness of postural extensors (trunk and hip muscles). **Kneeling, weight shifts (SRs—anterior/posterior shifts):** Controlled mobility. **Indications:** Weakness and incoordination of postural extensors (trunk and hip muscles).

- **OT 2:** The patient is able to assume kneeling. **T/MT:** Kneeling to heel-sitting; kneeling to side-sitting; kneeling to heel-sitting (ARs). **Rationale for Selection: (1) Kneeling to heel-sitting. (2) kneeling to side-sitting: Both movement transitions focus on the problem of weak hip extensors. In addition, kneeling to heel-sitting provides the important advantage of isolating hip extension from knee extension. (3) Kneeling to heel-sitting (ARs):** This is an important lead-up activity for the patient with poor eccentric control who has difficulty sitting down slowly or going down stairs slowly. It is also an important lead-up to assumption of upright stance (floor-to-standing transfers). **Technique and GI: Agonist reversals (ARs):** Controlled mobility, static-dynamic control for UE patterns. **Indications:** Weakness and incoordination of postural extensors (trunk and hip muscles).

- **OT 3: The patient is able to move in kneeling using a reciprocal trunk and limb pattern. T/MT: Kneeling, weight shifting, slow reversals (SRs), diagonal shifts; kneeling, balance training activities; kneeling, manual perturbations. Rationale for Selection:** These activities provide inhibition to the spastic knee extensors while the patient is free to practice the elements needed for forward or backward progression. Dynamic balance is promoted. Proper timing of pelvic movements can be encouraged. Allows facilitation of appropriate compensatory responses. Important lead-up skills for normal gait. **Techniques and GI: Kneeling, weight shifting, slow reversals (SRs), diagonal shifts:** Controlled mobility. **Indications:** Weakness incoordination; an important lead-up activity to upright control in stepping and gait. **Kneeling, balance training activities and kneeling, manual perturbations:** Controlled mobility, static-dynamic control. **Indications:** Promotes dynamic balance.

- **OT 4: The patient is able to assume and maintain the half-kneeling position. T/MT: Movement transition into half-kneeling from kneeling; half-kneeling, holding (AI); half-kneeling, weight shifting (SRs, diagonal shifts). Rationale for Selection: Base of support (BOS) is increased over kneeling and occurs on a diagonal. Center of mass (COM) is intermediate, as in kneeling. Half-kneeling is more stable than kneeling so long as resistance or movements occur within the BOS (on a diagonal); the posture is unstable to resistance or movements outside the BOS.** Half-kneeling involves head, trunk and hip muscles for upright postural control. The head and trunk are maintained of the vertical in midline orientation, with normal spinal lumbar and thoracic curves. The pelvis is maintained in midline orientation, with the hip fully extended on the posterior (knee-down) limb. The hip and knee are flexed to 90 degrees, with slight abduction on the anterior (foot-flat) support limb. Normal righting reactions contribute to upright head position (face vertical, mouth horizontal); Balance reactions contribute to maintenance of upright posture. Holding in the posture and weight-shifting activities in half-kneeling provide early partial weight bearing for the foot and can be used to effectively mobilize foot and ankle muscles, for example, in the patient with ankle injury. Inhibitory influences are in effect for the knee-down support limb (as in kneeling). The half-kneeling position breaks up LE spasticity patterns. **Techniques and GI: Movement transition—half kneeling from kneeling:** Controlled mobility (active-assistive movements to active movements). **Indications:** An important lead-up skill to independent floor-to-standing transfers. **Half-kneeling, holding (AI):** Stability. **Indications:** The more unstable patient may benefit from training in half-kneeling first before kneeling, due to the wider BOS. **Half-kneeling, weight shifting (SRs, diagonal shifts):** Controlled mobility, static-dynamic control. **Indications:** Promotes control in a stable posture (wide BOS).

- **OT 5: The patient is able to assume and maintain upright standing. T/MT: Movement transition: Half-kneeling to standing; modified plantigrade, weight shifting. Rationale for Selection: Functionally, this activity is important to ensure that the patient who has fallen can get up independently. Modified Plantigrade: Base of support (BOS) is wide—hands on treatment table and feet in a symmetrical-stance position. Center of mass (COM) is high. Posture is more stable than standing owing to the four-limb support.** Involves head, trunk, UE and LE muscles for upright postural control. The head and trunk are maintained forward with weight over extended UEs; the shoulders are flexed (typical ranges are 45 to 70 degrees). The hips are flexed with knees extended; ankles are dorsiflexed. Normal righting reactions contribute to upright head position (face vertical, mouth horizontal). BOS can be varied. **Techniques and GI: Movement transition: half-kneeling to standing:** Controlled mobility (active-Assistive movements progressing to active movements). **Indications:** Practicing half-kneeling to standing; dependence in floor-to-stand transfers. **Modified plantigrade, holding (AI, RS):** Stability. **Indications:** An initial standing posture for the patient who lacks the stability control needed for free standing. **Modified plantigrade, weight shifting (SRs; SRs, diagonal shifts):** Controlled mobility (weight shifts). **Indications:** An important lead-up activity for bipedal gait.

CASE STUDY 8: UPPER EXTREMITY TRAUMA

1. *Prioritized Physical Therapy Problem List and Terminology:*
   1. **Diminished right shoulder stability:** *composite impairment.*
   2. **Diminished strength and control of right UE muscles:** *composite impairment.*
   3. **Diminished strength and control of right UE grasp:** *composite impairment.*
   4. **Decreased ROM of right UE:** *indirect impairment.*
   5. **Diminished sensation adjacent to scar area (secondary to surgical intervention):** *indirect impairment.*
   6. **Inability to use right UE for functional activities:** *functional disability.*

2. *Patient Asset List:* **(1) Early intervention of physical therapy following cast removal; (2) maintained a home program of active-assistive exercises while immobilized; (3) motivated to increase strength and ROM of right UE, compliant; (4) identified goal of improving functional use of right UE; and (5) would like to return to high-intensity sport activities.**

3. *Functional Outcome(s) of Physical Therapy (Long-Term Goals):* **The patient has full functional use of the right UE, including postural stabilization; protective extension and fine motor skills.**
   - *Outcomes of Treatment (Short-Term Goals):*
     1. **Able to stabilize the right shoulder in all positions needed for UE function;**
     2. **Independent in basic activities of daily living with the right UE (bathing, grooming, dressing), FIM level = 7.**
     3. **Independent in instrumental activities of daily living (IADLs) with the right UE (writing, meal preparation, housekeeping, tasks, money management, and so on), FIM level = 7.**

4. *Formulate and Justify Physical Therapy Plan of Care:* Problem; Outcome of Treatment (OT), or short-term goal; sequential order of the three advanced therapeutic exercise procedures (A, B, or C). For each procedure, describe the Position or Activity (P/A) and Movement Transition (T/MT); for movement transitions, describe the method of assistance and teaching strategy; describe Techniques (with Motor Control Goals and Indications) and include rationale for selection.
   - **Problem 1: Diminished right shoulder stability. OT: The patient is able to stabilize the shoulder in all positions needed for UE function.**
     A. *First Intervention*—**P/A: Proximal stabilization activities: Shoulder stabilization; active holding:** Initial training should address the problems of postural stability and proximal UE control before focusing on difficulties with reach and grasp activities. The patient is positioned in supine. The elbow is extended and the UE passively positioned at 90 degrees of shoulder flexion. The patient is asked to actively hold this position. The patient is then asked to maintain the position of the shoulder while flexing and extending the elbow. These simultaneous movements increase the difficulty of the task. The therapist can provide initial support (assistance) and remove support as soon as the patient is able to assume voluntary control. **Techniques:**
       1. **Rhythmic stabilization (RS):** The patient is positioned in supine and instructed to move in the PNF D1 flexion pattern (the UE moves up into flexion, adduction, and external rotation with the elbow held straight). As the UE moves up and across into D1F, the patient is asked to hold at approximately 90 degrees of flexion. The therapist applies isometric resistance to shoulder flexors, adductors, and external rotators. The therapist then switches hands to the opposite side of the limb to resist the D1E pattern (resistance is now applied to shoulder extensors, abductors, and internal rotators). A **verbal command** ("Now hold here—don't let me move you up and across") is given before resistance is applied. Resistance is gradually built up; the patient is expected to hold the UE steady. The technique is continued for several repetitions. The patient is then asked to complete the D1E pattern and push the arm down and out to the side. Isometric training is specific to the range of joint motion where it is applied. The therapist, therefore, must vary the shoulder joint angle and apply resistance using RS to the UE at various points in the range in order to ensure shoulder stability throughout the entire range of motion. Rhythmic stabilization (RS) can also be applied in sitting position with the shoulder extended. **Alternating isometrics (AI)** is another technique that can also be used to promote shoulder stabilization. The difference between the two techniques is the absence of isometric resistance to rotators in AI.

2. **Hold-relax active motion (HRAM):** The patient is positioned in supine, with the limb positioned in D1 extension, with the shoulder holding at approximately 30 degrees of shoulder flexion. The patient is asked to hold while the therapist applies gradually increasing isometric resistance to shoulder extensors, abductors, and internal rotators. The patient is then asked to actively relax. The therapist moves the UE quickly in the opposite D1 flexion pattern and provides a quick stretch and a **verbal command** to "Push the arm down and out" back to the original start position. The patient actively contracts and pushes the arm down. The sequence is then repeated.

> **Rationale for selection of proximal stabilization activities: Shoulder stabilization, active holding** (90 degrees shoulder flexion): **This is an important initial position for stabilization training of the shoulder owing to the minimized influence of gravity. Another advantage is that the position can be modified to promote active holding in alternate positions: sidelying, sitting, or standing.** Upright positioning with the shoulder holding at 90 degrees of flexion with the elbow extended imposes a greater challenge due to maximum effects of gravity acting on the shoulder and the increased demands for upright trunk stability. **Techniques and GI: Rhythmic stabilization (RS): Promotes co-contraction of opposing muscle groups; emphasizes rotational control; allows grading of resistance. Alternating isometrics (AI): Used here to promote shoulder stability; allows application of resistance in a variety of directions (anterior/posterior, medial/lateral, or diagonal). Hold-relax active motion (HRAM): This is an effective procedure to improve shoulder stabilization within a functional position needed for weight bearing; it is also useful for strengthening the latissimus dorsi, teres minor, and triceps.**

B. *Second Intervention*—**P/A: Weight-bearing activities:** Weight-bearing activities can be initiated with the elbow flexed (forearm weight bearing). With gains in ROM, the elbow can then be extended (extended UE weight bearing). The patient is asked to actively hold the position or may be passively assisted to hold the position. Joint compression (approximation) facilitates action of the shoulder stabilizers. The patient can actively shift weight onto the weight-bearing arm to increase proprioceptive loading or the therapist can apply approximation force down through the top of the shoulder. The therapist needs to assist the patient in correct alignment of the trunk and scapula during all weight-bearing activities.

1. **Forearm weight bearing:** Table-top forearm weight bearing can be achieved with the elbow positioned on a table top in front of the patient or on a stool placed at the patient's side. This functional position can be used to gain stability for tasks such as eating, to use the limb to stabilize paper during a writing task or a book while reading. The height and proximity of the table should be adjusted for comfortable weight bearing.

2. **Extended elbow weight bearing:** As gains in ROM are achieved, a progression is made to extended-elbow UE weight bearing activities. Sitting, extended-elbow UE weight bearing, with the right hand still positioned anteriorly on a table top, the patient actively extends the elbow while keeping the hand stationary. This movement into a modified plantigrade position can be a useful lead-up activity to promote functional use of the right UE in movement transitions.

3. **Extended UE weight bearing:** Sitting with an extended UE bearing weight at the side is useful activity for this patient. The right UE can be positioned in weight bearing. Demands for upright postural control are increased from the previous activity (forearm weight bearing) and extension of the trunk is promoted, especially with both hands positioned to the side of the hips or behind the hips. This can be a useful to promote shoulder stability (inherent in approximation) and ROM.

4. **Weight shifting:** Weight shifts (medial/lateral, anterior/posterior, rotational) increase the stability demands on the right UE. Dynamic patterns with one limb (the dynamic limb moves in D1F and D1E) also increase the stability demands on the static limb, as does reaching forward toward the support surface.

5. **Standing, modified plantigrade, extended elbow UE weight bearing:** The patient is standing with the hands open on an anteriorly placed treatment table, with shoulders flexed and elbows extended. The amount of weight bearing through the UE and range of shoulder flexion can be controlled by the position of the feet (close to the table decreases UE loading and shoulder flexion range; placement farther from the table increases UE loading and shoulder flexion range). The patient can also be positioned directly facing a wall, either in sitting or standing. The shoulder is positioned in flexion and external rotation with the elbow extended and the hand rests anteriorly on a wall. The patient partially supports the body by leaning onto the UEs. The shoulders stabilize in a range that may be initially difficult to control (90 or 120 degrees of shoulder flexion). The therapist can assist upward rotation of the scapula and stabilization of the elbow in extension. The patient can also practice modified push-ups in this position to improve elbow extension

control. An alternate position is to have the patient face sidewards to the wall, stabilizing the right UE in elbow extension with the shoulder in abduction.

> **Rationale for selection of weight-bearing activities: Forearm, extended elbow, extended UE, weight shifting, standing, modified plantigrade, extended elbow UE weight bearing—Goals and Indications: Weight-bearing activities are used here to increase the challenge to shoulder stabilizers.** An initial sitting position is used to reduce the degrees of freedom and overall challenges to upright posture; the positions allow the therapist to superimpose approximation to facilitate action of the shoulder stabilizers; weight shifting increases proprioceptive loading; modified plantigrade allows increased UE loading.

   C. *Third Intervention*—**P/A:** Prone-on-elbows, quadruped:

   1. **Weight bearing:** The most difficult weight-bearing positions for shoulder stabilization are prone-on-elbows and quadruped. Both positions require maximum loading on the shoulder at 90 degrees of shoulder flexion. The patient should be challenged in postures with decreased stabilization requirements prior to attempting these postures. **Note:** Scapular winging with movement of a portion of the scapula off the thorax is an indication of serratus weakness and scapulothoracic instability. This situation must not be allowed to persist, as it will likely further increase weakness and instability. The therapist must recognize the posture in which scapular winging is occurring is too stressful; the patient's position should be modified immediately. Weight-bearing demands should be reduced by selecting a less challenging posture.

   2. **Rhythmic stabilization (RS):** This technique can be applied directly to the UE with the elbow holding in slight flexion (hyperextension is avoided). This technique is used to facilitate stability control of the elbow. The therapist can also provide manual assistance to stabilize the position of the shoulder and elbow (generally by gripping in the axillae).

   3. **Weight shifting:** Weight shifting during UE weight bearing can be used to increase glenohumeral range of motion and scapulothoracic mobility. Weakness of elbow extensors can be problematic in maintaining an extended elbow UE weight-bearing position. The triceps can be facilitated by tapping directly over the muscle belly.

   > **Rationale for selection of prone-on-elbows, quadruped: weight bearing, weight shifting, rhythmic stabilization (RS): These procedures place additional demands on shoulder stabilizers; weight shifting is used here to promote increased ROM at the glenohumeral joint and scapulothoracic mobility: RS facilitates stability control of the elbow. This patient will require a high level of shoulder stability to return to competitive gymnastics. This selection of treatment positions and activities has important implications as lead-ups to functional upper extremity (UE) tasks.** Performing gross motor tasks includes stabilization and support of body weight (for example, crawling and movement transitions). Progressive challenges are placed on proximal stabilizers to support body weight using prone-on-elbows, table-top forearm weight bearing, and quadruped positions. Postural stabilization demands vary according to the task. Training activities should reflect the high variability of demands required of the proximal stabilizers during functional use. Selective movements of the upper extremity (UE) are also dependent upon stabilizing action of proximal shoulder girdle muscles. **Techniques and GI: Shoulder stabilization, active holding: rhythmic stabilization (RS), alternating isometrics (AI); hold-relax active movement (HRAM):** Stability. **Indications:** Weakness, instability of shoulder and UE stabilizing muscles.

- **Problem 2: Diminished strength and control of right UE muscles. OT: The patient is independent in basic activities of daily living (BADLs—bathing, grooming, dressing) with the right UE; FIM level = 7.**

   A. *First Intervention*—**P/A: Reach Training Activities—Initial Practice of Reach Without Grasp:** Practice is directed toward different excursions and ranges such as forward reach, sidewards reach, backward reach, reaching across the midline, and away from the midline. Practice is also directed to different combinations of shoulder and elbow motions, such as reach with shoulder and elbow flexion (close to the body), reach with shoulder flexion and elbow extension (away from the body), reach with shoulder extension and elbow flexion, reach with shoulder external/internal rotation, and reach with forearm pronation/supination.

   > **Rationale for practice of reach without grasp:** Initial training for reaching is practiced without grasp. The patient moves through different UE excursions and ranges while practicing maintenance of postural alignment. This allows the therapist to ensure normal trunk, scapula, and shoulder alignment during all movements (different excursions and ranges). Postural instability may need to be addressed by using supported positioning of

the trunk. Progression is then made to sitting unsupported. **Motor control goal:** Controlled mobility. **Indications:** Impaired control of UE muscles.

B. *Second Intervention*—**P/A: Reach Training Activities—Practice of Functional Tasks:** Practice addresses different functional tasks such as reach and lift, reach and move toward body, reach to the top of the head (needed for BADLs), and reach to the opposite arm (also needed for BADLs). The therapist must ensure normal trunk, scapula, and shoulder alignment during all training activities. Difficulty in control of UE movement patterns can be reduced by controlling the degrees of freedom present with multijoint control; manual assistance is given as needed to promote optimal limb function and reduce errors. Guided movements should be eliminated as soon as the patient is able to assume voluntary control of the movement.

Rationale for practice of functional tasks: Rehabilitation of upper limb function requires repetition and practice of functional tasks. The therapist can assist in re-establishing desired patterns through optimal positioning and structuring of the desired movement patterns. The patient should be instructed in the elimination of undesired or unnecessary movement components. A direct hands-on approach (guided or active-assistive movements) and/or facilitated movements should be limited in favor of a focus on active learning. Upper limb tasks involve complex, combined movements and necessitate training using a variety of movement combinations. Early practice of daily life tasks and situations is important to ensure desired functional outcomes. **Motor control goal:** Controlled mobility. **Indications:** Impaired control of UE muscles.

C. *Third Intervention*—**P/A: Reach Training Activities—Resistive Patterns:** The patient can be positioned in sitting, plantigrade, or standing, depending upon the degree of postural control present. The following synergistic PNF patterns can be lightly resisted to promote improved control in reaching:

1. **PNF UE D2F** (shoulder flexion, abduction, external rotation) with the elbow straight or extending promotes overhead reach out to the side of the body, which is useful, for example, in reaching for overhead cabinets during instrumental activities of daily living (IADLs).
2. **PNF UE D2F** (shoulder flexion, abduction, external rotation) with the elbow flexing promotes overhead reach to the top of the head, which is useful, for example, in reaching the top of the head for basic grooming tasks.
3. **PNF UE D1F** (shoulder flexion, adduction, external rotation) with the elbow straight or extending promotes overhead reach across the midline of the body.
4. **PNF UE D1F** (shoulder flexion, adduction, external rotation) with the elbow flexing promotes reach to the mouth or opposite shoulder, which is useful, for example, in many basic activities of daily living (BADLs) such as feeding and grooming.
5. **PNF UE Dl thrust** (shoulder flexion, adduction with elbow extension and forearm pronation) promotes forward reach, which is useful, for example, in bringing the hand in front of the body to protect the face with elbow extension.
6. **PNF UE D1 reverse thrust** (shoulder extension, abduction with elbow flexion and forearm supination) promotes scapula adduction with shoulder extension, which is useful, for example, to bring the hand flexed and close to the body in a withdrawal pattern or pulling motion.
7. **Bilateral patterns:** bilateral symmetrical and asymmetrical patterns combine to allow for many different functional tasks, such as raking or shoveling snow and sports-related activities.

Rationale for resistive PNF patterns: Resistance can be used to increase proprioceptive loading and kinesthetic awareness of limb movements; resistance also improves strength and synergistic action (coordination) of shoulder and elbow muscles. **GI: Resistive PNF patterns:** Controlled mobility. **Indications:** Impaired control of UE muscles; weakness. **Note:** Two additional techniques that are useful for this patient are: (1) slow reversals (SRs): slow isotonic contractions of first the agonist, then the antagonist patterns, using grading of resistance and optimal facilitation, reversal of antagonists, and progression through increments of range; and (2) slow reversal-hold (SRH): an isometric contraction added at the end of the range or at a point of weakness.

- **Problem 3: Diminished strength and control of UE grasp. OT: The patient independently performs instrumental activities of daily living (IADLs)—writing, meal preparation, housekeeping, tasks, money management, and so on) with the right UE; FIM level = 7.**
  A. *First Intervention*—**P/A: Grasp Training Activities:** Training activities for the grasp component of functional activities are task dependent, shaped by the size, weight, shape, and use of the object. The therapist may need to initially guide the movements and verbally cue the desired movements (for example, "Open your hand and grasp this object.") Initial

pre-positioning of the limb may be necessary; for example, supination is combined with an open hand to facilitate function. Practice is directed toward everyday objects with varying sizes, shapes, weights and textures, such as grasping a cup or a ball. Practice is directed toward different functional tasks such as drinking from a cup or mug, eating with a spoon or fork, and so on. Grasp is initially isolated from reaching; for example, the object is positioned close to patient's body or on a table top.

B. *Second Intervention—P/A:* Reach and grasp training activities:

1. **Training using both reach and grasp:** The object is positioned away from the patient's body. The patient must reach toward the object and grasp the object (for example, pick up an object and reposition it; pick up an object and throw it; pick up an object and manipulate it). Practice is directed toward transporting an object (for example, picking up an object and moving it toward the body; bringing an object to the mouth (for example, eating or drinking); bringing an object to the head (comb hair, wash face).

2. **Training using resistive patterns:** Hand opening with reach can be promoted with use of PNF UE D2F or D1E patterns. Hand closing with reach can be promoted with use of PNF UE D1F and D2E patterns.

C. *Third Intervention—P/A:* **Reach and grasp training activities:**

1. **Bimanual tasks:** Training activities that involve simultaneous use of both upper extremities (bimanual tasks) should be introduced as soon as possible. The patient is instructed to: (1) grasp onto a wand or cane and raise it to the forward horizontal position, overhead, or out to the side (cane exercises); the range can be varied to increase difficulty; (2) catch and throw a ball: the size and weight of the ball can be varied to increase or decrease difficulty (for example, a kickball to a weighted medicine ball); (3) pick up an object (for example, a plate or box) with both hands and reposition it; size and weight can be varied to increase difficulty; (4) pour from one cup to another; (5) use a knife and fork to cut up food.

2. **Reach and grasp activities with trunk movements:** Training activities involve simultaneous use of UE reach and grasp with trunk movements. In sitting, the patient bends forward and pick up an object off the floor (trunk flexion and extension). In sitting or standing, the patient turns and reaches to one side or behind to grasp an object (trunk rotation). In standing, the patient stoops and picks up an object off the floor (trunk and LE flexion and extension).

   Rationale for using reach and grasp training activities: The activities presented were selected on the basis of their lead-up features to functional activities. Manipulation skills require accurate sequencing and timing. Manipulation skills consist of two independently controlled components: (1) reach (transport); and (2) grasp. The activities selected allow practice in sequencing the reach and grasp components of manipulation skills within the context of functional activities.

   1. **Reach (transport) component requires practice with:** reaching movements to elevate the UE to position the hand for function; coordinated, synergistic patterns of movement (for example, shoulder abduction and external rotation with elbow flexion to position the hand close to the body); rotational components of normal patterns of UE movement (for example, external rotation with supination, internal rotation with pronation; combining reaching movements across the midline of the body with trunk rotation to the same side; overhead reaching movements (requires rotation of the scapula on the thorax with humeral elevation); reaching and pulling movements; and coordination of reaching movements with movements of the eye and head.

   2. **Grasp component requires practice with:** use of the hand to capture and grip the object, forearm rotational movements (pronation or supination) to orient the hand for grasp; must be sequenced simultaneously with reaching movements, stabilizing the wrist in slight extension in preparation for grasp, opening and closing the fingers around a variety of objects (finger opposition and flexion), adapts the hand to the size, width, and shape of the object, and use of hand and fingers to manipulate an object to determine its spatial characteristics. **Techniques and GI: Grasp training activities: PNF UE patterns: D2F, D1E; D1F, and D2E patterns:** Controlled mobility and skill. **Indications:** Impaired control of the UE muscles; weakness.

CASE STUDY 9: LOWER EXTREMITY AMPUTATION

1. *Prioritized Physical Therapy Problem List and Terminology:*
   1. **Upright balance compromised on uneven terrain:** *composite impairment.*
   2. **Diminished protective steps sideways (stepping strategy) to regain balance:** *composite impairment.*

3. **Diminished protective steps forward (stepping strategy) to regain balance:** *composite impairment.*
4. **Decreased awareness and control of center of mass and limits of stability:** *composite impairment.*
5. **Diminished musculoskeletal responses needed for balance:** *composite impairment.*
6. **Weakness of hip extensors and abductors:** *indirect impairment.*
7. **Gait deviations: decreased forward pelvic and lower trunk rotation; asymmetrical weight distribution; diminished overall timing and sequencing of gait pattern:** *composite impairment.*

2. *Patient Asset List:* **(1) Independent in BADLs and IADLs (FIM level = 7); (2) strength of right (R) lower extremity, both upper extremities, and trunk = WNL; (3) young, healthy, no medical complications; (4) independent in ambulation without an assistive device on level surfaces and stairs; (5) patient has identified specific goals to include in developing plan of care; (6) motivated/compliant; willing/able to follow through with home exercise program.**

3. *Functional Outcome(s) of Physical Therapy (Long-Term Goal):* **The patient is able to ambulate using appropriate functional balance and weight bearing on all surfaces.**

   • *Outcomes of Treatment (short-term goals):*
   1. Able to ambulate using appropriate timing and sequencing.
   2. Able to ambulate sideways.
   3. Able to ambulate using complex stepping patterns.
   4. Able to control center of mass (COM) within limits of stability (LOS) during standing and walking.
   5. Able to ambulate with appropriate musculoskeletal responses necessary for balance.

   • *Projected Number of Visits:* Expect some variation in your selection of time interval to accomplish your outcomes (goals). It is often difficult to make such projections from hypothetical cases. However given the case data, it appears that outpatient intervention over a 6-week period would be sufficient. Since this patient is functioning at a relatively high level initially, the therapist would want to observe progress over a reasonabel period of time. During the first 2–3 weeks of intervention, visits twice a week would be appropriate. Once the patient is competent with a home exercise program, visits could be reduced to one per week (for a total of 8–9 visits).

4. *Formulate and Justify a Physical Therapy Plan of Care:* Problem; Outcome of Treatment (OT), or short-term goal; sequential order of the three advanced therapeutic exercise procedures (A, B, or C). For each procedure, describe the Position or Activity (P/A) and Movement Transition (MT); for movement transitions, describe the method of assistance and teaching strategy; describe Techniques (with Motor Control Goals and Indications) and include rationale for selection.

   • **Problem 1: Upright balance compromised on uneven terrain. OT: The patient will be able to ambulate using appropriate timing and sequencing.**
   A. *First Intervention*—**P/A: Standing, stepping:** This activity is initiated with the LEs in step position. The patient weight-shifts diagonally forward over the anterior support limb (stance limb) and takes a step forward with the dynamic (swing) limb. The movements are then reversed: the patient shifts diagonally back and takes a step backward using the same dynamic limb. **Technique: Slow reversals (SRs), stepping:** The therapist is in front of the patient, either sitting on a rolling stool or standing. Manual contacts are on the pelvis. The therapist applies light stretch and resistance to facilitate the forward pelvic rotation as the swing limb moves forward. Approximation can be given as needed over the top of the pelvis as the dynamic limb comes into extension and weight bearing. **Verbal commands** are "Shift forward and step; now shift back and step."
   B. *Second Intervention*—**P/A: Walking forward, backward. Techniques:**
   1. **Guided movement.** Starting in the parallel bars, the patient practices walking forward and backward. The therapist focuses on the proper timing and sequencing, beginning with the sequencing of the weight shift diagonally forward (or backward) onto the stance limb and pelvic forward rotation with advancement of the opposite limb. The movements are repeated to allow for a continuous movement sequence. **Verbal commands** are used to assist the patient ("Shift forward, and step, step, step . . ."). Manual contacts can be used to guide movements and facilitate missing elements. For example, the therapist can assist forward pelvic rotation during swing by placing the hands on the anterior pelvis. For backwards progression, the therapist's hand can be placed posteriorly over the gluteal muscles to facilitate hip extension and weight acceptance on the stance leg. As training progresses, the therapist can alter: Level of assistance: progressing from walk-

ing in the parallel bars to unassisted walking; step length, from reduced to normal. Speed of walking: from reduced to normal to increased; base of support: feet apart to feet together; acceleration or deceleration: the patient practices stopping and starting on command. Of particular importance for this patient is to vary the support surfaces from flat to carpeted to irregular (outdoors) and to include anticipatory timing demands: walking a distance within a specified period of time (for example, crossing at a street light).

2. **Resisted Progression (RP):** The therapist is in front of the patient, either in standing or sitting on a rolling stool. As the patient moves forward, the therapist also moves in a reverse or mirror image of the patient's movements. The therapist provides maintained resistance to the forward progression by placing both hands on the pelvis. Resistance should be light (facilitatory) to encourage proper timing of the pelvic movements. Approximation can be applied down through the top of the pelvis to assist in stabilizing responses as weight is taken on the stance limb. Stretch to pelvic rotators can be added as needed to facilitate the initiation of the pelvic motion. Resistance can also be applied with manual contacts on the pelvis and contralateral shoulder. The position and movements are reversed for backwards walking. Resistance can also be applied using surgical tubing or Theraband. The tubing can be wrapped around the patient's pelvis. The therapist then holds the tubing from behind and provides light resistance to the forward progression of the trunk.

Rationale for Selection—Standing, Stepping: Slow Reversals (SR), Stepping. Walking Forward, Backward: Guided Movement; Resisted Progression (RP): (1) Standing, Stepping: Slow Reversals (SR), Stepping: promotes dynamic standing; important lead-up activity for gait. (2) Walking Forward, Backward: Guided Movement: promotes pelvic rotation; allows facilitation of hip extension and weight acceptance on the stance leg. (3) Walking Forward, Backward: Resisted Progression (RP): promotes appropriate timing and sequencing of gait; decreased effort of gait; allows therapist to use manual contacts to facilitate pelvic motion; approximation can be used down through the top of pelvis to facilitate stabilizing responses; allows tracking resistance to be used to encourage proper timing of pelvic motions. **GI:** Standing, Stepping: Slow Reversals (SR), Stepping: static-dynamic control; **Indications:** Lead-up activity for bipedal gait; community ambulation. Walking Forward, Backward, Guided Movement: active control; effective problem solving; promotes early learning. Walking Forward, Backward, Resisted Progression (RP): Skill. **Indications:** To promote timing and sequencing of gait.

- **Problem 2: Diminished protective steps sideways (stepping strategy) to regain balance. OT: The patient will be able to ambulate sideways.**
  A. *First Intervention*—**P/A: Walking, side-stepping, crossed-stepping. T/MT: Guided Movement.** The patient practices walking sideways. The side-step involves abduction and placement of one LE to the side. The remaining limb is then moved parallel to the first. Abductors are active on both the dynamic (moving the limb) and static limb (maintaining the pelvis level).
  B. *Second Intervention*—**P/A: Walking, crossed-stepping. Technique: Guided Movement:** The patient begins with a side-step, followed by movement of the opposite lower extremity crossing over and in front of the other. **Verbal commands** are "Step out to the side, now step up and across . . ." The movements are then repeated to allow for a continuous movement sequence.

  Rationale for Selection—Walking, Side-Stepping, Crossed-Stepping; Guided Movement: These activities allow the therapist to facilitate movements with manual contacts placed lightly on the patient's pelvis. Particularly important for this patient are the demands the activities place on the hip abductors. Also important is the therapist's ability to displace the body unexpectedly (manual perturbations) in order to promote protective stepping strategies. The patient responds with automatic steps in the direction of the displacement. Hip abduction movements can be resisted, either manually or with surgical tubing or Theraband. **GI:** Walking, Side-Stepping, Crossed-Stepping; Guided Movement: Skill. **Indications:** Hip abductor weakness; facilitation of the protective steps sideways (stepping strategy) to regain balance.

- **Problem 3: Diminished protective steps forward (stepping strategy) to regain balance. OT: The patient will be able to ambulate using complex stepping patterns.**
  A. *First Intervention*—**P/A: Braiding. Technique: Guided Movement:** The patient begins with side-step, followed by a crossed step up and over in front (PNF: LE D1F pattern). This sequence is followed by a side-step, then a crossed-step, backwards and behind the first limb (PNF: LE D2E pattern). The movements are repeated to allow for a continuous movement sequence. The therapist can facilitate learning by standing in front of the patient,

modeling the desired steps. Additional support can be provided by having the therapist place both hands directly in front of the patient, forearms supinated and having the patient lightly place the hands on top of the therapist's hands. The patient and therapist then move together. **Verbal commands** should be well timed and include "Step out to the side; now step up and across, and step out to the side; now step back and across."

B. *Second Intervention*—**P/A: Braiding. Technique: Resisted Progression (RP):** The therapist is behind the patient, standing slightly to side in the direction of the movement. As the patient moves sidewards in braiding, the therapist moves in the same sequence and timing with patient. The therapist provides maintained resistance to the sideward progression by placing one hand on the side of the pelvis. The other hand alternates, first on the anterior pelvis resisting the forward pelvic motion and crossed step in front. It then slides to the posterior pelvis to resist the backward pelvic motion and crossed step behind. Resistance should be light (facilitatory) to encourage proper timing of the pelvic movements. A stretch to pelvic rotators can be added as needed to facilitate the initiation of the pelvic motion.

Rationale for Selection—Braiding: Guided Movement; Resisted Progression (RP): These activities promote: lower trunk rotation; lower extremity patterns with upright postural control; protective stepping strategies for balance; complex stepping patterns. These activities also provide variety to training activities. As balance is highly task and context specific, balance control should be practiced using many different functional tasks and environments. Variety will improve effectiveness of practice schedules and improve responsiveness of postural muscles and overall balance performance. **GI:** Braiding: Guided Movement; Resisted Progression (RP): Skill. **Indications:** Facilitation of lower trunk rotation, lower extremity patterns with upright postural control; protective stepping strategies for balance.

- **Problem 4: Decreased awareness and control of center of mass and limits of stability. OT: The patient will be able to control of center mass and limits of stability during standing and walking.**
  A. *First Intervention*—**P/A: Standing. Technique: Guided movement.** Exaggerated arm swings; functional reach activities; reduced BOS: feet together; eyes open to eyes closed; marching in place, high stepping: holding on with light touch-down support (both hands to one hand).
  B. *Second Intervention*—**P/A: Gait.** Guided movement. Gait with narrowed BOS; gait with wide turns to right and left; side stepping: holding on with light touch-down support of both hands, progressing to one hand. **Technique: Guided movement. P/A: Standing, partial squats; ball activities: kicking a ball.** *UE Ball Activities:* Bouncing ball; catching or throwing a ball: vary weight and size of ball; hitting a balloon, hitting a foam ball with a paddle; games that involve stooping, aiming: bowling, shuffleboard; and floor-to-standing transfers: UE support on chair to no support.

- **Problem 5: Diminished musculoskeletal responses needed for balance. OT: The patient will be able to ambulate with musculoskeletal responses necessary for balance.**
  A. *First Intervention*—**P/A: Gait activities. T/MT: Guided movement. P/A:** Unassisted walking forward; backward near a wall (eyes open to eyes closed); while moving head left and right: slow movements to fast; side-stepping (without arm support); crossed step walking, braiding; gait with small turns to right and left; walking in circles: first one direction, then reverse direction; walking in a figure-of-eight pattern; stopping and starting; turning on command; stepping through a grid walking; bouncing or tossing a ball while walking through an obstacle course; and walking while conversing with a patient: divert the patient's attention away from the activity; balance should be automatic.

  Rationale for Selection: Advanced and intermediate level balance activities provide higher levels of challenge to balance; promote reeducation of limits of stability and centered limits of stability; improve responsiveness of postural muscles and overall balance performance; provides feedback about sensory information, postural patterns, muscle recruitment and coordination. The selected activities continue to appropriately varying challenges to balance, combining some activities that are relatively easy for the patient, and some that are more difficult. Effective motor learning strategies ensure the patient experiences success. The variety of activities presented, allows the therapist to alternate activities, and begin and end each treatment session with activities the patient can successfully complete. **GI:** Gait, Standing: Guided Movement: Skill. **Indications:** Provide high level challenges to sensory systems for balance (somatosensory, visual, and vestibular).
  B. *Second Intervention:* **P/A: Community activities. T/MT:** Guided movement. Unassisted walking in a community (open) environment walking on uneven terrain; finding solutions to real-life functional problems pushing or pulling open doors; pushing a grocery carts; car-

rying a bag of groceries; and anticipatory timing activities: getting on an escalator, elevator; crossing at busy intersection or at a traffic light.

Rationale for Selection: Advanced and intermediate level balance activities provide progressively higher levels of challenge to balance; allow focus on safety awareness and compensation; provide opportunity for patient to practice functional balance requirements within the context in which they will be used. As balance skills are both task and context specific, balance control should be practiced using a variety of different functional tasks and environments; Activities allow patient to practice in an open (variable) environment. **G/I:** Gait Activities; Community Activities: Guided Movement: Skill. **Indications:** Provide high level challenges to musculoskeletal responses necessary for balance in community, work, and leisure environments.

CASE STUDY 10: ACHILLES TENDON RUPTURE

1. *Prioritized Physical Therapy Problem List and Terminology:*
   1. **Diminished medial/lateral right foot/ankle control:** *direct impairment.*
   2. **Diminished anterior/posterior and diagonal foot/ankle control:** *direct impairment.*
   3. **Diminished static-dynamic control of right foot/ankle:** *direct impairment.*
   4. **Diminished static weight-bearing capability of right ankle/foot:** *direct impairment.*
   5. **Decreased ROM in right ankle:** *composite impairment.*
   6. **Decreased strength of right ankle:** *composite impairment.*
   7. **Decreased balance:** *composite impairment.*

2. *Patient Asset List:* **(1) Knowledgeable about injury and surgical intervention; (2) motivated to make functional gains; (3) high physical activity level prior to injury; (4) able to identify specific goals for seeking physical therapy; (5) without any apparent complicating factors which might hinder progress; (6) compliant with home exercise program; (7) BADLs: Independent (FIM level = 7); IADLs: Independent (FIM level = 7).**

3. *Functional Outcome(s) of Physical Therapy (Long-Term Goals):* **The patient will be able to ambulate independently on all surfaces.**
   - *Outcomes of Treatment (Short-Term Goals):*
     1. Able to stabilize the ankle/foot in a medial/lateral direction in bridging.
     2. Able to shift weight forward, backward, and diagonally in half-kneeling.
     3. Able to shift weight in modified plantigrade.
     4. Able to shift weight in standing.
     5. Increase strength in ankle muscles from F−to G−.
     6. Increase dorsiflexion ROM from 0–5 to 0–15 degrees.
     7. Increase plantarflexion ROM from 0–10 to 0–20 degrees.
     8. Increase inversion ROM from: 0–10 to 0–20 degrees.
     9. Increase eversion ROM from 0–5 to 0–10 degrees.

   - *Projected Number of Visits:* Expect some variation in your selection of time interval to accomplish your outcomes (goals). It is often difficult to make such projections from hypothetical cases. However given the case data, it appears that outpatient intervention over a 4-week period would be appropriate. During the first 2 weeks, the patient could be seen 3 times per week and once or twice per week for the last 2 weeks (for a total of 8–10 vistits).

4. *Physical Therapy Plan of Care:* **Problem; Outcome of Treatment (OT), or short-term goal; sequential order of the three advanced therapeutic exercise procedures (A, B, or C). For each procedure, describe the Position or Activity (P/A) and Movement Transition (MT); for** Movement transitions, **describe the method of assistance and teaching strategy; describe Techniques (with Motor Control Goals and Indications) and include rationale for selection.**
   - **Problem 1: Diminished medial/lateral right foot/ankle control. OT: The patient is able to stabilize the ankle/foot in a medial/lateral direction in bridging.**
     A. *First Intervention*—**P/A: Bridging, holding. Techniques: Alternating isometrics (AI):** The patient is asked to hold the bridge position while resistance is applied. Manual contacts are placed at the knees. Resistance is applied at the knees to increase the length of the lever arm. This recruits more lower limb muscles, especially foot and ankle muscles. The position of the therapist will vary according to the line of force required.

B. *Second Intervention*—**P/A: Bridging, weight shifts. T/MT: Slow reversals (SRs).** The therapist is positioned in kneeling at the side of the patient. The movement of the hips is assisted a few repetitions to ensure the patient knows the expected movements. Manual contacts are placed at the knees. Side-to-side movements are then lightly resisted. This again increases the length of the lever arm and recruits medial and lateral ankle and foot muscles to shift the body from side to side.

C. *Third Intervention*—**P/A: Bridging, advanced stabilization. Technique: Bridging, leg lifts:** Manual contacts are placed at the knees. The patient is asked to lift one leg up while maintaining the bridge position using single-limb support. This is a particularly important activity for this patient because of the challenges placed on the static limb. Lifts can include knee extension or marching in place (hip and knee flexion). The patient is asked to alternate limbs, lifting first one LE, then the other. Movements can be assisted with tactile or verbal cueing. The patient should be started with UE stabilization (abducted and extended on mat) during initial training; as control progresses, difficulty can be increased by reducing the UE support (increasing shoulder adduction or crossing the arms over chest).

Rationale for Selection: Bridging, holding; bridging, weight shifts; bridging, advanced stabilization. Alternating isometrics (AI); slow reversals (SRs); bridging, leg lifts. **Base of support (BOS) in bridging is large. Center of mass (COM) is low. Posture is very stable.** Following foot/ankle injury, bridging activities are an important lead-up for gait and stair climbing. Bridging allows for early weight bearing through the foot and ankle without the body-weight constraints of a fully upright posture. Greater demands can be focused on a single limb with static-dynamic activities. **T/MT: Alternating isometrics (AI):** Stability. **Indications:** Instability of medial/lateral foot/ankle muscles. **Slow reversals (SRs):** Controlled mobility. **Indications:** Instability of medial/lateral foot/ankle muscles. **Bridging, leg lifts:** Controlled mobility: diminished medial/lateral foot/ankle control.

- **Problem 2: Diminished anterior/posterior and diagonal foot/ankle control. OT: The patient is able to weight-shift forward, backward, and diagonally in half-kneeling.**
  A. *First Intervention*—**P/A: Half-kneeling, holding:** The patient is half-kneeling with weight borne equally on the posterior (knee-down) and anterior (foot-flat) support limbs. The head and trunk are upright. The therapist is also in half-kneeling in front of the patient, in a reversed (mirror-image) position. During initial training, the patient with instability may benefit from support provided by forward placement of the UEs on the therapist's shoulders. Alternately, both hands can be positioned on the patient's elevated anterior knee for support. **T/MT: Alternating isometrics (AI):** The patient is asked to hold the half-kneeling position while the therapist applies resistance to the pelvis, first pushing the pelvis diagonally back toward the posterior (knee-down) limb, then pulling the pelvis forward toward the anterior (foot-flat) limb. The resistance is built up gradually, starting with very light resistance and progressing to the patient's maximum. The isometric contraction is maintained for several counts. Resistance is applied only diagonally, in the direction of the BOS. The therapist must give a transitional command ("Now don't let me move you the other way") before sliding the hands to resist the opposite muscles. This allows the patient an opportunity to make appropriate preparatory postural adjustments.
  B. *Second Intervention*—**P/A: Half-kneeling, weight shifting: diagonals. Technique: Active movement:** The patient is the half-kneeling position with the right LE forward. The therapist is diagonally in front of the patient. The therapist guides the movement from the pelvis, first moving the pelvis diagonally back toward the posterior knee down limb, then moving the pelvis forward toward the anterior (foot-flat) limb. The therapist again uses a transitional command when changing direction ("Now get ready to move the other way") before sliding the hands to guide movement in the opposite direction. The therapist removes guidance when the patient is able to take over the movement. The patient actively shifts weight diagonally forward over the foot-flat support limb; then diagonally backward over the knee-down support limb.
  C. *Third Intervention*—**P/A: Half-kneeling, weight shifting:** The patient actively shifts weight diagonally forward over the foot-flat support limb; then diagonally backward over the knee-down support limb. **Technique: Slow reversals (SRs), diagonal shifts:** The patient is positioned in half-kneeling. The therapist is diagonally in front of the patient. Light resistance is applied to the pelvis as the patient weight-shifts diagonally forward over the support foot, then diagonally backward over the support knee. **Verbal commands** are "Shift forward and toward me; now shift back and away from me."

  Rationale for Selection: Half-kneeling, holding: alternating isometrics (AI); half-kneeling, weight shifting, diagonals: active movement; half-kneeling, weight shifting, slow reversals (SRs), diagonal shifts. Holding in the posture and weight shifting activities in half-kneeling provide early partial weight bearing for the foot and can be used to effectively mobilize foot and ankle muscles following injury. **GI:** (1) **Half-kneeling, holding (AI):** Stability. **Indications:** The more unstable patient may benefit from training in half-kneeling first before kneeling due to the wider BOS. (2) **Half-kneeling, weight shifting, diagonals (active movement):** Controlled mobility, static dynamic control. **Indications:** Guidance reduces error during early learning; active control of movement is overall goal; diminished movement capabilities, reduced kinesthetic inputs that normally guide movement. (3) **Half-kneeling, weight shifting, diagonals (SRs, diagonal shifts):** Controlled mobility, static-dynamic control. **Indications:** Promotes control in a stable posture (wide BOS).

- **Problem 3: Diminished static-dynamic control of right foot/ankle. OT: The patient is able to shift weight in modified plantigrade.**
    - A. *First Intervention*—**P/A: Modified plantigrade, holding:** The patient is in modified plantigrade, with weight borne equally on both UEs and LEs. The LEs can be positioned in a symmetrical-stance position or in step position. During initial training, the patient will benefit from bilateral upper limb support. As control develops the patient can be progressed from bilateral to single-limb support to free standing. **Technique:**
        1. **Alternating isometrics (AI):** The patient is asked to hold the plantigrade position while therapist stands behind the patient and applies resistance to the trunk. Hands can be placed on the pelvis, pelvis/contralateral shoulder, or both shoulders. Resistance is applied first in one direction, then the other (anterior/posterior, medial/lateral, or diagonal with the LEs in the step position). The position of the therapist will vary according to the direction of the line of force. Resistance is built up gradually, starting from very light resistance progressing to the patient's maximum. The isometric contraction is maintained for several counts. The therapist must give a **transitional verbal command** ("Now don't let me move you the other way") before sliding the hands to resist the opposite muscles; this allows the patient an opportunity to make appropriate preparatory postural adjustments.
        2. **Rhythmic stabilization (RS):** The patient is asked to hold the plantigrade position while the therapist stands behind the patient and applies rotational resistance to the trunk. One hand is placed on the posterior pelvis on one side, pushing forward, while the other hand is on the anterior upper trunk on the contralateral side, pulling backward. **Verbal commands** are "Don't let me twist you—hold, hold; now don't let me twist you the other way."
    - B. *Second Intervention*—**P/A: Modified plantigrade, weight shifting. Technique: Guided movement to active movement:** The patient actively shifts weight, first forward (increasing loading on the UEs), then backward (increasing loading on the LEs). Weight shifts can also be performed side to side (medial/lateral shifts) with the LEs in a symmetrical-stance position, or diagonally forward and backward with the LEs in a step position.
    - C. *Third Intervention:* **P/A: Modified plantigrade, weight shifting. Technique:**
        1. **Slow reversals (SRs):** The therapist is standing at the patient's side (for medial/lateral shifts), or behind (for anterior/posterior shifts). Manual contacts are placed on the pelvis. The movement is assisted for a few repetitions to ensure the patient knows the movements expected. Movements are then lightly resisted. The therapist alternates hand placement, resisting the movements first in one direction, then the other. Smooth reversals of antagonists are facilitated by well-timed **verbal commands** ("Pull away; now push back.")
        2. **Slow reversals (SRs), diagonal shifts:** The patient is positioned in plantigrade with the LEs in step position. The therapist stands diagonally behind the patient. Resistance is applied to the pelvis as the patient shifts weight diagonally forward over the more advanced LE, then diagonally backward over the other LE. **Verbal commands** are "Shift forward and away from me; now shift back and toward me."

        Rationale for Selection: Modified plantigrade, holding: alternating isometrics (AI), rhythmic stabilization (RS); modified plantigrade, weight shifting: guided movement to active movement; slow reversals (SRs); slow reversals (SRs), diagonal shifts. The plantigrade position offers several important advantages for the patient with an ankle injury (weight bearing to tolerance). The patient is standing with both elbows extended, hands open and bearing weight on a treatment table or plinth. This allows the patient to gradually become acclimated to weight bearing on the ankle. Weight bearing is shared through both upper and lower extremities. The wider BOS as compared to standing make this a safe posture for initial training in the fully upright position. Another primary benefit for this patient is that weight-shifting activities in plantigrade can be used to obtain ROM in ankle dorsiflexion (shifts forward). **Techniques and GI: modified plantigrade, holding: alternating isometrics (AI), rhythmic stabilization (RS):** Stability. **Indications:** An initial standing posture for the patient who lacks stability control for free standing. **Modified plantigrade, weight shifting: guided movement to active**

movement; **slow reversals (SRs); slow reversals (SRs), diagonal shifts:** Controlled mobility (weight shifts), static-dynamic control (stepping). **Indications:** Increase ankle mobility; an important lead-up activity for gait.

- **Problem 4: Diminished static weight bearing capability of right ankle/foot. OT: The patient is able to weight-shift in standing.**

    A. *First Intervention*—**P/A: Standing, holding:** Initially, the patient may require UE support by placing the arms forward with the hands on the therapist's shoulders. The patient is standing, with equal weight on both LEs. The feet are positioned parallel and slightly apart (a symmetrical-stance position); knees are slightly flexed, not hyperextended. Pelvis is in neutral position. An alternate standing position is with one foot slightly advanced of the other in a step position. **Technique:**

    1. Alternating isometrics (AI): The patient is asked to hold the standing position while therapist applies resistance to the trunk. Manual contacts can be placed on the pelvis. Resistance is applied first in one direction, then the other (anterior/posterior, medial/lateral, or diagonal with a progression to the LEs in the step position). The position of the therapist will vary according to direction of the line of force applied. Resistance is built up gradually, from very light resistance to the patient's maximum. The isometric contraction is maintained for several counts. Light approximation can be given to the tops of the shoulders, hips, or the head to increase stabilizing responses. The therapist must give a **transitional verbal command** ("Now don't let me move you the other way") before sliding the hands to resist the opposite muscles; this allows the patient the opportunity to take appropriate preparatory postural adjustments.

    2. **Rhythmic stabilization (RS):** The patient holds the symmetrical standing position while the therapist applies rotational resistance to the trunk. One hand is placed on the posterior pelvis on one side, pushing forward, while the other hand is on the anterior upper trunk on the contralateral side, pulling backward. **Verbal commands** are "Don't let me twist you—hold, hold; now don't let me twist you the other way."

    B. *Second Intervention*—**P/A: Standing, weight shifts:** The patient actively shifts weight, first forward, then backward. Weight shifts can also be performed side to side (medial/lateral shifts) with the LEs in a symmetrical-stance position, or diagonally forward and backward with the LEs in a step position. Active reaching activities can be used to promote weight shifting in all directions. The therapist provides a target ("Reach out and touch my hand.") **Technique: Slow reversals (SRs):** The therapist is standing at the patient's side (for medial/lateral shifts), or behind (for anterior/posterior shifts). Manual contacts can be placed on the pelvis. The movement is assisted a few repetitions to ensure the patient knows the expected movements. Movements are then lightly resisted. The therapist alternates hand placement, resisting the movements first in one direction, then the other. Smooth reversals of antagonists are facilitated by well-timed **verbal commands** ("Pull away; now push back.")

    C. *Third Intervention*—**P/A: Standing, weight shifts.**

    Slow reversals (SRs), diagonal shifts: The patient is in standing with the LEs in step position. The therapist is diagonally in front of the patient, either sitting on a stool or standing. Resistance is applied to the pelvis as the patient weight-shifts diagonally forward over the more advanced limb, then diagonally backward over the opposite limb. **Verbal commands** are "Shift forward and away from me; now shift back and toward me."

    Rationale for Selection: Standing, holding: Alternating isometrics (AI), rhythmic stabilization (RS); standing, weight shifts: slow reversals (SRs): Useful activities to promote ankle strategies required for gait (important for maintaining upright stability and balance). BOS can be varied to decrease or increase difficulty. A decreased stance (feet together) can be used to increase the challenge to postural control. Asymmetric standing can promote additional challenges to a single limb. Action of the foot/ankle muscles and balance reactions can be facilitated. Promote anticipatory postural responses (especially those involving ankle strategies). **Techniques and GI: Standing, holding: alternating isometrics (AI), rhythmic stabilization (RS):** Stability. **Indications:** Stabilization control in standing is an important lead-up activity to unilateral stance and bipedal gait.

REFERENCES

1. O'Sullivan S, and Schmitz T (1994). Physical Rehabilitation: Assessment and Treatment, ed. 3. Philadelphia: FA Davis.
2. Voss D, Ionta M, and Myers B (1985). Proprioceptive Neuromuscular Facilitation—Patterns and Techniques, ed. 3. Philadelphia: Harper and Row.
3. Bobath B (1990). Adult Hemiplegia: Evaluation and Treatment, ed. 3. London: Wm. Heinemann Medical Books Ltd.
4. Sawner K, and Lavigne J (1992). Brunnstrom's Movement Therapy in Hemiplegia, ed. 2. Philadelphia: JB Lippincott.
5. Smith L, Weiss E, and Lehmkul D (1995). Brunnstrom's Clinical Kinesiology, ed. 5. Philadelphia: FA Davis.
6. Rood M (1954). Neurophysiological reactions as a basis for physical therapy. Phys Ther Rev 34: 444–449.
7. Schmidt R (1988). Motor Control and Learning, ed. 2. Champaign, IL: Human Kinetics Publishers, Inc.
8. Carr J, and Shepherd R (1987). A Motor Relearning Programme for Stroke, ed. 2. Rockville, MD: Aspen.
9. World Health Organization (WHO) (1980). International classification of impairments, disabilities, and handicaps. A manual of classification relating to the consequences of disease. Geneva, Switzerland: WHO.
10. Guccione A (1991). Physical therapy diagnosis and the relationship between impairments and function. Phys Ther 71: 499.
11. Nagi S (1969). Disability and Rehabilitation. Columbus, OH: Ohio State University Press.
12. Schenkman M, and Butler R (1989). A model for multisystem evaluation, interpretation, and treatment of individuals with neurologic dysfunction. Phys Ther 69:538.
13. Uniform Data Set for Medical Rehabilitation (UDSMR^{SM}), a division of UB Foundation Activities, Inc. (1996). Guide for the Uniform Data Set for Medical Rehabilitation (including the FIM^{SM} instrument), Version 5.0. Buffalo, NY: SUNY Buffalo.
14. Guccione A (1994). Functional assessment. In O'Sullivan S, and Schmitz T (eds): Physical Rehabilitation: Assessment and Treatment, ed. 3, p. 193. Philadelphia: FA Davis.

Supplemental Readings

American Physical Therapy Association (1997). A Guide to Physical Therapist Practice. Phys Ther 77:1–1.

Ball Dynamics (1991). Orthopedic, Sports Medicine, and Fitness: Exercises Using the (Swiss) Gymnic Ball, videotape. Denver, CO: Ball Dynamics International.

Basmajian J, and Banerjee, S (eds.) (1996). Clinical Decision Making in Rehabilitation. New York: Churchill Livingstone.

Carr J, Shepherd R, Gordon J, et al. (1987). Movement Science Foundations for Physical Therapy in Rehabilitation. Rockville, MD: Aspen.

Creager, C (1994). Therapeutic Exercises Using the Swiss Ball. Boulder, CO: Executive Physical Therapy.

Davies P (1985). Steps to Follow. New York: Springer-Verlag.

Davies P (1990). Right in the Middle. New York: Springer-Verlag.

Davies P (1994). Starting Again—Early Rehabilitation after Traumatic Brain Injury or Other Severe Brain Lesion. New York: Springer-Verlag.

Davis C (1994). Patient Practitioner Interaction: An Experiential Manual for Developing the Art of Health Care, ed. 2. Thorofare, NJ: Slack.

Duncan P, and Badke M (1987). Stroke Rehabilitation: The Recovery of Motor Control. Chicago: Yearbook Pub.

Duncan P (ed.) (1990). Balance. Alexandria, VA: American Physical Therapy Association.

Edwards S (1996). Neurological Physiotherapy—A Problem-solving Approach. New York: Churchill Livingstone.

Foundation for Physical Therapy (1991). Contemporary Management of Motor Control Problems: Proceedings of the II Step Conference. Alexandria, VA: Foundation for Physical Therapy.

Goldstein T (1995). Functional Rehabilitation in Orthopedics. Gaithersburg, MD: Aspen.

Granger CV, Cotter A, Hamilton BB, et al. (1990). Functional assessment scales: A study of persons with multiple sclerosis. Arch Phys Med Rehabil 71:870–875.

Herdman S (1994). Vestibular Rehabilitation. Philadelphia: FA Davis Co.

Higgs J, and Jones M (eds.) (1995). Clinical Reasoning in the Health Professions. Boston: Butterworth Heinemann.

Hypes B (1991). Facilitation Development and Sensorimotor Function—Treatment with the Ball. Hugo, MN: PDP Press.

Johnston M (1991). Therapy for Stroke. New York: Churchill Livingstone.

Johnston M (1995). Restoration of Normal Movement after Stroke. New York: Churchill Livingstone.

Johnston M (1996). Home Care for the Stroke Patient, ed. 3. New York: Churchill Livingstone.

Keith RA, Granger CV, Hamilton BB, et al. (1987). The Functional Independence Measure. Adv Clin Rehab 1:6–18.

Kisner C, and Colby L (1996). Therapeutic Exercise Foundations and Techniques, ed. 3. Philadelphia: FA Davis.

Kucera M (1993). Gymnastik mit dem Hupfball (Swiss Ball Exercise Book). English transl. by Joanne Posner-Mayer. Denver, CO: Ball Dynamics.

Magill R (1993). Motor Learning Concepts and Application, ed. 4. Dubuque, Iowa: Brown and Benchmark.

Norkin C, and Levangie P (1992). Joint Structure and Function, ed. 2. Philadelphia: FA Davis.

O'Sullivan S (1995). Functional Training for Physical Rehabilitation, videotapes. Philadelphia: FA Davis.

Palmer L, and Toms J (1991). Manual for Functional Training, ed. 2. Philadelphia: FA Davis.

Posner-Mayer J (1995). Swiss Ball Applications for Orthopedic and Sports Medicine. Denver, CO: Ball Dynamics International.

Purtillo R (1993). Ethical Dimensions in the Health Professions, ed. 2. Philadelphia: WB Saunders.

Ryerson S, and Levit K (1997). Functional Movement Reeducation. New York: Churchill Livingstone.

Shumway-Cook A, and Woollacott M (1995). Motor Control—Theory and Practical Applications. Baltimore: Williams and Wilkins.

Sullivan P, and Markos, P (1995). Clinical Decision Making in Therapeutic Exercise. Norwalk, CT: Appleton and Lange.

Sullivan P, and Markos, P (1996). Clinical Procedures in Therapeutic Exercise, ed. 2. Norwalk, CT: Appleton and Lange.

Visual Health (1993). Therapeutic Ball and Closed Chain Exercises. Tacoma, WA: Visual Health Information.

Wolf S (1985). Clinical Decision Making in Physical Therapy. Philadelphia, PA: FA Davis.

INDEX

Note: Page numbers followed by *f* indicate figures.